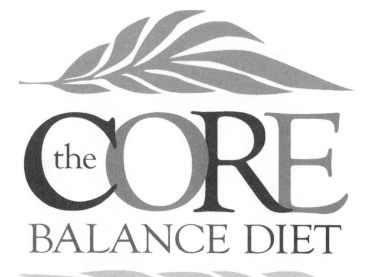

the CORE

BALANCE DIET

the CORE
BALANCE DIET

4 Weeks to Boost Your Metabolism
and Lose Weight for Good

MARCELLE PICK, MSN, OB/GYN NP
co-founder of Women to Women

with GENEVIEVE MORGAN

HAY HOUSE, INC.
Carlsbad, California • New York City
London • Sydney • Johannesburg
Vancouver • Hong Kong • New Delhi

> **A Word to the Wise:** *No book can take the place of a caring medical professional's advice. If you are currently under a practitioner's/doctor's care, taking a prescription medicine, or working with a chronic disease such as diabetes, please check with your healthcare practitioner before starting this program. Most of my patients have easily incorporated* The Core Balance Diet *into their self-care routines, but it is always prudent to discuss any changes in diet and lifestyle with a caring medical professional, preferably one who understands both traditional and alternative methods of care—an approach we call "integrated medicine." If you are pregnant or breastfeeding, I advise you to reconsider any weight loss program—now is not the time.*

ISBN: 978-1-4019-2201-6

Printed in the United States of America

For my children, Joshua, Micah, and Katya, and their future.

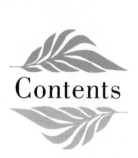

Contents

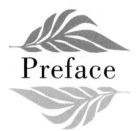

Preface

At one point in my life, I was as much as 40 pounds overweight—and up until relatively recently I carried 15 to 20 stubborn extra pounds. From my early teens until my fifties, I was in a constant battle with my weight fueled by a lot of confusion and self-doubt. As a girl growing up in Australia, I never thought about my body. I ran and played and worked happily; I was healthy and strong and ate regular, home-cooked meals made from food my parents were able to grow, gather, or purchase for our home in the Outback. When I was 10 years old, my family moved to the States, and for the first time in my life I became body-conscious. Girls at school teased me for being bigger then they were (though I was hardly overweight) and I began to obsess over my size. Our diet changed as we began to integrate into American culture, though my mother still cooked for us every day. I was never overweight as a child, but I was never skinny. And boy, did I want to be skinny!

It was the 1960s and all of the cultural icons were sticks—like Twiggy. Through high school, I engaged in all the typical skirmishes we women do to lose weight: I starved myself, I ate only grapefruit for a week, I yo-yoed back and forth between fad diets, and I stayed active on the pep team; but I never got really skinny, no matter how hard I tried. During my twenties and thirties, as I started my family, extra pounds crept on and I spent huge amounts of energy trying to lose them. I went on Weight Watchers, measured every ounce of food I ate, and oh-so-slowly lost weight at the agonizing rate of about a half a pound a week. I was stupefied when others in my group who were doing the exact same program would lose two to five in the same time period! It took me a year to lose 15 pounds, and it came right back on the moment I started eating normally again.

Had I known then what I know now, I would have immediately suspected some underlying issues that were getting in the way of my weight loss. But I didn't know—so I simply ate less, went to the gym early in the mornings, and blamed myself for not being disciplined enough to lose the weight. The silver lining to this experience was that I began to tune in to my diet and learn more about the importance of optimal nutrition and eating organically. I also began to explore holistic and then functional medicine. My weight was stable (even though I was heavier than I wanted to be) and I was healthy and full of energy. It was around then that three partners and I began Women to Women, one of the first medical clinics in the States to practice holistic healing for women by women, with a mission to change women's health for the better.

Things percolated along for a decade. My family and the medical clinic were thriving; I had a group of supportive and loving friends; and I was living my dream—albeit with 15 extra pounds. I was frustrated by my inability to lose this weight. I felt as if I was doing everything right, but nothing really worked for very long. And then, in my late 40s, things went haywire. My body began to rebel. My mother (with whom I'd always had a complicated and unresolved relationship) fell ill and eventually passed away. At the same time, I began to undergo premenopausal hormonal shifts and packed on a mysterious additional 20 pounds—even though I had not changed a thing in my diet or my exercise patterns. Shocking as it was, I look back now and realize that the sudden weight gain was a kind of gift, because it forced me to finally look beyond outdated "diet" thinking and pay real attention to what I, as a unique individual, needed to do. It was my wake-up call.

As a medical practitioner who has treated women for almost 30 years, I have seen up close the miraculous transformation that can occur when a woman finally begins to take care of herself on every level. Many of the diet and lifestyle guidelines I have set out for you here have been culled from decades of medical experience—and a few "aha" moments—with real patients. In these pages you will read some of their stories and share in their successes. During all those years, I strove to be a good example of my own teachings and I was able to design the physically supportive concepts set out in *The Core Balance Diet*. By practicing them myself, I successfully kept myself well and eventually lost the weight I put on at menopause—but continued to struggle with those intractable 15 unwanted pounds that had bothered me since early adulthood.

The sea change finally came a couple of years ago when I began to delve into my past, specifically into my relationships with my mother and my father, as well as their legacy to me. When I engaged in this work, I truly began to feel on an emotional level the new direction I needed to take. For this, I must thank the Quadrinity Process and my teachers at The Hoffman Institute (which I'll tell you more about later on when we talk about your emotional work). There, I was finally able to integrate all the aspects of my true self. I finally became whole and balanced—to my core—and almost magically that stubborn, resistant weight that had plagued me all those years simply came off. It has never come back. This was the last piece of my own puzzle that fell into place, and this book just flowed from there. This has been my journey—you are now about to set off on your own. And it is your very own. It won't look like anybody else's. I am happy to offer you my story as proof that the ideas behind this book are valid and effective if you are serious about putting the energy into following them. They worked for me, they've worked for hundreds of women just like you, and they can work for you.

Marcelle Pick
Yarmouth, Maine
July 1, 2008

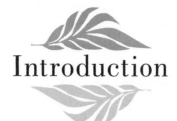

Introduction

Why is it so hard to lose weight? And why is it often harder for women, especially around and after menopause? Most of the women I know try anything and everything: They count calories, cut out fat, reduce carbs, and eat only certain combinations of food; they work out more; they even take diet aids such as ephedra, Dexatrim, and ma huang to rev up their metabolisms. And they still can't lose weight.

The fact is I've seldom had a new patient who's been able to lose weight and keep it off by dieting. This is the unhappy truth, though I know many of you won't want to hear it. Over 95 percent of traditional dieters find themselves at their starting weight or heavier a year later—and that's not because they are lazy or lack willpower. Many of the patients I see have a tremendous desire to lose weight; they just can't, no matter what they do. Some have starved themselves on 1,000 calories a day and gone to the gym religiously just to maintain a weight they aren't even happy with. Those who have managed to lose unwanted pounds inevitably experience "scale creep" even when they eat well. Not only is this incredibly frustrating, it's also bad for women's long-term health: excess weight is a proven risk factor for a host of chronic illnesses, including diabetes, arthritis, obesity, depression, infertility, hypertension, and heart disease.

As a women's health care practitioner, I see that we've been trained—mostly by advertising and the fashion industry—to think of weight loss as the end that justifies *any* means. We've set it up as a goal that pits us against the natural need to eat and makes us tune out our physical instincts and emotional health when the real answer depends on us tuning in. Weight is not a mystery, but it *can't* be reduced to one simple equation: eat less + exercise more = weigh less. That may work in a laboratory setting, but not in real life, for real women. If it were that simple, we'd be a nation of skinny-minnies. But we're not. We're a nation of individuals, and lasting weight loss is an individual process.

So I'd like you to think about your weight in relation to *you*—your individual height, frame, and musculature. One of the most important indicators of a healthy or unhealthy weight is how much weight you have gained since your 20s. Another is your waist-to-hip ratio. I like to see some waist definition in women at every age: In a perfect world, one's hips will measure about 10 inches wider than one's waist. For example, if your waist measurement is 30 inches or less, a healthy hip measurement would be about 40 inches. Once your waist measurement outgrows your hip measurement—the difference between them is less than 10 inches—the health risks mount. (Still another indicator is your body mass index, or BMI, which you can easily calculate or look up in a chart; see the Appendices.) But here's an even simpler way to think about it: if you are 30 pounds or more overweight or find that you are a good 10 to 20 pounds heavier than you were at 18, that your belly appears to have a life of its own, or that you feel lethargic, moody, and sick most of the time, there's a good chance that something has gone awry with your biochemistry—that you've lost what I call your Core Balance—and no amount of willpower will help you lose weight until you find it again.

What Is Core Balance?

Think back to the last time you felt good from the moment you opened your eyes in the morning to the minute you closed them to sleep. This doesn't mean no aches and pains and hassles, but the feeling that life is good, that you can cope, that you have the energy, stamina, and resilience to deal with whatever the day—or the future—has in store. You feel content with the way you look. Even your hair looks great. You're on top of the world.

I sincerely hope that you have experienced this at some point in your life. If so, you have an idea of your potential. If not, you have a lot to look forward to.

When your biochemistry and your metabolism are in good working order and your core physiology and emotional health are balanced, your body has a natural optimal weight and biomass that is self-sustaining and incredibly efficient. You feel energized, clear, and fit. Your mood is great and you easily shake off viruses. Your appetite is regular, without cravings or binges, and you feel great inside your skin (and your clothes). You have a sense of lightness that persists no matter how much you actually weigh.

This is the goal of the Core Balance Diet. My weight loss plan is actually a plan to create physical and emotional *wellness,* from the inside out. By wellness, I mean feeling great—in body, mind, and spirit. Real, permanent weight loss can only be achieved if you are well. Period. And being well is the sum of many parts that overlap and interact with one another in a balanced and healthy fashion—or the reverse. It's a puzzle made up of all the pieces of your own personal history, both physiological and emotional, that make you the person you are. You may be able to trick your body (and your mind) into losing weight for a little while by starving it or following some fad diet, but until you restore your Core Balance, the weight *will not* stay off.

The Core Balance Diet is a program that targets wellness as its goal and weight loss as a happy side effect. I've written this book to help you achieve it, no matter what the scale says or how you feel right now. I can say with confidence that you will achieve this goal because I've seen it happen over and over again with my patients. And it will happen for you.

Who Will Benefit from the Core Balance Diet?

The short answer is: anyone. Any woman who is struggling to lose weight will find in these pages the solution that—finally!—takes the pounds off and keeps them off. And there are many ways a woman can benefit from the Core Balance Diet even if excess weight isn't her main complaint. If you're wondering whether this book will work for you, take a minute to listen to your body and truthfully answer the following questions.

Please check the appropriate box

Statement	Yes	No
I'm unhappy with the way I look or feel.		
I'm on a diet and not losing weight.		
I lose weight, only to gain it back.		
I can't lose my pregnancy (or menopausal) weight.		
I often have strong food cravings.		
I often feel sick after I eat and I don't know why.		
I'm prone to colds/flu/viruses/injury.		
All my fat is moving to my middle.		
I feel forgetful and foggy most of the time.		
I'm having a lot of health issues or chronic pain.		
Being overweight is normal in my family.		
I'm exhausted, irritable, and/or miserable most of the time.		

If you answered yes to any of the above, the Core Balance Diet will help you.

And the first thing we are going to do together is congratulate you for being honest about the way you really feel. The women I see in my practice put on a brave face a lot of the time, as we all do so that we can do what needs to be done. We power through our days and ignore what our bodies are desperately trying to tell us. The cost of this performance is high, and all too often it comes out of our long-term health and our daily sense of well-being. So many accomplished, apparently cheerful and confident women sit in my office and fall apart after they do what you've just done—answer these questions honestly. They crumble under the relief of finally being able to confess that they feel anxious, ill, fat, hormonal, depressed, exhausted, fuzzy, aching, angry, or all of the above most of the time! But I know—and my patients at Women to Women quickly learn—that you don't have to feel that way anymore.

Entering the Conversation

I am a functional medical practitioner, and I've created the Core Balance program on the principles of functional medicine, recognizing that every person is unique, that health is not merely the absence of disease, and that we can use the body's wisdom to heal. Functional medicine is an integrative model that focuses on patient care, rather than disease care, and uses research from various disciplines to treat complex, chronic health concerns. Even though my specialty is obstetrics and gynecology, as a functional practitioner I have a responsibility to understand the body in its entirety. Like practitioners in many other holistic traditions that stretch back for millennia, I look at the totality of the individual patient—her biology, her emotional life, and her history—and intervene at various levels, using the most appropriate methods available, starting with the least invasive and most natural alternatives, to promote lifelong health and balance.

My practice is based on the principle that the human body functions as an orchestrated network of interconnected systems, rather than individual systems functioning autonomously. So when I talk about your "core physiology," I mean all the organs and systems in your body, together with the fluctuating sea of chemicals and hormones they produce, which control metabolism, appetite, sleep, mood, pain, immunity, bone growth, detoxification, and a myriad of other functions. Human beings are always adapting, not only as a species, evolving over millennia, but as individuals: every minute of every day, our bodies scan our internal and external environments and respond with infinitesimal adjustments to our biochemistry. Think of it as a conversation of mythic proportions that connects your mind to your body, your body to your spirit, and—ultimately—your diet, lifestyle, thoughts, and feelings to the biochemicals that communicate with your DNA and determine the long-term state of your cellular health.

I first began to understand this phenomenon during the controversial days of the diet supplement Phen-Fen. So many of my patients who could never stop binge eating, who could never lose weight, did lose weight when they took Phen-Fen. Now, I don't in any way encourage Phen-Fen use—it's been found to be extremely taxing on the heart, and the drug has been taken off the market. But before that happened, it was used successfully to treat some patients for obesity, and the way it worked was revealing. The chemicals in Phen-Fen, fenfluramine and phentermine, act on important brain chemicals: *fen* increases levels of serotonin and the feeling of fullness and contentedness; *phen,* an amphetamine-based appetite suppressant, activates the same neurotransmitters involved in the fight-or-flight stress response, which short-circuit hunger signals. Many of the patients I saw had dieted all their lives, restricted calories, and exercised regularly—and were still 20 to 30 pounds overweight until they took Phen-Fen. It all clicked for me then. I realized that for many people, weight loss is not related to calories, but to something deeper and more personal—in this case, to these patients' neurotransmitter levels. I then set out to look at the specific balances (or imbalances) in individual patients' core physiology and see how I could regulate them naturally, through nutrition and lifestyle. My treatment protocols—and this book—grew from there.

I'm not the only one who has been treading this path. The field of nutrigenomics, which studies how nutrients and lifestyle choices interact with genes and influence cellular activity, is proving that your cells respond to everything that enters your body, whether you eat, drink, breathe, touch, or bathe in it.[1] That's because nutrients and chemicals in food and in the environment are ingested and broken down by your system, where they serve either as building blocks for your biochemicals or as active chemicals themselves. This is why scientists always say "you are what you eat." Moreover, there's increasing evidence that your feelings trigger specific biochemical reactions in the body that can strongly influence your internal conversation—so it's equally true to say that you are what you think and feel.

Toxic Weight

What does this mean for your waistline? In practical terms, nutrient-dense food and supplements, adequate sleep, activity, and healthy detoxification (including exhalation, perspiration, and excretion) enable the conversation between your biochemicals and your cells. Conversely, empty calories, prolonged stress, lack of exercise, emotional burdens, and too many body toxins disrupt and confuse the conversation. Over time, this confusion throws off your body's Core Balance, and the disruption starts to cause noticeable problems—one of which is that you put on weight and the weight sticks.

All humans have this in common: when the body is under threat or not functioning well, it communicates that fact by way of physical symptoms. And the one irritating symptom that is most common is stubborn weight gain—weight that just won't budge, no matter what you do. In fact, weight gain as a symptom of a body out of Core Balance is so ubiquitous that I've coined my own term for it: toxic weight. You gain toxic weight when your body and mind are overburdened, and you won't ever lose it permanently until you unburden yourself.

As The Core Balance Diet will show you, your body is hardwired to insulate itself from stress by putting on weight—storing reserves of nutrients against hard times, a genetic holdover from our hunter-gatherer days.[2] This is a biological reality, one that impacts both men and women, but because of differences in our physiologies tends to affect women more. And no amount of willpower can deny it. Extra weight is not a sin, it's a symptom—a sign of a core imbalance, an injury that must be healed before the body will feel safe enough to let go of its reserves. Remove the imbalance and the body will begin to function more efficiently. It will come back into balance, and the weight will come off.

Our job over the next month is to figure out what factors in your diet, your life, and your emotional background are causing you to gain toxic weight. Over the years I've identified six major biochemical imbalances that seriously impede weight loss. They are:

- Digestive imbalance
- Hormonal imbalance
- Adrenal imbalance
- Neurotransmitter imbalance
- Inflammatory imbalance
- Detoxification imbalance

All of these imbalances create extremely powerful obstacles to weight loss, no matter how few calories you consume. That's because they have a harmful effect on your metabolism—the rate at which your body converts food into usable energy. You've probably heard a lot of talk about metabolism and how to boost it, because a higher metabolic rate enables you to burn more calories more efficiently—a primary goal when you are trying to lose weight. But my goal is to teach you how to heal your metabolism first by fixing your core imbalance. There's no point in trying to get an injured runner to run faster; she'll only hurt herself and have to drop out of the race!

The core imbalances I've identified often overlap, so you may have more than one affecting you at once. But don't let that discourage you: I've found that when you begin to restore balance in one area, other imbalances get easier to address and sometimes even correct themselves. The Core Balance Diet will help you identify for yourself the imbalance that is impacting you most right now and give you a customized eating and action plan designed to heal it.

Over the next month, we'll work on clearing away the clutter that's disrupting your internal conversation, and we'll restore support in the areas that are overburdened, thereby removing the most obvious obstacles to your weight loss. At the same time, we'll begin to explore the emotional patterns that may be keeping you from letting go of your protective weight. We'll be taking a month-long class in you: what makes you feel good, what stresses you out, what inspires you, what holds you back. You will learn how your long-term physical and emotional health depends on your body's ability to deal with stress as it affects you personally. This is really what we talk about when we talk about wellness: How do you cope with the bad stuff? What are your burdens? Where do you find support?

Your answers will define the pieces of your individual health puzzle; they'll explain why you can eat and do the same things as your best friend, and she won't gain a pound but you'll gain five! Weight and weight loss are different for everyone, and they're different for you at different stages of your life. That's why cookie-cutter diets don't work. The Core Balance Diet is different, because it understands that you are not a lab experiment, but an ever-changing, constantly adapting, glorious woman who needs to eat! And because you are all that, you always have the potential to make different choices that result in a better and healthier future. This doesn't mean you will eliminate burdens and threats from your life—stress is part of being human—but you will learn how to provide yourself with the right support to keep you lean and resilient, even in the worst of times. Believe it or not, your body already possesses almost everything it needs to heal. You just need to give it a little nudge in the right direction.

If The Core Balance Diet can do one thing for you, I hope it's to convince you that the old way of thinking about yourself and your weight is over. The time has come to get off the diet merry-go-round. You can stop treating your body like a bad boyfriend (one you'd love if only he would change)—you're about to start a whole new relationship with yourself. Soon—in a month, in fact—you'll be sprinting toward the lean, fit body that will see you into your (very) old age. And you've just taken the first step by reading these lines.

How the Program Works

The Core Balance Diet is a medically based strategy for wellness and weight loss that has proven successful for hundreds of patients at my clinic as well as hundreds of members enrolled in my online health service, the Personal Program. The method is divided into four stages to help you assess your needs; calm down your stressed-out system; clear the clutter from your diet, lifestyle, and emotions; and then identify and treat the main core imbalances that are getting in the way of your weight loss right now.

Stage I—Tuning In: As we lay the groundwork for your month-long journey to balance, you'll learn about the science behind the Core Balance method and the reasons why it works. I will briefly explain the nuts and bolts of your core physiology, the key components of your food, and how the physical body and the emotions are interwoven. And we'll examine the four corners of health that create a stable foundation on which to build a lifetime of healthy habits.

Stage II—The Core Balance Essential Plan: Here you'll learn the basic eating and action plan that forms the backbone of the Core Balance method. This is the plan you'll follow for the first 14 days of the program. Its guidelines, the same recommendations I give to all my patients, are designed to clear away the most offensive and distracting clutter from your diet and lifestyle. After two weeks, you may be happy enough with the results to simply continue with this plan for the rest of the month. If you haven't seen the results you want, you can move on to Stage III.

Stage III—The Core Balance Custom Plan: This stage of the program targets the individual core imbalances that are making it hard for you to lose weight and keeping you from getting the results you want. You'll take my Core Imbalance Quiz to discover which of the six major imbalances is affecting you most significantly right now. Then you'll find a customized eating and action plan to follow for the next 14 days of the program, complete with suggestions for nutritional supplements, physical activity, and additional diagnostic testing you may need, as well as easy-to-use shopping guides, menu suggestions, and recipes to help you adapt the eating plan to your lifestyle.

Stage IV—Core Balance for Life: Here is where you'll find the key to keeping weight off: the integration of your physical self with your inner life. In this stage, which you should read during the first two weeks of the Core Balance Program, we'll explore how to celebrate the natural wisdom of your body and the healing capacity of your heart—at any age. You'll discover the powerful influence that your emotional health has on long-term weight loss and well-being; you'll learn how to shift self-sabotaging emotional patterns, and you'll get advice on how to find professional help if you want to look deeper. This stage of the program will also help you look and feel your best no matter what the scale says.

Some Food for Thought

Many of my patients are so overwhelmed with conflicting information about diet and health—all the things they think they're supposed to limit or avoid—that they throw up their hands and ask me, "What can I eat?" Well, while you are on this program, I really, really want you to eat—often and well. Food is medicine, and in my practice I consider nutrition and hydration to be the first line of defense in healing core imbalances and removing the obstacles to weight loss. Depending on your core imbalance, you may be asked to restrict certain foods for a period of time, but you will never feel deprived or ravenous, because you are going to eat!

The meals and snacks I've planned for you are delicious, filling, and flexible—you can easily adapt them if you're feeding a family, or if you don't like to cook—and most of the recipes can be made in 30 minutes or less. The menu plans are based on quality whole foods in combinations that closely follow the healthiest diet in the world, the Mediterranean diet.[3]

Over the next month, you may be trying out some new foods, and you may be eating more than you are used to (or maybe you'll be eating less). Remember, we are trying to remove stress, not pile it on, so I'd like you to focus less on the amount of food you are eating (or its quantity of carbs or fat) and focus more on its quality and variety. For that reason, I haven't included calorie counts or nutrient breakdowns in my recipes, though I have paid attention to it for you in putting the recipes together. *Willpower* is not a word I like to use—or a quality I admire—when it comes to women and food. So take all that willpower from your former, failed diets and channel it into carving out time for yourself, for the important self-care elements of the program. For the next month, allow yourself to move beyond default behavior like wishful thinking (*I'll only eat 750 calories a day for a week*) and simple equations (*If I go to the gym and spend an hour on the elliptical machine every day, I'll get my body back*) and follow the comprehensive, combination approach laid out in these pages. If you do this for a month, I promise you'll be well on your way to a lifetime of healthy leanness.

The Core Balance Diet is designed to help you lose weight safely and permanently. A safe rate of weight loss—one in which you are losing fat, not muscle or water—is one to two pounds per week. Some women may lose a bit more on this program, some a bit less. Because many toxins are stored in fatty tissue and get released into your bloodstream as your body metabolizes fat, I don't advise trying to lose more than two pounds per week; that way, your liver has ample time to detoxify your system. While you are losing fat and bloat, you will also be gaining muscle, so your jeans may feel quite a bit looser even if the scale doesn't show a dramatic shift.

Over the next month, weigh yourself twice a week, at the same time of day each time. Remember that a woman's weight can go up or down as much as five pounds in a day, depending on the time of the month. So use the scale judiciously, just to keep yourself motivated and accountable. If you start to obsess about the numbers or beat yourself up, put the scale away! Instead, rely on the measuring tape, the way your clothes fit, and the way you feel. By the end of a month, you can expect to experience a remarkable shift in energy, well-being, and mood—and drop a dress size in the process, without having to live on lettuce!

The Five T's

Your goal for the next month can be summed up in a little thing I like to call the five T's, which describe the positive changes that will occur if you follow the advice and guidelines in this book. During the next month, you will learn to:

1. Tune in to your wisest teacher, your body.

2. Turn down physical and emotional stress, both of which make it harder for your body to feel safe enough to let go of extra weight.

3. Treat yourself to deliciously yummy food and supplements that will ensure you are getting optimal nutrition to restore balance and health to your physiology and help you lose weight.

4. Tune out negativity in the form of self-sabotaging thoughts and actions.

5. Take care of yourself on every level: body, mind, and spirit.

By the end of this next month, you should be on your way to feeling totally, tremendously, top-of-your-game, tantalizingly terrific! (That's another five T's, just for good measure.)

I hope you will take heart from the truth that losing weight is not as simple as you've been led to believe. But it is doable—infinitely doable. And it all starts with a month of your attention.

So now you need to ask yourself: do you think getting healthy and fit for the rest of your life is worth a month of your attention?

I hope you do, because I certainly do.

So let's start now!

STAGE I

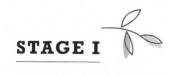

Tuning In

chapter one

YOUR BALANCING ACT

Do you ever feel like a juggler in the center ring of a circus? You do your best to keep your balance, draw on your available resources, and manage your responsibilities like so many plates spinning in the air. If you're like many of my patients at Women to Women, you rush from one thing to another, grabbing a meal here, a coffee or a nap or a sugary snack there—whatever it takes to keep you going—hoping the whole time that your juggling routine won't come to a dramatic, crashing halt.

Every woman has her own set of plates in the air and her own way of managing them—her own personal balancing act, you could say—that works for her. Until it doesn't work anymore. Women these days are taking on, and succeeding at, so many things: raising families, rising in careers, caring for elders, owning businesses, volunteering, and running increasingly complex households. At the same time, the information revolution has moved our entire society into the fast lane, plugging us in 24/7 and allowing us precious little downtime. In the 21st century, everyone's having a harder time keeping the plates in the air.

As a species, too, we seem to be struggling to maintain our balance. While modern medicine has vanquished most of the acute infectious diseases that were once our greatest threat, chronic conditions are on the rise: obesity, diabetes, depression, heart disease, cancer, anxiety disorders, allergies, chronic pain syndromes, autoimmune disorders, autism, and Alzheimer's disease, to name a few. And I know that many of you may have an intimate relationship with these concerns. If you're like me, you may find it's easy to get overwhelmed by the statistics, by all the bad news.

But here's some good news: statistics are averages in the population. They may represent trends, but they tell only one part of the story, and they do not necessarily tell your story. Only you can do that. And your story does not have to be like anyone else's—no matter what gene pool you're born into, what diagnosis you have, or how much weight you've gained.

The Power of You

Do you want to know the real reason why it's so hard to lose weight, and why, when we do lose it, most of us gain it all back within two years? It's because we keep trying to solve the problem with simplistic, one-size-fits-all solutions. But you can't fix an individual problem with a one-size-fits-all solution. Creating a healthy, lean body depends on how well your body copes with the demands made on it. This is very personal: what works for you may not work for your friend. The important thing is that you understand what works for you. I wrote *The Core Balance Diet* to help you figure out what your body needs, both physically and emotionally, to thrive.

A well-functioning, balanced body will naturally maintain a normal body weight without requiring epic demonstrations of discipline and deprivation. But most popular diet plans today are still touting the outdated, oversimplified equation: calories in = calories out. In other words, to lose weight you must decrease your input of calories and increase your output of energy. This may have worked well for you in the past, when your body was younger and your metabolism was in high gear, but not so well now. You may be one of the many women I see who, at midlife, are eating very few calories but still gaining weight. There are women who overeat, don't get me wrong, but in my experience there are many more who don't—without seeing the smallest dip on the scales.

In the reductive atmosphere of a laboratory (that is, where things are reduced to the simplest of equations), if a test subject uses up the same number of calories that it takes in, there is a zero net; there aren't any calories left over to store in muscle tissue or fat cells, so, voilà, no weight gain. This has been the golden rule of weight loss for as long as I've practiced medicine, and it has meant more miserable women dragging themselves to the gym at 5 ᴇ. than I can count, not to mention a ridiculous amount of time spent counting calories. Now, it is true that if you consistently eat more calories than your metabolism can burn, the extra will be stored as fat and you will gain weight. But everyone has a different metabolism that burns at a different rate, and some may be genetically predisposed to burn one nutrient or another more efficiently.

A Calorie Is a Calorie Is *Not* a Calorie

Some of you may have seen the movie *Super Size Me!*, in which a young film-maker, Morgan Spurlock, spent 30 days eating all of his meals at McDonald's, keeping physical activity to a bare minimum and never turning down an offer to "super-size" his meal. At the end of the experiment, Spurlock had gained more than 20 pounds and his cholesterol had skyrocketed, in direct contrast to his mood, which had plummeted. More seriously, he was on his way to clinical liver damage—in just a month. (I keep telling you, a lot can happen in a month!) Spurlock's experience inspired another researcher, a man named Fredrik Nystrom at Linkoping University in Sweden, to conduct a similar experiment of his own, using a group of 18 college-student volunteers.[1] These students were asked to double their usual caloric intake, eating anywhere from 5,000 to 6,000 calories in junk food a day, and to avoid physical activity as much as possible.

Based on the film and our current ideas about weight control, you would probably expect all the volunteers—after doubling their caloric intake and reducing their caloric output—to be well on their way to obesity, like Spurlock. But that wasn't what happened at all! Now, each of the volunteers did gain some weight. Some gained almost as much as Spurlock, others only a few pounds, and at least one gained half of his additional weight in muscle. More surprisingly, many of the subjects saw no change in their cholesterol levels (one student's actually went down), and none of them had liver problems. What Nystrom discovered was what I've been telling you: everyone responds differently!

The bottom line is, most of the science telling us that input must equal output—or that "a calorie is a calorie is a calorie"—doesn't adjust for a person's individual metabolism, nor does it take into account the various other physical and emotional factors that may be creating obstacles to weight loss. The truth is actually quite simple: a calorie is a calorie is a calorie . . . until it enters your mouth. What happens next—the way your body burns, stores, or excretes that calorie—is specific to you, and specific to where you are right now. A woman's physiology isn't static; it's a reflection of her biochemistry, her nutrition, and all the things she's doing, thinking, and feeling—consciously or unconsciously—at a particular time in her life. Learning how these factors work in tandem is like trying to fit together the pieces of a jigsaw puzzle.

There's a fascinating experiment I'd like to tell you about. In 2007, a Harvard University researcher, Ellen Langer, studied 84 hotel housekeepers to gauge the impact of what they were thinking—to see how their perception of how much exercise they were getting would impact their actual body mass.[2] Langer found that, despite a workday that consisted of almost nonstop physical activity, 67 percent of the women she interviewed did not believe they exercised enough, and their bodies appeared to bear this out with extra weight. After measuring the women's body fat, waist-to-hip ratio, blood pressure, weight, and body mass index, she found that their body types largely matched their perceptions of how much they exercised. Langer then split the women into two groups; her team took one group aside, told them how many calories each housekeeping task burned, and explained that their daily activity already met the U.S. surgeon general's definition of an active lifestyle. The other group was left in the dark.

Guess what?

After a month, Langer and her team measured the women again and found that in the group that had been educated, there was a decrease in systolic blood pressure (the upper number in a blood pressure reading, which interprets how hard the heart is working under stress), weight, and waist-to-hip ratio, and a 10 percent drop in overall blood pressure, which includes the lower number, or diastolic reading, indicating how hard the heart is working at rest. (A low diastolic number is a good sign of physical fitness.) Now, it's possible that the education changed the way the women did their jobs, but neither the subjects nor the hotel managers reported a significant difference in their activity— the difference was in how they thought about their activity. This is, in effect, the same placebo response medical researchers see when they study drug treatments: half the time, placebos are as effective as drugs.

What it really tells us is that your thoughts are extremely powerful and that they manifest in your physical reality. On some level, whether scientists can prove it empirically or not (and they are proving it), we've always known that we are one body, not disconnected at the neck. Why else do we describe things that happen to us as "mind-bending," "gut-wrenching," and "heartbreaking"?

Your Body and Your Mind

In the 1970s, Dr. Candace Pert proved, with her groundbreaking work on endorphins, that emotions and thoughts translate into measurable biochemical molecules in the body and vice versa. Her book, *The Molecules of Emotion*, shows that the body and the mind are one. Another movie you may have seen, *What the Bleep Do We Know?*, explores this topic further, showing how quantum theory is being used to prove mind-body concepts through biological physics. In this field of study, scientists are working on building simulations of neurons and brain circuitry that learn from both top-down and bottom-up experiences. In other words, there's strong evidence that your brain and cellular DNA learn by conscious experience (like weight training or learning a musical instrument) or, more startling, by unconscious experience (like a low-grade immune reaction, trauma, or negative thought patterning). Health pioneers Louise Hay and Deepak Chopra, M.D., have been instrumental in explaining how this kind of responsiveness—or "quantum healing"—lends our physiology and brain function a plasticity we never before imagined. What this means for you and me is that the potential for physical and emotional regeneration is always at hand.

Repetitive stress can teach one's cells to react in a certain way, and then condition them to keep reacting that way, à la Pavlov, learning some "behaviors" and forgetting others. Once cells are conditioned—which can happen slowly over time or quickly in one life-altering trauma, as in post-traumatic stress disorder—a cycle is under way in which experiences and thoughts trigger certain biochemicals that target certain cells and cause them to act in an abnormal fashion, which in turn influences their cellular activity and sends the wrong message back to the brain. The most extreme example of such conditioning is drug addiction, but cells can become conditioned to many abnormal states, such as allergies, hyperanxiety, low-grade pain, and bacteria overgrowth. When cells are conditioned to accept these abnormal internal states as normal, a woman may be able to function but in the long term will not feel well. Interestingly, negative life experiences may condition certain extreme responses: for instance, if a woman has been sexually abused in the past, she may experience vaginal pain with intercourse or during her annual exam that has no known physical cause but is no less real. To a lesser degree, loading everyday experiences with negativity influences biochemical activity, which over time can condition cells to behave abnormally. Take, for example, the guilt and conflict many women feel when they eat. Physically speaking, eating is a relaxing activity (see pages 35–36 for an explanation of what happens when you eat), but our culture has loaded food with so many negative connotations that eating has become a very stressful act for some women. How many times have you thought *I shouldn't be eating this* or *I'm so bad* as you swallow? This thought eventually becomes your reality! Soon enough, eating ceases to soothe your body and becomes another threat. The simple truth is that your body and your mind are intrinsically linked at a cellular level—and the same is true of your physical and your mental health. Learning how they all work together is like trying to put together pieces of a jigsaw puzzle.

I see the synergistic qualities of body and mind play out every day in my patients. I can't tell you how many women come into my office after spending years in conventional medical treatment who are surprised to learn that thoughts and feelings don't stop at the neck. It is always a joy for me to introduce them to the power of the mind and how quickly that power manifests in the body. To demonstrate this, I often have a patient stand up with one arm extended. I ask her to think of a happy memory—something really delightful—as I press down lightly on her extended arm. Her arm usually lowers slightly, if at all. Then I ask her to think of a sad memory or a painful event. I press down again, the same pressure, and her arm almost always lowers to her side. The connection is that distinct and that immediate.

The ancient concept of body-mind-spirit that inspires all Eastern healing modalities is slowly making headway here in the West (albeit a thousand years late). In the simplest terms, the mind-body connection recognizes that you can't separate thoughts and emotions from the body—the body is a mirror for our psychological state. Some people may find this talk a little too out there, but Western medical practitioners have been quantifiably proving the connection for decades, even though opposition from the medical establishment has made change in this country slow in coming. After all, Dr. Thomas Holmes and scientist Richard Rahe created the Holmes-Rahe stress scale in 1964.[3] This scale, which is still a standard test, rates over 40 stressful life events, from the death of your spouse to the size of your mortgage, and calculates how much each increases your chances of developing a related physical illness! The mainstream may have been reluctant to admit the deeper implications of the connection, but clearly it's been long accepted that life stress contributes to the risk of chronic disease.

Dr. Herbert Benson, who helped bridge the mind-body divide in the 1970s with his best-selling book *The Relaxation Response,* was a pioneer in the field of behavioral medicine at Harvard Medical School.[4] With his use of the electrocardiogram, he proved that the heart responds measurably and predictably to emotion-related neuron impulses transmitted by the nervous system. This discovery encouraged others to look further into the relationship between psychological factors and chronic illness. From there, several effective therapies emerged to treat physical concerns by using the mind, such as biofeedback, guided visualization, and hypnotherapy.

Forty years later, MRIs and PET scans are providing further evidence that certain sections of the brain light up or trigger the release of different biochemicals in response to thoughts and emotions.[5] And as we know from Candace Pert's work, these agents communicate information through cell receptors across the vast landscape of the body to initiate change at a cellular level. She proved, in short, that what we call consciousness is the body. We experience this instinctively: anyone who has blushed with embarrassment, blanched in fear, felt her knees knock from nervousness or her heart skip a beat with anticipation, shaken with fury, or had an orgasm in her sleep has known the mind-body connection firsthand. These responses are your real-life proof that your thoughts, memories, and emotions manifest in the physical—and biochemical—realm.

Pieces of the Puzzle

Let's say we really are going to put together a jigsaw puzzle. Usually, we have some idea of what the finished product should look like, such as a picture on the lid of the box. We need to clear a space to work, and we need to lay the pieces out in some organized fashion, facing up so we can see what they are. Then we need to start somewhere. Most of us begin with the four corners, then complete the edges, before we start filling in the center. That way, we get a sense of the size and shape of the whole thing. As the picture slowly emerges, we are better able to fit in difficult pieces and make sense of where we are. Sometimes we need to work on one section at a time; other times we step back and look at the whole table. Either way, we are always working with the finished picture in mind.

Restoring wellness and losing weight the Core Balance way is not so different. Your health puzzle has four corners, four essential elements of your self that take part in your internal conversation. They are: your physical body, everything from your DNA to your nutrition; your instincts, including your spiritual impulses and your reactions to pain and pleasure; your emotions, all your feelings, moods, and memories; and your intellect, your thinking self. If you don't work on all the corners of your puzzle, your picture will never be complete. So as we move through the next month, try to keep all four corners of your health in mind, even when we're focusing on only one.

Every Symptom Tells a Story

Have you ever woken up with a scratchy throat and a runny nose and thought, *Uh-oh, I've caught a cold?* In this scenario, it's pretty easy to make a connection between your physical symptom and a potential cause. The common cold and its telltale signs are, well, common, so you know what to look for. But what if I told you that being overweight is not so different?

Scientifically speaking, it's true. Unexplained weight accumulation, especially in middle age, can be a physical indication of a body under prolonged stress—stress that topples your balancing act by creating more demand for support than you've provided. And by support I mean nutrients, physical activity, sleep, fresh air, sunshine, play, relaxation, and self-care. It's a symptom, just as a runny nose is a symptom of your immune system fighting off a virus. That's it. Stubborn weight gain is not the result of

As we go on, you'll hear me mention the waist-hip ratio more than once. Simply put, this ratio is a measure of the difference between your waist circumference and hip circumference—and a strong indicator of heart health. To find yours, simply take a measuring tape and measure around the widest part of your hips, then measure your natural waist, and compare the two numbers. There should be a difference of 10 inches or more. Keep in mind that regardless of hip size, a waist measurement of over 35 inches for women (especially if our hips aren't correspondingly wide) has been linked to a higher risk of metabolic syndrome and cardiovascular disease as we age.

you being lazy or bad. It's not a demon lurking inevitably in middle age to grab you no matter what you do. It's a biological reaction to a body out of Core Balance. And going on a crash diet or an exercise binge, depriving your body of nutrients, or yo-yoing between eating extremes only exacerbates the stress by putting you that much more off balance.

Every woman who comes into my practice has a different set of factors, internal and external, at work in her mind and her body at any time. Remember those plates spinning in the air? Those are the external factors—the stress on you from sources outside you. Some of them are obvious, like your workload or the amount of exercise you get. Others are less obvious, like the chemicals in your environment or the lack of nutrients in your diet. How your mind and your body process those factors is entirely individual. But one thing is certain: when the demands on you are more than you can meet, your body will let you know.

One way it may let you know is unmistakable. I call it the Curse of the Muffin Top. You know, that extra belly fat that bulges over the waist of your jeans—formally known as visceral abdominal tissue (VAT). VAT is quite hormonally active and, though it tends to be most common among older women, it can spark a mutiny in your biochemistry at any age: It creates its own hormones (specifically, the "satiety" hormone leptin and small amounts of estrogen) that override the normal hormonal signals and sabotage your appetite controls, putting more pressure on your liver and your heart.[6] The more belly fat you have (especially if your waist-to-hip ratio is too high, that is, there's less than 10 inches difference between the two measurements) the harder you'll have to work to put down the insurgency and restore normal lines of biochemical communication. You will also be at greater risk of developing metabolic syndrome (see page 126), a spectacularly vicious cycle. Your fat cells, unlike most of your body, do not have your best interests at heart: Researchers have drawn enough evidence to conclude that VAT is a "unique, pathogenic fat depot."[7] Translation: "extraordinary disease-causing dump." Well, okay. At least we know.

So how does stress translate into unwanted weight gain? Stress wears down the immune system, which translates into a host of illnesses and accelerated aging. Scientifically speaking, stress has a deleterious effect on the tiny clock inside each of our cells called a telomere.[8] Telomeres get shorter each time a cell divides, aging the cell (and, ultimately, you). An enzyme called telomerase keeps immune cells young and active by protecting their telomeres. Cortisol, the hormone that's released when we're under stress, suppresses the immune cell's ability to make telomerase, thereby increasing the rate at which immune cells age and weakening the body's defenses. The more stress, the higher the levels of cortisol, the lower the levels of telomerase. If stress is unremitting, one of the ways your body compensates is to go into self-protection mode by switching metabolic gears (a trait stemming from our feast-or-famine past). Like laying in a lot of wood in anticipation of a cold winter, your body protects itself from long-term stress by storing potential energy as fat instead of burning it. This weight is protective, insulating weight meant to carry you through tough times.

In my opinion, our biochemistry simply has not evolved fast enough to handle the burdens of a postindustrial, technology-saturated world—in particular, a world of highly processed and overly refined nutrition. It's quite possible that in the next ten thousand years, our systems will evolve to allow us to metabolize all the processed sugar and artificial compounds in our food and our environment without gaining body fat, but that hasn't happened yet. In the meantime, we are paying the price. We're a remarkably resilient and adaptive species, and our brains calibrate our biochemistry to survive under even the most harrowing conditions (think starvation, chronic pain, chronic abuse), but never without some long-term cost.[9]

So, if you're facing a weight gain that has no direct cause—that is, weight gain you cannot attribute to a recent or significant change in your diet, habits, medication, or health—or weight that won't come off even though you're eating well and exercising, it's a signal that your body has taken out an insurance policy against stressful times.[10] It's a natural response, and particularly so for women, who are designed to need more of this "insurance" over time as they take responsibility for carrying and nurturing other lives besides their own. In our time, we may not have to hunt and hoe and fight for every morsel, but we face some pretty staggering stressors ourselves. (Take a look at my list of possible stressors on pages 24–25. I'll bet you can add some of your own.)

Stress is a very small word for an enormous variety of events that means something different to every woman. In medical terms, however, stress is simple. It is any action or emotion that triggers a response from the sympathetic nervous system. The sympathetic nervous system, which comprises your brain and your gut, is part of your central nervous system, which manages every other function in your body; it's the woman behind the curtain, orchestrating everything, protecting your survival at a very primitive level and initiating the "fight or flight" response in the face of danger.

Stress can be real (a car speeding at you) or perceived (watching a movie of a car speeding at you). It can be subtle, taking the form of burdens placed on your physiological systems—for instance, illness and injury on one end of the spectrum and lack of sleep or proper nutrients on the less severe end. And then there's emotional stress. This may be obvious, as in the case of abusive or taxing relationships, overwork, or life crises, or it may be hidden, stemming from deep-seated issues that originate in half-forgotten childhood traumas. Emotional stress may not trigger an instant survival response, but over time it too will topple your Core Balance.[11] More and more scientific evidence shows that chronic stress—real or perceived, physical or emotional—takes a tremendous toll on the body, tamping down the immune system, piling on the pounds for protection, and even accelerating the aging process.

A Message from Your Body

In order to counteract all this stress and allow your body to feel safe enough to let go of toxic weight, you need to listen to your body's signals and respond to them with the right kind of support. Remember, restoring your Core Balance means entering into a whole new relationship with your body—one based on dialogue. Your body speaks a primitive language—the language of physical symptoms—and your wellness depends on your ability to understand what it's telling you.

In bits and pieces, or sometimes all at once—all the plates tumbling down in that shattering crash we're so afraid of—your body will eventually revolt if it cannot process the stress that you unwittingly place on it. Think of it as supply

Common Stressors

- Allergies
- Pollution—indoor, outdoor, or noise
- Chemicals—in food, air, drinking water, or personal products
- Chronic disease
- Growing up in a dysfunctional home
- Less than eight hours of sleep per night
- Living in an urban area
- More than a 20-minute commute to work or school
- Currently (or constantly) dieting
- Excess sugar, salt, or animal products
- Processed foods and trans fats
- Excess alcohol (more than one glass, three times a week)
- Nicotine
- Overwork, working without breaks, or multitasking
- Excess caffeine (more than 2 to 3 cups a day)
- Drugs (pharmaceutical or recreational)
- Infections, viruses, or parasites
- Injuries, chronic pain, or major surgery
- Depression
- History of trauma or physical or emotional abuse

and demand—that eternal balancing act. You have a variable amount of resources that can meet a certain amount of demand. If you increase the demand without increasing the supply, you'll lose your balance. The tricky part here is that your brain will try to buy you extra time by convincing you to turn to cheap and easy forms of support, like lattes and candy bars. But living on these quick and easy energy supplies is like paying all your bills with a credit card: At some point those debts must be paid, and if you don't have enough money in the bank, you'll be in for a whole lot of trouble.

Good thing you have a built-in ally: your body. As demand starts to outweigh supply, your body throws up red flags in the form of physical symptoms. These symptoms can range from insomnia to worsening PMS and menopausal symptoms to digestive difficulties to mood and skin disorders—it's different

Common Stressors, cont'd.

- Tension at work or in a relationship
- Hormonal shifts (PMS, perimenopause, menopause)
- Caring for children or elders
- Boredom
- Insomnia
- Death of a loved one
- Divorce or separation
- Anxiety, guilt, or fear

for every woman. But for most women, the first sign of the struggle is the symptom we've already seen: stubborn weight gain. No matter what they do, they either keep gaining weight or can't lose it. And many women respond by placing more demands and more stress on the body—by fad dieting, over-exercising, or using more caffeine or nicotine—without adding any more support. Is it any wonder that the body reacts by holding on to that weight, plus some?

You may not think of your body as an ally when you're watching the numbers on the scale creep up. But take your body's point of view for a second: it's just been doing its job all these years in the only way it knows how. To your body, those extra pounds are a very good thing. Just the thing, in fact, to keep you standing tall in the face of all that stress! After all, your body is not setting its standards by watching *America's Next Top Model* or flipping the pages of *Vogue* (it's your mind that does that). Your body is operating on ancient hardwired instructions encoded in your DNA from our hunter-gatherer days. It's insulating you (perhaps too literally) from real and perceived danger. While you may be ready to trade it in, your body is as loyal to you as ever.

chapter two

YOUR CORE PHYSIOLOGY

Every major biological system in your body is a piece in your health puzzle, and all these systems work together to influence your Core Balance. The six major imbalances we'll tackle later in this book impact all of these systems in one way or another. The good news is that when you fix one system, it tends to have a beneficial effect on all the others.

You don't have to become a medical practitioner to understand your body's signals and address your core imbalances, but it does help to have a basic understanding. When it comes to weight loss, the systems outlined in the following pages are the major players.

Your Body's Systems

Your Digestive and Elimination System

The digestive system includes the tongue, the salivary glands and their enzymes, the esophagus, the stomach and its enzymes, the small intestine, the large intestine (or colon), the gall bladder, the pancreas, and the liver. It's your first line of defense when it comes to health and weight, and it can break down anywhere along its considerable length.

Your digestive system works hand in hand with your immune system and your ability to detox. The lymph tissue surrounding your intestines is where much of your immunity originates. When you're allergic to a food, the diarrhea, nausea, and other symptoms you feel are initiated by this tissue. But you don't have to have a full-blown allergy to experience a low-grade immune reaction.

The digestive tract is a main path of entry for offensive substances—bacteria, allergens, heavy metals, molds, fungi, chemicals, trans fats—that can get past the gut's defenses and blossom into an undiagnosed food sensitivity or allergy. Many of my patients who are struggling with weight gain actually have one or more digestion-related issues: food sensitivity, low gastric acidity, yeast overgrowth, parasites, an imbalance of digestive enzymes and gut bacteria, or an overburdened liver and immune system.

Your Endocrine System

This system includes your hypothalamus, pituitary, and pineal glands, your thyroid and parathyroid glands, your adrenal glands and pancreas, and your ovaries and fat cells—and, of course, all the hormones these glands produce. Hormones are the chemical messengers of your body; when they work in your brain, they are called neurotransmitters. Sex hormones and adrenal hormones are fat-soluble and derived from cholesterol. Other hormones are built from varying chains of amino acids, called peptides, which are considered to be the basic building blocks of all life.

Hormones are very impressionable, and they have the greatest impact on how you feel from day to day. (Any woman who has suffered from PMS or menopausal symptoms knows the power of hormones.) What's more, they connect every system in the body to the brain and every organ to all the others. So many external factors influence your hormones—from age to diet to chemicals in the environment to the way you process stress—that it's safe to say they are the difference between feeling in balance and feeling out of control.

Your Nervous System

The nervous system comprises your brain, your spinal cord and peripheral nerves, your neurons and the synapses that connect them, and your neurotransmitters. As we go on, we will often refer to the central nervous system (CNS), which is thought of separately from the peripheral nervous system (PNS). Peripheral nerves are the ones that take in information from the outside, such as sight, hearing, smell, taste, and touch, and signal voluntary actions (for instance, raising your hand). The autonomic nervous system, part of the central nervous system, is more concerned with receiving stimuli that you are rarely aware of on a conscious level, such as the amount of light in a room. It is orchestrated by the brain, specifically the hypothalamus, which can rev us up or calm us down. (More on this powerful gland later.) Sympathetic reactions prepare us for action by elevating heartbeat, constricting blood flow, and dilating the pupils; parasympathetic reactions return the body to normal by slowing down the heartbeat, increasing blood flow, and enabling peristalsis in the digestive tract. As we'll see, one of the most important tools for healing core imbalances involves learning to activate the parasympathetic response and counteract stress.

Your Neuroendocrine System

This is the system that connects your brain and your hormones. Hormones and neurotransmitters are the same chemical messengers; their names differ, confusingly, depending on where they do their work. A hormone is called a neurotransmitter when it relays messages between neurons via synapses in the central nervous system. For example, let's say you slip on a banana peel in front of a lot of people and fall down: the embarrassment you experience in your mind is accompanied by a hormone-induced flushing of cheeks, an elevated heartbeat, and a surge of adrenaline (as in, *Get me out of here!*). That's the neuroendocrine system at work. It is very important to your stress response and your immune system, and thus to your Core Balance. Dr. Candace Pert is one of the leading scientists to make the biochemical connection between your endocrine system, your immune system, and your emotions—a field called psychoneuroimmunology. Her work with endorphins (pain-reducing chemical messengers that we call "bliss-inducing") helped prove that all the systems in the body are connected through our hormones.

Your Immune System

Your immune system includes the thymus, bone marrow, spleen, lymph and associated lymph tissues, as well as white blood cells, B cells, and T cells. Also part of this system are the biochemicals involved in the cycle of inflammation and healing: the pro-inflammatory messengers (prostaglandins, cytokines, and histamines) and anti-inflammatory hormones, such as steroid hormones.

The immune system defends you against injury, as well as viruses, bacteria, and other pathogens. It's woven like a tightly knit web throughout your digestive system, and it patrols other systems as well to enable your body to respond rapidly to a threat. When you catch a cold, eat something you're allergic to, or sprain your ankle, your immune system puts on its riot gear. Infection, allergy, or injury triggers a chain of events called the inflammatory cascade, which is accompanied by telltale signs—fever, pain, and swelling. A healthy immune system is one that rallies for every skirmish, then recedes when the danger is neutralized.

Your Detoxification System

Made up of your liver, skin, lungs, kidneys, and lymph ducts, nodes, and fluid, this system is your body's cleanup crew: it flushes and filters toxins and debris from cells for elimination as breath, sweat, urine, and stool. Your skin is your largest detox organ, with the liver and spleen working about as hard: the kidneys filter your blood, while your liver and spleen cleanse your blood and lymph fluid of excess hormones, neurotransmitters, dead and damaged cells, bacteria, and body toxins.

The often-overlooked lymph system is like your body's sanitation department: it cleans up the mess made by virtually all the other systems of the body. Widely regarded as a lesser sister to the circulatory system, it has no dedicated muscle (such as the heart) to pump lymph fluid, yet every cell in your body is continuously bathed in lymph fluid, which circulates through a vast network of capillaries and ducts, pulsing with motion and breath. Like a river of fluid, the lymph system sweeps debris from the shores of your cells and filters it through the appropriate receptacles (your lymph ducts and nodes, spleen, and liver) for removal. If your lymph stopped moving, you would die of toxicity in a matter of hours.

Your Circulatory System

The circulatory system is made up of the vessels that contain and control the flow of blood around the body—your heart, arteries, capillaries, and veins—as well as the muscles that assist the flow. Healthy circulation is crucial for stabilizing body temperature and pH; for moving nutrients, biochemicals, immune cells, and oxygen throughout your body; for removing the byproducts of metabolism, such as extra hormones, toxins, and damaged or dead cells; and for fighting off disease.

Your Musculoskeletal System

This system, which includes the structure and alignment of bones and muscle tissue, is especially important for women as they get older. Cultivating strong, healthy bones and maintaining lean muscle is a crucial part of aging well. Bones and muscle are constantly regenerating—as much as 5 to 10 percent per year— and as such the process of building bone and muscle is intrinsically woven into your digestion and absorption capabilities. Muscles require protein, among many other nutrients. Healthy bones store about 99 percent of the body's calcium, 85 percent of the body's phosphorus, and 50 percent of the body's total sodium and magnesium. It requires a lot of digestive teamwork, including the presence of stomach acid, a whole alphabet of vitamins, magnesium, other essential minerals, and a well-functioning GI tract, to deliver calcium's many benefits. Your blood pH and your hormone balance also play a role here—an imbalance in either place can impede the regeneration process. Bones and muscles get stronger with use. Exercise and physical stress naturally build new bone and muscle, even when you're older. Spinal injury, misalignment of bones, and other musculoskeletal problems can fire up the immune system, cramp digestive organs, and impede good circulation and detoxification.

By the time you reach age 35 or so, and certainly as you approach menopause, it is common for one or more of these systems to get overloaded, confused, or imbalanced, causing a disruption in the lines of communication that allow your body to create and store energy efficiently—in other words, your metabolism.

Your 250,000-Year-Old Metabolism

For most of human history—until relatively recently, in evolutionary terms—food was hard-won. We walked or ran to get everywhere; we struggled to track and kill, or find and gather, enough sustenance to survive; and we became masters at storing nutrients in the form of body fat to get us through the lean times and to give us energy for long hours of physical effort.[1] Our DNA has changed little since those days; only a small fraction of the genes that make up the human genome show evolutionary change over the past 5 to 15 millennia.[2] When you consider how much our diet, habits, and environment have changed in only the last 250 years, it's hard to believe we're walking around in virtually the same bodies we had when our ancestors roamed the earth 250,000 years ago.

This DNA orchestrates the chemical processes in your body that allow you to digest food and make energy—the processes known collectively as your metabolism. When it comes to energy production, your metabolism has three basic settings: burn immediately; store for short-term use in your muscles in the form of glycogen; and store for long-term use in the form of fat. In the modern, developed world, we have far less need than we did in the past for long-term storage to see us through lean times; nonetheless, it's in our genes (and our jeans).[3]

Stoking the Fire

Your metabolism acts like a furnace in a house, burning fuel in the form of food and oxygen to make energy and release heat as a byproduct in a process called thermogenesis (that is, heat creation). You perform thermogenesis all the time, just by breathing, eating, drinking, and moving, because your metabolism is always converting calories to energy. The act of eating increases your metabolic rate, and some foods increase it more than others because they require more energy to digest, such as foods high in fiber. In contrast, skipping meals actually decreases your metabolic rate so that whatever fuel is available can be burned more slowly. That's why depriving yourself always backfires: When you don't eat, your brain sends out signals to cool your metabolism down, readying your body for starvation. Your cells get the message to store calories, rather than burn them, and your metabolism shifts into lower gear.

How Food Becomes Energy

Most of the food you eat gets broken down into three nutrient forms your cells can use for fuel: glucose, fatty acids, and amino acids. Glucose, a blood sugar made from the starch in your foods, is the primary source of direct energy for your cells— it can cross cell membranes without further digestion and be used immediately for energy. Fatty acids, derived from the fat you eat, enter your system as triglycerides, which are too big to be utilized directly by cells. They are further broken down into "free fatty acids" (lipids) to fit through the cell membrane and be used for energy. Amino acids, which come from ingested protein, not only provide energy but are the building blocks of blood protein and the basis of the peptides.

These fuel molecules travel via the blood and through the liver, where they are either stored for later use, broken down further for transport to cells, or cached in the large intestine for elimination. The stored molecules are either converted into glycogen, which can be used quickly in the near future, or put into deep storage in the form of body fat—your body's insurance policy against future starvation.

Once inside the cell, food molecules are transformed into accessible energy by your mitochondria. Mitochondria are microscopic structures in every one of your cells that have their own independent DNA, inherited from your mother. They act like mini-combustion engines in cars, turning food into fuel in the presence of oxygen. The rate at which your cells create energy is your metabolic rate. How fast this rate is depends on how many mitochondria are present within a cell and how efficiently they burn oxygen and food molecules.[4]

Your metabolism has priorities, and number one is the brain (it's the master organ, after all), so your body always tries to have a ready supply of brain food on hand: glucose and oxygen. Oxygen travels to the brain via the respiratory system; glucose comes primarily from sugars and carbohydrates in your diet and is easily metabolized. Appetite and all its attending signals—growling tummy, hunger pangs, cravings—are regulated by a number of hunger hormones to provide the mechanism by which your body tries to ensure its consistent supply of glucose. The protein and fat that feed all the other systems are important, too, but metabolism will always protect the brain first, even at the expense of other organs and tissue.

If this continues for an extended period of time—as it does for many women who've dieted since they were teenagers—it can be challenging to shift the metabolism back into high gear, but it can be done.[5] Clearly, though, simply reducing calories is not the answer. Think about it: If you wanted to build a strong, hot blaze, would you stop feeding fuel to your fire? Or would you make sure that you had the best-quality wood, in abundant supply, and stoke your furnace on a regular basis? Your body is no different. To operate at its best, it needs abundant high-quality fuel. That's why, on the Core Balance program, you'll eat—abundantly and well.

Metabolic rate differs for everyone, as we saw in Chapter 1, and is largely inherited. If you have obesity in your family, you may be dealing with a genetic predilection for the "store" setting, though that doesn't mean the switch is stuck there. Different researchers and nutritionists have reported that distinct groups of the population are hardwired to metabolize certain nutrients (protein, carbohydrates) more efficiently than others in subtle variations of the "thrifty gene" hypothesis, which suggests that different strains of genes that direct metabolism evolved over time in different populations to successfully deal with long-term nutritional deficits.[6] While I agree that it's important to ferret out any genetic quirks and/or family legacies influencing your individual health picture, I take this premise one step further: when it comes to metabolism, it's not population, it's *personal*. Nature may deal you a stacked deck, but nurture—in the form of optimal nutrition, healthy activity, and self-care—can turn the tables.[7] If your metabolism is injured—a common side effect of a core imbalance—there can be confusion in the calorie-storage conversation that makes it even harder to lose weight. Identifying and healing the core imbalance helps reopen the proper lines of communication and restore metabolic health. No matter what you've been told, you can heal your metabolism; you can improve your mood and energy; and you can transform your body, all by clearing up the interference in the conversation. I know because my patients show me this truth every day. I know because I've experienced it myself. And I know because the body has shown me the place where all those lines of communication meet.

The Hypothalamus—Center of the Conversation

The hypothalamus is an amazing, complicated piece of tissue that is part of the limbic brain. A remnant of our mammalian past, the limbic system resides deep in your skull, between your ears, and supports the functions of instinct, behavior, emotion, and long-term memory. The limbic system and the cerebral cortex (the largest, "thinking" part of the brain) collaborate in the processing of emotions, primarily through structures called the thalamus and the amygdala, the part of the brain responsible for triggering fear. The hypothalamus, which sits just below the thalamus and above the brain stem, connects the nervous system to the endocrine system through the pituitary gland, making it the controller of the neuroendocrine system, the conductor of your biochemistry, and the master of Core Balance.[8] It monitors vital behavioral and hormonal functions, including appetite, thirst, libido, fertility, circadian rhythm, the stress response, thyroid function, immune response, and many autonomic functions such as breathing and blood pressure; in addition, it influences the hormones that contribute to feelings of anger, depression, maternal affection, and joy.[9]

I like to think of the hypothalamus as a switching station standing at the crossroads of two major systems, registering information and calibrating your physical response— all at the most basic, reflexive level. It is the primitive you, able only to register a need (for food, drink, sleep, warmth, sex) and call out the appropriate hormones to disperse the information to your cells. But it is crucially important to how your cells have become conditioned to react. Each and every moment, your brain and your cells are talking to each other, via the hypothalamus and your biochemistry. If you understand that you are always sending messages to your body this way by what you eat, think, and do, you see that you can change the message anytime.

Study after study since the 1940s has shown that a dysfunctional hypothalamus causes extreme shifts in internal homeostasis, damaging the body's ability to balance caloric energy conversion and impairing metabolism on all fronts.[10] Depending on the region of the hypothalamus affected, the result may be extreme hunger and weight gain or, conversely, appetite loss and starvation. In fact, many women may think their thyroid is underactive, when it's actually the hypothalamus that is under- or overperforming. Yet in all the discussions concerning diet and weight loss, very little attention is paid to the importance of the hypothalamus and how it relates to your impulse to eat a bag of chips when you're stressed.

The Hypothalamus and the Cookie

When it comes to appetite and eating—two important contributors to weight gain and loss—the hypothalamus plays a powerful part that begins the moment we smell food. As an example, think of chocolate-chip cookies baking in the oven. Say it's 10 o'clock in the morning and you haven't eaten since 7. Assuming your metabolism is well and all your systems are communicating, the pancreatic hormone glucagon is keeping your blood sugar steady by stimulating the liver to make glucose out of any remaining fats or carbohydrates from breakfast. When your nose picks up the cookie scent, the hypothalamus registers it, and a call goes out to specific organs: food is near! Depending on your habits and associations with the smell of chocolate-chip cookies—this is where intellect and emotional history come in—this call may be soft or it may be loud, like

Cookie Monster loud! Glucagon levels begin to dip, instructing the pancreas to secrete more of its sister hormone, insulin, which regulates the cells' uptake of glucose from the bloodstream. This is important: the hypothalamus can trigger the rise in insulin in anticipation of the glucose hit, before the food actually reaches your mouth.[11] So the hypothalamus translates a sensory message and initiates a biochemical reaction before any physical activity has even taken place.

The smell of the cookie also activates digestive enzymes in your saliva, as well as the stomach hormone ghrelin, and you get a rumbling tummy and hunger pangs. At the same time, an impulse is being transmitted to the cerebral cortex, which coordinates action, so you set out to find the source of the smell. Cookie in hand, you bite, and pleasure centers in your brain light up as you anticipate a rush of glucose. Your synapses release serotonin, while levels of cortisol and adrenaline (the stress hormone) ebb. Your breathing slows, your blood pressure drops slightly, and your muscles relax—all functions of the parasympathetic nervous system, coordinated by the all-important HPA, or hypothalamus-pituitary-adrenal, axis (which you can explore in more detail in the Appendices).

As digestion occurs, cookie molecules are transported into the blood for use as energy or to the large intestine and bladder to be excreted as waste. Your cells absorb the fuel from the bloodstream, and mitochondria go to work turning it into energy. Any nutrients left over are transported to your fat cells. When the fat cells are, for lack of a better word, "full," they secrete leptin, the satiety hormone, which tells your hypothalamus to relay a "no more" message to your brain. You stop eating and go back to what you were doing before you smelled cookies, and your metabolism continues to burn along with you until your body works through your stomach contents and any ready supplies of glucose. Then the whole cycle starts again. For some, even just one cookie increases the desire for sugar; if you have a core imbalance this can lead to a binge that doesn't end.[12]

You may have noticed from this description that when you eat, your body shifts into a more relaxed state. So the act of eating counteracts stress. That's why it's such a great comfort—and can be so addictive—to so many of us. Of course, your body can only relax while you're eating if you limit the other stimuli it has to process at the same time. Scarfing breakfast as you drive to work, eating lunch at your desk, or having dinner in front of your favorite TV crime drama can counteract the soothing effect on the nervous system.

Conditioned to Balance

A thriving hypothalamus is one that is functioning well, receiving and sending out signals without interference or confusion. In the many layers of your emotional self, the hypothalamus—metaphorically speaking—is like the permanent newborn inside your grown-up shell: the reflexively needy part that the cerebral cortex has to parent. Like a newborn, the hypothalamus can survive on the bare necessities, but it needs nurturing to thrive.

In book after book, the hypothalamus is cited as a master gland, but there's little advice given on how to support and maintain its function—or on how you can rewire your impulses and influence your biochemistry simply by changing the signals you send it. For the most part, this is because the hypothalamus is still a bit of a mystery to scientists. It's my belief that you can "teach" your hypothalamus to initiate healthier responses by changing what you yourself do and think. On a psychological level, this means learning how to discern and meet your own emotional needs, which we'll tackle in Stage IV of the Core Balance program. On a physical level, it means bringing your body back into balance—which we'll start to do very soon in Stage II.

chapter three

YOU ARE WHAT YOU EAT

In the last chapter, we looked at your metabolism as a furnace that you need to stoke with the best fuel available to keep it burning well. So what, exactly, do you use to feed the fire? In this chapter, we'll take a closer look at what's in the food you eat and how it functions once it gets into your body.

You're probably familiar with the term *nutrients,* but you may be confused about what it really means, so let me give you a quick overview. First of all, nutrients are food! Sometimes, in the tidal wave of nutritional information that we get from TV, radio, and magazines, we forget that nature has provided almost everything a body needs to be well and fit. Consuming the right active nutrients, in sufficient amounts, is the first line of defense when it comes to achieving Core Balance (followed closely by fresh water, sunshine, and rest). Nutrients are divided into two groups, macronutrients and micronutrients, which Nature, in her wisdom, bundles conveniently for us in the perfect delivery system: a balanced meal.

Macronutrients

Macronutrients are the substances you need to take in each day in relatively large amounts: protein, fat, and carbohydrates. I'm going to include fiber in this group, too, even though fiber, which is indigestible, is not strictly speaking a nutrient. If your body were a house, macronutrients would be its major building materials—the beams, plaster, insulation, plumbing, wiring, floors, and walls.

Protein

Protein is what our own tissue is made of. It builds and repairs our bodies—bones, muscle, hair, nails, cells, enzymes, hormones, neurotransmitters. So it's literally essential for life.

If you don't get enough protein—a common risk on low-fat diets—your body will begin to break down the protein in your muscles. This reduces lean muscle mass and slows down your metabolism, since muscle cells convert food into energy more efficiently than fat cells. Eating protein in lieu of carbohydrates, on the other hand, has the bonus effect of stimulating the synthesis of muscle and the breakdown of fat. Here's how that happens: When protein enters the bloodstream, particularly if the level of glucose in the blood is low, a process called lipolysis takes place in fat cells. In lipolysis, free fatty acids are released into the bloodstream for transport to muscles and other tissues that need energy. But don't forget, you still need carbohydrates, just less of them.

The most convenient, densest sources of protein are meat, fish, poultry, dairy products, nuts, legumes, and tofu, but you can also get complete protein from certain complex grains, like quinoa, or by mixing two incomplete proteins, such as rice and beans. As an alternative, you can also add soy, whey, or rice protein powders—available at natural-food stores—to drinks and smoothies. The body should have a daily ration of protein, about 60 to 70 grams a day for most women. The usual rule of thumb is that you need 1 gram of protein for about every 2.2 pounds of body weight, but this calculation doesn't take into account your individual needs or activity level (which is what this book is all about!). I've found that my patients are successful using the following guide as a base and then adding or subtracting based on their own weight.

Protein requirements for a 130-pound woman based on activity level:

- Sedentary (less than 3 hours of physical activity a week): 60 grams per day
- Moderate (3–6 hours of physical activity a week): 70 grams per day
- Active (more than 6 hours of physical activity a week): 80 grams per day
- Athlete (training 4 or more days a week): 90–100 grams per day

How much protein is too much? If you find that your breath is sour, or if you're very thirsty for an extended period (48 hours or more), you may be eating too much protein and not enough complex, unrefined carbohydrates. The bad breath is a side effect of a metabolic process called ketosis, in which the liver breaks down fat into fatty acids and ketones to be used by the brain as a substitute for glucose. A little ketosis is a desired effect to help you shed toxic weight, but too much—enough to change your breath and raise your thirst—is a sign that your brain has switched to starvation mode. Other signs of too much protein are stomachache, too-rapid weight loss, sleeplessness, irritability, and sudden onset of joint or arthritic pain. One way to ensure that your diet stays balanced is to always eat a complex carbohydrate, like a vegetable or an unrefined grain, with your protein.

Carbohydrates

Low-carb, high-carb, no-carb—it's no surprise if you're confused about what's best for you! I like to call my nutritional plans carb-controlled, which means lowering carbs with room for flexibility depending on individual needs. If you are struggling with toxic weight, reducing your daily carbohydrate intake will significantly improve how you feel.

It's true that the body can exist primarily on protein and fat (as some indigenous peoples do, such as the Masai in Africa), but I don't recommend it. Carbohydrates are your body's main source of glucose—brain fuel. They are readily broken down, and they provide a relatively quick source of energy and an increase in serotonin, the body's feel-good neurotransmitter. The problem with carbohydrates today is that most of us get them from the wrong source—from refined grains and sugar, instead of whole grains, fruits, and vegetables. Eating refined sugar and grains causes a huge spike in glucose and insulin (and serotonin) followed by a precipitous blood-sugar and serotonin crash that triggers a craving for another hit.

Your brain loves it when you eat simple carbs and sugar, because they're cheap and easy (and often tasty) sources of glucose—and it has trouble telling you when to stop. Unlike protein or fat, you can eat far too many carbohydrates before your brain realizes you're full. Think of it: how many bowls of cereal can you eat in one sitting? How many chips? Now think how many hard-boiled eggs or tablespoons of vegetable oil you could eat in that same time. Food manufacturers have spent decades distilling wholesome food into mouthwatering simple-carb delivery systems—they know they can keep you coming back for more!

Sugar is a little like nature's heroin: It trips the same pleasure centers in the brain and leaves us always wanting more. Unlike heroin, sugar is not addicting in reasonable amounts, but our culture is sugar-crazed! Soda, candy, breakfast cereal, pasta sauce, even mustard, all have sugar now—or sugar's more potent cousin, high-fructose corn syrup. Overconsumption of sugar is at the center of many core imbalances because it ambushes your insulin levels, takes your neurotransmitters on a wild ride, and fires up the immune system. Shifting your sugar intake to safe alternatives will go a long way in restoring your Core Balance.

Refined carbs were a good idea when the Romans first began the practice of refining grains into flour for transportation across their Empire. It was an efficient way to feed multitudes (requiring far fewer man-hours than hunting and foraging), and it improved overall nutrition by making needed calories more readily available. In other words, it helped keep people from starving—and still does in parts of the world. But in the industrial world, where food is plentiful, an excess of refined carbs has set off a kind of glucose frenzy. This is because refinement strips grains and natural sugars of their chewier, more nutrient-dense casing and leaves a simple carbohydrate chain that the body basically mainlines as glucose. Daily overconsumption of simple carbohydrates without enough protein or fiber wreaks havoc on metabolism by seriously throwing off the insulin/glucagon balance and all subsequent cellular activity—an imbalance that can have far-reaching implications, including increased cortisol production, VAT (visceral abdominal tissue), inflammation, and hormonal imbalance. You'll get off this health-defeating roller coaster in the first 14 days of the Core Balance program by limiting carbohydrates to 66 grams per day, derived from complex sources.

Because they are a primary source of energy, complex carbohydrates are abundant in nature—they do not need to come out of a package. They're found in vegetables, fruit, legumes, and grains. Complex carbs are best consumed with protein and/or fat, which will leave you feeling fuller longer. Protein and fat take longer to metabolize, so they have a kind of time-release effect on carbohydrates, which helps keep blood sugar stable. So go ahead and put sour cream on your potato or butter on your green beans!

Glycemic What?

There are several terms you may have heard that describe different carbohydrates, and you may find them more than a little confusing. Glycemic index (GI), glycemic load (GL), net carbs—what do they mean, and how much do you need to know? In brief, glycemic index measures how rapidly a carbohydrate is turned into glucose, causing a spike in insulin (white table sugar is the fastest, with the highest GI, 100). Over time, eating foods with a high GI sustains high insulin levels and disrupts other hormonal cross talk, encouraging the body to put on fat. Glycemic load, on the other hand, takes into account the amount of carbohydrates in a single serving of a food, so it's a more practical measure of how high the insulin spike might reach with a single portion of a certain food. For example, rice has a high GI (81) but a moderate GL (28). And net carbs considers the carb/glucose content of food alongside its content of protein and fiber, which slow glucose absorption. The net carb content of a serving of rice and beans would be 20: 32 grams of carbohydrates minus 12 grams of fiber. What this means is that you don't have to avoid all carbohydrates, but you should pay some attention to the GL and net carbs of a certain food. Complex carbs naturally have low net carbs compared to refined and processed foods, because there are so many other nutrients involved (that's why they're complex!). If you find yourself having a sugary snack, dessert, or drink, try to eat some protein with it—a practice that lowers the net carbs of the dessert and decreases the accompanying insulin spike. You'll find a chart of glycemic index and glycemic load values for some common foods in the Appendices.

Fat

We love to eat it, hate it in the mirror. But dietary fat is essential for life, just like glucose and protein. In fact, if glucose is unavailable, the body will break fat down by ketosis as a backup brain fuel. Fat is crucial to maintaining cell membranes, brain tissue, and nerve sheaths, increasing immunity, maintaining energy reserves, stabilizing blood sugar, and controlling hunger. Digestion breaks fat down into fatty acids and lipids, one of which, cholesterol, forms the basic building block of our sex hormones.

A couple of fatty acids that we cannot synthesize ourselves—omega-3 (linoleic acid) and omega-6 (alphalinoleic acid), called the essential fatty acids (EFAs)—have been linked with decreases in inflammation, hypertension, and LDL cholesterol and improvements in mood, cognition, and hormonal balance. More important than the EFAs themselves are the components they break down into, many of which serve as precursors to our all-important hormones. Since we don't make them, we must get these EFAs in our diet. The ratio between them is important: in our Westernized diet, we tend to get too much omega-6, found in many common vegetable oils like soybean, safflower, and corn, compared to our intake of omega-3, which is found abundantly in fatty and freshwater fish and in primrose, flaxseed, and hemp. (You can read more about EFAs in the Appendices.)

When cells have easy access to glucose in the blood, they rely less on the long-term stored energy in fat. Instead of flowing in and out of fat cells, then, fatty acids accumulate there as triglycerides, forming tissue called white adipose tissue—body fat. The kind we love to hate. When one fat cell is full and you still have extra energy to store, your body makes another, and so on until you can't zip up your skirt. But the key thing to realize here is that it's extra glucose making you fatter faster, not extra dietary fat. Dietary fat has more calories per gram than protein or carbs, but it is metabolized differently. And you can't eat as much in one sitting as you can of carbohydrates, so you often end up eating fewer calories overall (not that we're counting calories).

Does this mean you can march right out and order a triple bacon cheeseburger with fries? No, because the dietary fat I'm talking about is healthy fat—real fat, found in organic dairy products, fish, vegetables, nuts, seeds, and their oils. Depending on the structure of the fat molecule, it is monounsaturated, polyunsaturated, or saturated. All three types are fine to eat in moderation. These healthy fats, found in nature, are made of long chains of carbon molecules bonded together. Fats become unhealthy—damaged— when these bonds are broken, which occurs during cooking, charbroiling, artificial processing, or poor storage. Next time you're in a fast-food restaurant, take a whiff—that smell is rancid, damaged fat!

You've probably heard about the dangers of trans fats—artificially hydrogenated oils used mainly to extend the shelf life of food. To make these substances, extra hydrogen is pumped into polyunsaturated vegetable oils to saturate the carbon molecules in them. Margarine, butter substitutes, and any foods containing hydrogenated or partially hydrogenated oils have trans fats in them, even if it's not listed on the label. (The government allows products with less than 0.5 percent trans fat per serving to be labeled trans-fat-free. The problem, of course, is that most people don't eat just one serving.)

The USDA can't determine a healthful limit for trans-fat intake, because even very small amounts appear to be harmful. Researchers are now in nearly universal agreement that trans fats and damaged fats, rather than saturated fats, are the culprits in atherosclerosis and high cholesterol in most healthy individuals. Studies indicate that if we didn't eat these fats, more than 30,000 deaths from cardiovascular disease could be avoided every year.

Fiber

Fiber, simply put, is roughage: the stuff your mother told you to eat. It's not really considered a classic macronutrient, but I think it's so important that I'm ranking it as such.

In fact, fiber is nutrient-neutral; it is the indigestible parts of vegetables and grains that act as a cleanup team for your digestive tract. It absorbs extra cholesterol and bulks up and softens stool, which shortens transit time in the bowel and limits your potential exposure to toxins.

Fiber can be soluble or insoluble. Soluble fibers, such as inulin, fructans, xanthan gum, cellulose, guar gum, fructooligosaccharides, and oligo- or polysaccharides, are found in grains, vegetables, nuts, seeds, and some fruits. They bind with fatty acids and undergo a kind of fermentation that feeds the digestive flora in your intestine and helps slow the metabolism of carbohydrates into glucose. Insoluble fiber, such as bran, fruit skins, seeds, nuts, and whole wheat, expands in your digestive tract to make you feel fuller longer. It also promotes regular bowel movements and helps remove toxins from the gut.

Most of us get too little fiber in our diets—a problem that is easily remedied by filling your plate with veggies at every meal, even breakfast. And just to be sure you're getting enough, I'll include an easy-to-make fiber shake as part of the Core Balance eating plan.

Micronutrients

Macronutrients may be the walls of the house, but micronutrients, though needed in smaller amounts, are essential as well. They are vitamins and minerals, including antioxidants, that protect and maintain your body. Without them, your "house" would fall into serious disrepair and age far too quickly.

Essential Vitamins

These building blocks are the ever-busy worker ants of the metabolic process. They are numerous and their functions on the verge on the miraculous, from protecting eyesight to scrubbing cells to repairing DNA.

Vitamins work hard with the help of enzymes to activate (catalyze) body functions. As co-enzymes, they regulate metabolism and help in myriad biochemical processes that release energy from food. Most are water-soluble, so any excess is excreted in urine. Those that are fat-soluble—vitamins A, D, E, and K—are stored in tissue and can become toxic at high levels. For this reason, I do not recommend self-prescribing high dosages of fat-soluble vitamins beyond what's recommended in the Core Balance program. I do recommend a high-potency daily multivitamin and an EFA supplement during the first 14 days of the program. You'll continue this throughout the month, unless your customized Core Balance plan calls for something different in the next 14 days.

There are several subcategories of vitamins. Bioflavonoids, sometimes referred to as vitamin P, are not true vitamins, but are essential for the absorption of vitamin C. Carotenoids/carotenes, a subclass of vitamin A, are antioxidants thought to help prevent cancer, much like vitamin D. Beta-carotene and lycopene are two of the most widely known carotenes; however, there are as many as 600 and still more to be discovered. Finally, Co-enzyme Q10 is a vitaminlike substance that resembles the structure of vitamin E; it's a powerful antioxidant and mitochondrial helper.

Essential Minerals

Minerals are needed to protect the makeup of body fluids, blood, and bone and the maintenance of healthy nerve function and muscle tone. They also serve as co-enzymes and rely on enzymatic activity to function. Sufficient minerals are necessary for the full activation of vitamins, so a reputable multivitamin will also contain a full roster of minerals.

The essential minerals are boron, calcium, chromium, copper, germanium, iodine, iron, magnesium, manganese, molybdenum, phosphorus, potassium, selenium, silicon, sodium, sulfur, vanadium, and zinc. Essential minerals are found in our food, but it is still very common to see people suffering from certain mineral deficiencies.

Minerals are stored in bone and tissue, and it's possible—though exceedingly rare—to develop mineral toxicity if you ingest massive amounts. I do not advise self-prescribing large doses of minerals beyond what's recommended in the Core Balance plan. If you have questions about mineral therapies, talk to an integrative practitioner or naturopath.

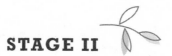

The First 14 Days: The Core Balance Essential Plan

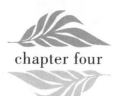

chapter four

GETTING STARTED

The first step of any journey is often the hardest, so I am going to try to make the next two weeks easy for you. You will not be making any radical changes (unless you are currently eating out all the time or getting your meals from fast-food restaurants). You will be making slow, subtle improvements to your nutrition and your habits. In particular, you will be eating more whole, unprocessed, undamaged foods and getting your carbohydrates primarily from vegetables and fruit and whole grains, not refined grains and baked goods.

Often when I first tell patients that they are going to have to change their diets, they start getting a panicked look in their eyes. More than a few have burst into tears at the thought of giving up their morning bagels or their daily dose of chocolate. If this is the way you're feeling, take a deep breath. Then consider: if you could help your partner to lose weight, or help protect your child's health, by changing what he or she ate for a month, wouldn't you try and do it? Now, aren't you worth that same amount of attention?

All I'm asking is that you do your best for a month. In my experience, once patients move past the shock factor and start following the Core Balance Diet, they look and feel so much better that they can't imagine eating any other way. For many women, eliminating refined carbs and sugar and watching overall carb intake is enough to restore Core Balance. Don't worry, I promise you will see your favorite sweet treat again—just not for the next month. And you may be surprised to find that when you and that sticky bun meet again, in your newly balanced state, you will feel very differently about it!

Over the next 14 days, you'll remove the most distracting clutter from your diet and lifestyle—the kind of clutter that gums up your body's signals, confuses your internal conversation, and creates toxic weight. Clutter, by definition, means extraneous items that we may like to have around, but that we don't need. The clutter in your diet and lifestyle is the snack you reach for when you aren't thinking; the habits and stimulants you fall back on when you're harried; the many ways you keep your hypothalamus and central nervous system on high alert and your intellect from paying attention to what's really going on inside you.

At the end of this chapter, you'll find my Core Balance Commandments, keys to making the program work for you. In the next two chapters, you'll find my guidelines for the Core Balance Essential Eating Plan and Wellness Plan—all you need to know about what to eat, what to do, and how to take the best care of yourself and your body for the next two weeks. I don't like absolutes, so I just ask you to work with these guidelines as best you can. Know that the more closely you follow them, the faster you will see results!

The organization of the Essential Eating Plan is the same as each of my custom plans, so you can get used to the format—except that here, where everything is laid out for the first time, I've split the nutrition and action plans into two parts so they won't be so cumbersome. In each plan you will find a handy "Marcelle's Prescription" that highlights the major points, a list of foods you can eat to your heart's content (and foods it's best to avoid), guidelines for supplements to support your healing, and a 14-day menu plan, as well as a "Day in the Life" rundown of what you can expect a day to look like while you're following a particular plan. Throughout, I've sprinkled information, hints, and tips to help you along. The Essential Eating Plan is the backbone of the Core Balance Diet. It's designed to teach you healthy eating and lifestyle habits that will sustain you for the rest of your life. It is also meant to form a firm foundation of health upon which the Custom Plans later in this book are built.

Before You Start

Most of my patients have easily incorporated the Core Balance Program into their self-care routines, but it's always a good idea to discuss any changes in diet and lifestyle with a caring medical professional, preferably an integrative practitioner who understands both traditional and alternative methods of care. This is especially true if you're currently taking medication or being treated for a chronic disease. And if you are pregnant or nursing a baby, I want you to stop reading and put this book on the shelf for the time being. Pregnancy and lactation are a time to nurture yourself and your baby with abundant nutrition and self-care, not a time for weight loss. There's plenty of time to revisit the Core Balance Diet when your baby is weaned. Here are a few elements of your health picture to consider before you start the program.

Prescription Medication

You may already be taking one or more prescription drugs or over-the-counter medications as part of your daily routine. And while my experience has shown me that certain medications may contribute to a core imbalance and thereby to your toxic weight gain, your health-care provider obviously thinks you are better off taking them, so don't go off them without consulting your practitioner.

Most of my patients don't want to take a pill for more than a few years at most, but no one's told them what else they can do. One of the travesties of our drug-saturated culture is that we have no endgame; people get on medications and stay on them. One of the goals of this program is to get you healthy, naturally, so that your body thrives on its own chemicals—not synthetic versions—and it should help you eventually eliminate the need for any medications you are on. In the meantime, all of the measures I prescribe over the next month are safe for the average healthy woman whether she is on a prescription or not. If you have any questions, ask your health-care practitioner. Show him or her this book and discuss the contents. At Women to Women, we are always happy to work with a patient's outside practitioners, and we have yet to see an adverse or dangerous reaction take place from combining prescription medications with the Core Balance plans.

Triglycerides

In the last chapter, we talked about healthy fat as an essential part of your nutrition picture. One important note: intake of healthy fat does increase blood levels of triglycerides, so if you already know that you have high triglyceride levels in your blood you will want to monitor your saturated fat intake carefully by watching your intake of animal fats and high-fat dairy products. At my practice, I consider a healthy triglyceride level to be any number under 100 milligrams; conventional practitioners will tell you 150 milligrams, so even if your number falls between the two you are probably okay. What I don't like to see is a rising trend if your triglycerides are already over 100 mgs or if high triglycerides are accompanied by high cholesterol and inflammation. If you are able to multiply your HDL number by 4 or 5 and get your triglyceride number, you are insulin resistant until proven otherwise. (For more on insulin resistance and metabolic syndrome, please read the Hormonal Imbalance Custom Plan.) But even if your tests do show high triglycerides, the right dietary changes can help. I had a patient who brought her triglycerides down from 450 to 104 with the Core Balance Diet, and her cholesterol went from 350 to 180 in the meantime. (I like to see cholesterol levels below 200.) If you are testing high, I recommend retesting your triglycerides every 3 to 4 months with a blood test, just to be safe.

If You Smoke

Later in this chapter, you'll find a list of things to avoid while you're following the Core Balance plan. I call these the Truly Toxic Ten—and nicotine is on the list. If you are interested in getting well and fit, you should try to stop smoking. But not now.

In my experience, making too many changes at once simply undermines women's confidence and commitment. So don't try to do it all at once. Instead, as you move through the next month, mark a date on your calendar—six weeks or two months from now—to quit. You'll be better able to do it successfully then: I have several patients who have stopped smoking with relatively little effort after following the nutrition and lifestyle guidelines in the Core Balance plan. Over the next month you'll be learning many new ways to support your body, mind, and spirit—making your need for nicotine a thing of the past.

You may be nervous about stopping, thinking it will cause you to gain weight. In the short term, it's true that nicotine is a stimulant to the HPA axis and a powerful appetite suppressant. Over the long haul, however, nicotine chews you up on the inside, damaging your cells and stressing every system in your body. And I've seen that women feel so much better and lighter after healing their core imbalances and shedding toxic weight that quitting smoking actually becomes doable without gaining weight!

A Word about Supplements

I've designed the Core Balance eating plan so you can give your body the nutrition it needs, mostly in the delicious form of real food. However, even when you are eating well, you may not be getting enough active nutrients to heal your core imbalances. Unfortunately, soil degradation and commercial farming, packaging, and transportation can sap live food of its inherent nutritional value.[1] According to a plethora of research, our food supply has approximately 25 percent less nutritional value than it did in 1977—and that's before it hits the truck, the plastic bag, or the refrigerator.[2] Freshly picked greens, vegetables, and fruit begin to lose their nutrient value the moment they're picked. Think of how quickly fresh produce goes bad. Would you eat lettuce after it had been in the crisper for two or three weeks? We actually do it all the time. Transportation in refrigerated trucks over long distances means that the greens you buy today may have been picked more than two weeks beforehand, frozen, and much of their nutrient value lost. The same goes for lettuce in a bag—even the organic varieties. Depending on the manufacturing process, the lettuce is picked early, frozen, jet-washed, bagged in a plastic film, and vacuum-sealed—sometimes with inert gases—to prevent oxidization that leads to wilting and browning. What's more, there's no knowing what else is in the bag. The process is very secretive and competitive and companies don't like to share their methods. The Dole Company recalled its packaged lettuce in 2006 after a mysterious E. coli scare; no one could explain how the bacteria got in the bags. Commercial farming and modern transportation means we can eat raspberries in winter, but we still haven't found a way to preserve their just-picked nutritional value. This sad truth is now so accepted that in 2002 the American Medical Association reversed its longtime stance on supplements and now recommends that all healthy adults take a daily multivitamin.[3]

So, in addition to all the good food you'll be eating, I will also be asking you to take some potent nutriceuticals—pharmaceutical-grade supplements that will ensure your body is getting enough nutrition to fill any holes in your diet. One important element of your supplement regime will be a probiotic: the opposite of an antibiotic, this supplement encourages the growth of beneficial microbes to help you fortify or rebuild the natural flora your body needs for health. (You'll learn more about probiotics later on when we discuss the special Core Balance program for digestive issues; you can also read more in the Appendices.) I also recommend that you take a high-potency daily multivitamin while you are on the Core Balance Essential Plan (Stage II) and continue it during your Custom Plan (Stage III), with one exception: when you are working with a specific core imbalance and using the full dosage of a medical food.

In a few different places in Stage III, you will hear me use that phrase, *medical food.* Medical foods are special nutrient combinations prescribed by healthcare practitioners (though they are available over the counter) to manage certain chronic conditions like hormone imbalance, joint pain, and inflammation and to provide support while a patient is undergoing a medical detox. I use medical foods in my practice, and I have found them to be hugely influential in healing core imbalances. Because the FDA prefers medical foods to be used under the guidance of a medical professional, the average consumer may not be aware of them. In the Appendices, I've included the basic formula for the medical foods I use at the clinic, but most women I know don't want to take a whole basket of individual supplements. For this reason, I prefer to use the premixed packaged medical foods. If you are interested, you—and your practitioner—can read more on my Website.

But for now, and perhaps for the entire month unless you decide to use a medical food (or an approximation of one), you'll take a daily multivitamin. I also recommend that you take a daily dose of calcium (about 800 mgs) and magnesium (about 400 mgs); women older than 50 should take 1200/600 mgs, respectively. You may take calcium and magnesium separately or bundled together for better absorption (magnesium helps calcium uptake). I also recommend an essential fatty acid supplement that contains about 600 mgs combined of both eicosapentaenoic acid (EPA) and docosahexaenoic acid (DHA) from fish oil. It can be taken in liquid form or pill form—preferable for most patients who did not grow up on a daily dose of cod liver oil. Later on, if your tests show that you have inflammation, you may want to increase the dose. If you are vegan or do not eat fish, you can get an EFA supplement made from flaxseed, borage, or evening primrose oil, but be aware that flax seed is an omega-3 and the others are omega-6s; our goal is to increase the ratio of omega-3s to omega-6s, so try to find a vegetarian EFA compound that accomplishes this.

Your daily multivitamin should contain these nutrients in the following approximate dosages:

- Vitamin A: 10,000 IUs, 85% betacarotene
- Vitamin B complex, including:
  - B1 (thiamine), 50–70 mgs
  - B2 (riboflavin), 25–35 mgs
  - B3 (niacin), 120–140 mgs
  - B5 (pantothenic acid), 225–270 mgs
  - B6 (pyroxodine), 25–35 mgs
  - B12 (methylcobalamin), 60–70 mgs)
- Biotin, 100–200 mcgs
- Choline, 100 mgs
- Folate (folic acid), 500 mcgs
- Vitamin C (ascorbic acid), at least 800 mgs
- Vitamin D, at least 400 IUs
- Vitamin E, at least 200 IUs
- Vitamin K, 35–45 mcgs
- Essential minerals
  - Iodine, 100 mcgs
  - Zinc, 10–15 mgs
  - Selenium, 100–135 mcgs
  - Copper, 1–2 mgs

- Manganese, 10–15 mgs
- Chromium, 100–135 mcgs
- Molybdenum, 100 mcgs
- Boron, 3–4 mgs
- Vanadium, 20–25 mcgs

Now, you should be aware that the FDA has not approved the use of supplements and herbs for medical conditions. There is plenty of evidence—empirical, circumstantial, and traditional—that backs up the use of herbs and nutrients for healing, but by their nature these substances are difficult and expensive to test under the Western medical standard we use for synthetic drugs: the double-blind placebo-controlled study. However, with interest in natural healing on the rise, more funding is available and more research into the synergistic effects of nutrients and herbs is getting underway—so stay tuned.

I have used supplements and medical foods for decades, personally and professionally, and have never seen a bad reaction. I am concerned, though, about the varying levels of effective ingredients in different brands on the market, so I encourage you to buy the best brand of supplement you can afford packaged in a way that makes it easy for you to remember to take. Make sure you know the brand and the company and where it makes its supplements. This is important because once you know a company is good at testing its product—or, as we say in the medical world, assaying—you can trust that what it says is in the product really is in the product. This may mean the product is more expensive, but also that it is more effective and not just filled with inactive ingredients (the ultimate waste of money).

The Truly Toxic Ten

As I've said, I don't like absolutes, but there are a few things out there in the world that I would like you to avoid over the next 28 days. I know it's hard. If you slip up, it doesn't mean you are naughty—the chemicals are the naughty ones! Do the best you can, and keep some activated charcoal tablets on hand to take as an antidote. Activated charcoal is available at natural-food stores; if taken as soon as you feel discomfort, it binds with the toxins in your gut and escorts them to your colon for elimination, thereby reducing any unwanted side effects, like bloating, nausea, headache, and gas. But I hope my guidelines will help you navigate the danger zones in your own life so you won't need these emergency countermeasures.

At the grocery store, steer clear of these nasties as much as you can. The chemicals on this list will impede the healing of your metabolism, slow your body's ability to metabolize fat and hormones, topple your blood sugar balance, and undermine your immunity by increasing inflammation. In short, they are the biggest sources of toxic weight that you can control. In the list on the right, they're shown in order from most harmful to least.

The Core Balance Commandments for Success

As you get ready to start the Core Balance Essential Plan, I know there's a lot to think about. I've given you a lot of information about your body, the nutrition it needs, and the ways to clear the clutter that's disrupting your internal conversation. And I'll be giving you more as we go along. So here's my list of the most important points to keep in mind—guidelines for the key elements of the Core Balance program and support for the efforts you'll be making.

- Consult with your health-care practitioner before beginning the program.

- Read the labels on food products and don't buy what you can't pronounce (you'll find more details on savvy label-reading in the Appendices).

- Try to eat foods that look like what they are (fish, not fish sticks; potatoes, not potato chips).

- Practice the rot rule: if it wouldn't perish on the shelf in three days, don't buy it.

- Avoid damaged fats, including trans fats.

- Avoid processed and packaged foods.

- Watch out for artificial preservatives, coloring, pesticides, and other artificial chemicals.

The Truly Toxic Ten

1. Recreational drugs/ narcotics

2. Tobacco/nicotine

3. Trans fats

4. Artificial sugars/ sweeteners–sucralose (Splenda), aspartame, acesulfame-K, saccharine, mannitol, and sorbitol

5. Refined sugars– sucrose, fructose, maltose, dextrose, maltodextrin, polydextrose, corn syrup, and high-fructose corn syrup

6. Chemical additives– artificial coloring, emulsifiers, thickeners, nitrates, monosodium glutamate (MSG), and preservatives

7. Alcohol

8. Over-the-counter medications–pain relievers, antihistamines, cough syrups, cold remedies, and so on

9. Caffeine

10. Too many prescription medications

- Eat slowly, savoring each bite.

- Disconnect from TV, the computer, phones, telephone, radio, and portable music players—particularly before bedtime.

- Avoid artificial sweeteners as much as you can; try a natural alternative like stevia or agave nectar.

- Don't quit any prescription drug cold turkey (or without discussing it with your health-care practitioner).

- Remember that baby steps will take you far if you keep taking them.

Above all, be patient and kind to yourself. Don't beat yourself up if you can't manage to do everything at once. Take your time and make changes slowly. As you move into the next two weeks, try for the 85-15 rule: 85 percent of the time, be as strict as you can, and don't worry about the other 15 percent. But realize that you will see success earlier the stricter you are with yourself.

At the end of two weeks, you may find that weight is dropping off (safely and slowly, I hope) and that your energy, mood, and resilience are much better. If so, feel free to continue with this plan for as long as you like, rotating the meals. This part of the program is meant to help you eat well for life, so there is no limit to how long it can be followed. If you aren't seeing the progress you'd like in these first two weeks, take my Core Imbalance Quiz on the morning of Day 14. Then we can go on to investigate any specific core imbalance(s) that may be getting in your way.

While you're on the Core Balance Essential Plan and beginning to restore balance in your body, please read Stage IV and start thinking about what's going on in the other corners of your health puzzle—your intellectual, emotional, and instinctual selves. In the next 14 days of the program, you can think about trying some of the techniques I suggest there for peeling back the layers to explore and heal your whole self.

While you're on the Core Balance program, check in with how you feel every day. In the beginning, you may feel a little worse before you feel better as your body begins to mobilize fat and the toxins stored there are released into your blood. This is why it's so important to drink lots of water and herbal teas to flush the kidneys and liver; to exercise moderately each day to pump the lymph system; and to not lose too much weight too fast. Otherwise your body will react to the influx of toxins by going back into defense mode, and you'll just gain the weight back.

chapter five

THE CORE BALANCE
ESSENTIAL EATING PLAN

Most practitioners have given up on counseling women to change their diets; it takes too much time, and it's far easier to write a prescription. But I've seen the beneficial effects that nutrition and positive lifestyle changes can offer—and they're far cheaper and longer-lasting than a prescription. Food is potent medicine on its own. And if you combine good nutrition with moderate daily exercise and safe supplements, you can and will make huge improvements to your health that will shrink inches from your waistline.

The guidelines I give you in this chapter are the same I give to all my patients. They are designed to clear away clutter from your diet, to stabilize your blood sugar and hormones, and to quiet the extraneous "noise" in your internal conversation so that you can listen to your core symptoms more clearly. For some women, this plan may be all it takes to allow their bodies to feel safe enough to let go of toxic weight.

So now it's time to figure out how you're going to eat all this yummy food!

Marcelle's Prescription for
CORE BALANCE NUTRITION

1. Eat three balanced meals and two snacks a day.

2. Eat adequate protein at every meal, especially breakfast.

3. Start the day with a cup of hot water, lemon, and a dash of cayenne pepper to stimulate the secretion of bile from the liver and rev up your digestion for the day.

4. Eat within an hour of waking; finish eating by 7 P.M. if you can.

5. Chew thoroughly so your saliva has a chance to work.

6. Eat as much as you want from my lists of leafy greens and non-starchy vegetables (page 70)—no limit!

7. Limit dairy products to four servings a day, and choose raw or lightly pasteurized milk or goat milk, yogurts, cheeses, and other organic products (and make them full or 2 percent fat unless you are watching your saturated fat because you have high triglycerides or cholesterol!).

8. Eat healthy fats, particularly foods rich in omega-3s, like deep-water fish, sardines in oil, and flaxseed, borage, hemp, sesame seed, and wheat germ oils.

9. Eliminate all "white" food—refined sugar, flour, and cereals.

10. Color your world—dark green, deep red, purple, orange, and blue—because colorful foods have a greater nutrient and enzyme concentration.

11. Remember to hydrate—drink at least eight 8-ounce glasses of filtered water or noncaffeinated herbal tea a day.

12. Limit caffeine to one or two cups a day, preferably from green tea.

13. Avoid soft drinks, including undiluted juice; drink herbal teas or bubbly water with lemon or lime instead.

14. Pay attention to portion size.

Eating for Essential Core Balance

It's best to get as many nutrients as you can by eating and enjoying real food—food that can be grown, hunted, or foraged without added chemicals. This means that on my program you will be cooking, perhaps more than you are used to. Since I know you are busy, I have tried to give suggestions to make cooking easier. I've also suggested a few pre-pared-food brands (in the Appendices) that I think are okay, particularly when it comes to specialty products and gluten-free foods. If you are getting most of your nutrition from real meals and snacks, I think it's fine to fill in gaps occasionally with high-quality nutrient bars. But these items should not take the place of real meals. When you skip real meals and forget to drink water you are depriving your body of the working materials it needs to function.

Each meal in the Core Balance Essential Plan is, well, balanced: approximately 30 percent protein, 30 percent healthy fats, and 40 percent complex carbohydrates, mostly from vegetables and complex grains (with a lot of fiber thrown in). You should eat these foods in combination, as they have synergistic effects that researchers are only now beginning to unravel. For example, fats seem to enhance the body's ability to access the antioxidants in vegetables; protein, which is digested more slowly than carbohydrates, works to slow the rush of glucose into the blood; and fiber helps absorb toxins and "indigestibles," such as fillers, nonnutritional additives, and chemicals unrecognized by the body, for easier elimination. I like a house analogy again: Think of your DNA as the architect, your brain as the general contractor, your biochemicals and cells as the day laborers, and your nutrients, including vitamins and minerals, as the building materials. If you want a sound and beautiful house, it makes sense to build it with the best materials and put them together in the best way.

You may want to follow a set menu—you'll find my Essential Menu Plan at the end of this chapter—or you may prefer to assemble each meal as you go. If you find you have some extra time—say, on the weekends—double a recipe and freeze the leftovers; that way you'll have a handy, quick, and healthy meal ready on a day when you have no time to cook.

The Core Balance Essential Menu Plan

The Essential Menu Plan will provide you with three balanced meals and two snacks per day for the next two weeks. Each meal has been designed to ensure that you receive optimal nutrition while your metabolism starts to recover. This is the first phase of your 28-day program, and it will help clear out an enormous amount of clutter in your diet—the reason you have toxic weight to begin with.

In all of the meals in the Essential Menu, I've figured out the proper proportions of nutrients for you. (If you decide to design your own meals, you can figure it out for your-self without much difficulty.) You can follow the menu plan exactly or substitute one similar meal for another (e.g., breakfast for breakfast). Because many women need a significant amount of protein to help heal their metabolisms, the menus are family-friendly and designed for omnivores. Most vegetarians and vegans can adapt these recipes to suit their individual requirements. And for every dish marked with an asterisk, I've included the recipe right here in the book. (Recipes start on page 259.)

In the last chapter, I told you that you'd get off the blood-sugar roller coaster by limiting your carbohydrates to 66 grams per day—that's 16 grams per meal and 9 grams per snack. For the next 14 days, I would like you to try to eat your 66 grams of complex carbs per day primarily from fresh vegetables, legumes, and fruits, with smaller portions of whole grain-based carbs thrown in. To make this a no-brainer, you can simply follow the Essential Menu Plan and avoid all baked goods, including bread; "instant" oatmeals; dried cereals and cereal bars; and all junk food, including candy and chips.

Foods for Core Balance

On the next couple of pages, you'll find lists of foods you should feel free to eat abundantly; foods it's fine to eat in moderation; and foods I'll ask you to limit or avoid. You'll also find a list of supplements I recommend you take during the next 14 days, along with some herbs and spices that will help maximize the benefits of your good nutrition.

Abundant Foods

- Leafy greens

- Nonstarchy vegetables

- Lean protein—turkey, chicken, duck, bison, tofu, soy protein, rice protein, whey protein

- Eggs

- Beans/legumes

- Wild and brown rice

- Complex grains—whole wheat, buckwheat, oats, groats, rye, spelt, amaranth, quinoa, millet, barley

- Berries

- Apples/pears/melon

- Nuts and nut butters

- Monounsaturated oils (see page 68)

Foods to Eat in Moderation

- Fish (because of high mercury levels, no more than once a week; for the same reason, smaller fish, such as tilapia, sole, and orange roughy, are preferable to larger fish, such as tuna or swordfish)

- Lean beef, pork, lamb (organic if possible)

- Dairy—hard cheeses, cottage cheese, ricotta, yogurt, cream, sour cream

- Polyunsaturated oils (see page 68)

- Saturated fats—butter, animal/poultry fat and skin, coconut and palm oils (see page 68); keep these to a minimum if you have heart disease, high cholesterol, and/or high triglycerides

- Starchy vegetables—artichokes, corn, lima beans, root vegetables (except celeriac and fennel, which you can eat in abundance)

- Citrus

- Celtic sea salt

- Maple syrup, brown rice syrup, honey, stevia

- Whole-grain breads and crackers, preferably gluten-free

- Kelp products (for iodine)

Foods to Limit or Avoid

- High-fructose corn syrup
- Trans fats, damaged and rancid fats
- Partially hydrogenated oils
- Artificial sweeteners
- Artificial chemicals/preservatives—BHA, BHT, MSG, food coloring, etc.
- Processed milk products (half-and-half, skim milk, low-fat milk)
- Smoked/preserved/canned meats

- Baked goods—cakes, cookies, pastries, scones, pancakes, waffles, etc.
- Candy and chocolate
- Refined-grain crackers
- Fried foods (potato chips, french fries)
- Alcohol
- Caffeine
- Refined sugar, white flour, white rice

Daily Supplements, Herbs, and Spices

- A high-quality multivitamin with calcium and magnesium

- Essential fatty acids

- A probiotic with Lactobacillus acidopholus and L. bifidus in the billions (take with water 5 to 15 minutes before eating)

- Seaweed or kelp

- Thermogenic spices—ginger, cayenne, mustard, cinnamon, turmeric—to season foods

A Good "Cuppa"

Spotting caffeine on the list of foods to limit or avoid may have given you more than a moment's pause. Many of us find it difficult to give up coffee and black tea—but the reason why may be more complex than just the daily buzz. An important part of the morning routine for many women is a hot "cuppa"—it's relaxing and warming and makes us feel comforted. And there's no reason to give this up. I'm okay with one cup of coffee in the morning while you are on the Core Balance Essential Plan, but know that weaning off caffeine for a period of time is always a healthy choice. If you need more than one cup, try changing what's in the cup! Herbal teas, decaf coffee, warm water with lemon, or even low-sodium chicken, beef, or vegetable broth sipped slowly in the morning are delicious alternatives.

If you're finding it really hard to stop drinking coffee and black teas, don't stress! Try to alternate cups of caffeinated coffee and tea with non-caffeinated varieties, or make your morning coffee with half decaf, half caf, slowly increasing the amount of decaf until you wean off caf completely. Always buy high-quality Arabica beans (which are lower in caffeine than robusta varieties) and really savor your cup; you may find you need only one.

As you wean off caffeine, experiment with herbal teas. Not only are they delicious, but they will help keep you hydrated. Many come in prepackaged tea bags, or you can buy loose-leaf tea and make your own infusion. See the list below for some ideas. If you are on prescription medication, diabetic, pregnant, or breast-feeding, do not ingest herbs or herbal teas without discussing them first with your medical practitioner.

Herbal Teas for All Reasons

- To invigorate and boost digestion: cinnamon, ginger, green teas, fennel, gentian, gotu kola, lemongrass, peppermint, red raspberry, sage, sarsaparilla, slippery elm, yerba maté

- To detoxify: alfalfa, anise, dandelion, fenugreek, gingko, licorice, nettle, parsley, red clover, uva ursi

- To boost immunity: birch bark, echinacea, elder, feverfew, garlic, goldenseal, horehound, hyssop, marshmallow, pau d'arco

- To calm and relax: borage, chamomile, dong quai, hops, kava kava, kudzu, passionflower, St. John's wort, valerian

To make a delicious infusion, preheat an 8-cup teapot and a mug with hot water. Fill kettle with cold water and heat just until boiling. Empty teapot and add 2–3 tablespoons herbal leaves or flowers (or to taste). Fill teapot with just-boiled water. Let steep for 3–4 minutes. Empty mug and pour infusion through a small, tight-mesh tea strainer. Serve with lemon.

Stocking Up

Sticking to the program is much easier when you keep a well-stocked Core Balance pantry and fridge: If you have good food available when you're ready to prepare a meal at the end of a tiring day, you won't feel tempted to default to something cheap and easy. Read on for some guidelines on grocery shopping, as well as staples to keep on hand to support your efforts.

Whenever possible, try to buy fresh local and organic produce and wash it thoroughly before consuming it. In a pinch, frozen or canned vegetables and fruit are also suitable, but check the label for additives and extra salt (sodium) and sugar. I know that buying organic can get expensive, so if you have to pick and choose, it's best to buy the foods that tend to be highest in pesticides from an organic source. Foods that are lower in pesticides can come from conventional sources, but try to buy local when you can; this supports your community growers and saves on all that energy it takes to ship produce internationally. See the list on the right for a breakdown.

I prefer to purchase organic poultry, fish, eggs, and meats to avoid ingesting additional antibiotics and hormones that accumulate in animal tissues. Whenever possible, buy grass-fed meats, as there is a lot of evidence that they produce fewer inflammatory acids in the blood than grain-fed meat.[1] Organic, grass-fed beef comes from cows that graze, as nature intended, not those who are grain-fed in a feed lot and pumped full of hormones and antibiotics. It is more expensive, but you will be eating it in moderation, so focus your dollars on quality, not quantity.

As often as you can, shop the outside aisles of the grocery story—where all the real food lives. Resist the temptation to browse the middle and fill your cart with boxes of fake food. Read the labels and don't buy anything that lists more than ten ingredients, or any ingredients you can't pronounce. Practice the "rot rule"—if it would keep more than three days on the shelf, pass it up—and think nature-made, not man-made.

Does It Have to Be Organic?

Try to buy organic

- Apples
- Bananas
- Bell peppers
- Celery
- Cherries
- Grapes
- Lettuce
- Nectarines
- Peaches
- Pears
- Potatoes
- Spinach
- Strawberries

Okay to buy conventional

- Avocado
- Broccoli
- Cabbage
- Corn (frozen)
- Eggplant
- Kiwi
- Onion
- Sweet peas (frozen)

How to Read a Label

I want you to become an expert at reading the label! If you have kids, teach them to do it, too. Know that the truth is in the fine print, not the big banners on the outside of the box (that's marketing). Don't be fooled by vague terms like *natural, pure,* and *enriched,* or even *organic, organically grown, pesticide-free, all-natural,* and *no artificial ingredients.* Trust only labels that say certified organically grown. These are the only words that mean the food was grown without chemical fertilizers and pesticides, in soil free of these substances.[2]

According to the USDA, all food labels must list the product's ingredients in order by weight. The ingredient the product contains in the greatest amount is listed first. Sometimes labels can be purposefully confusing; don't buy foods that play these tricks:

- Vague labeling. *Vegetable shortening* and *made from healthy fats* sound healthier than *lard* or *bacon fat,* but most shortenings are made with hydrogenated oils, which are trans fats—far worse than lard. Look for a more explicit label, such as *trans-fat-free.* Also beware of the tricky *no trans fats* claim. Manufacturers are allowed to claim this if there is less than 0.5 gram of trans fat per serving. Many of us eat more than one serving in a day, so the half-grams can add up.

- *Natural* claims. *Made from (or made with) natural ingredients* can be a big red herring. Most processed foods begin with natural ingredients—it's what happens to them on their way into the box that should concern you. For example, a lot of sugar cereals are now boasting that they are *made with whole grain*—but who cares when they also contain so much sugar?

Buy certified organic when you can, or shop at a trusted natural food store or farmer's market for local produce. For a list of healthy prepackaged brands that I have worked with successfully, see the Appendices.

The Core Balance Pantry

Some of these items may be new to you. Experiment with them, then keep your favorites on hand.

- Whole-grain flours (to be used in moderation): amaranth, arrowroot, brown rice, buckwheat, corn, cornmeal, potato, soy, triticale, whole wheat (durum)

- Condiments: apple cider, balsamic and other vinegars (if digestive issues aren't a problem), Bragg liquid amino acids, natural mustard, olives, home-made sauces, salsa (without added sugar), peanut sauce (without added sugar), low-sodium tamari (if wheat is okay for you), tahini, non-iodized sea salt, Celtic sea salt, kelp salt, black pepper

- Seaweeds (dried): dulse, hiziki, kelp, wakame, kombu, nori

- Sweeteners: organic honey, organic grade A maple syrup, blackstrap molasses, brown rice syrup, unsweetened applesauce, stevia, xylitol, agave nectar

- Fats and oils (store in refrigerator):
  - Saturated—butter and coconut and grapeseed oils
  - Monounsaturated (always buy cold-pressed varieties)—almond, avocado, canola, high oleic safflower and sunflower, olive, and peanut oils
  - Polyunsaturated—corn, cottonseed, sesame, sunflower, salmon, flaxseed, borage, evening primrose, cod liver, grapeseed, and wheat germ oils

- Spice rack:
  - Fresh—basil, dill, tarragon, rosemary, chives, cilantro, thyme, sorrel, parsley
  - Dried—basil, dill, rosemary, thyme, parsley, cumin, cinnamon, nutmeg, turmeric, cardamom, pepper, garlic salt, bay leaves, paprika, garam masala
  - Juices (to be used sparingly; store in refrigerator): unsweetened cherry, carrot, unsweetened cranberry, tomato, orange, mixed vegetable, apple, pomegranate

---

Healthy Oils

One thing you should know about cooking and storing fats and oils: they can go rancid if left in the cabinet or out on the counter. Rancid fat is damaged fat and very bad for your health. Throw out any rancid-smelling oils, stock up on fresh oil, and store it in the refrigerator. The more saturated the oil, the more solid it will become in the fridge.

Be careful when cooking with fats, too. Monounsaturated fats should never be used with heat; it alters their chemical structure and they, too, become damaged. As for polyunsaturated and saturated fats, it all comes down to how much heat you use. Olive oil is safest when cooking with medium-high heat. Butter, primarily a saturated fat, contains some polyunsaturated fat, so I advise my patients to use it with low heat. And for high-heat cooking? Grapeseed oil. It can tolerate high temperatures without damage.

How Much Should You Eat?

I realize I've said that counting calories isn't important—and I'd rather you eat more protein and fat and not worry about the calories in them—but you need to be reasonable when it comes to portion size. Eat slowly, taking time to chew and swallow, and give your brain time to register the contents of your stomach. This takes about 20 minutes. So stop before you feel stuffed! One way to measure your full portion of food per meal is to cup your hands together in a bowl. That's about how big your stomach is. Serve yourself that amount of food, then wait 20 minutes. If you are still hungry, help yourself to more. Your stomach can stretch to accommodate a lot of food at one time, but overeating shocks your metabolism and sends your insulin into hyperdrive. Our goal is to soothe your body, not keep it in high gear.

Here's a more detailed list of the foods you'll be eating in moderation or in abundance. Use it as a guide to serving sizes, as well as a reference for your shopping list. (All carbohydrate/serving information is based on data published in The Nutrition Almanac, 5th Edition, Lavon J. Dunne; McGraw-Hill, 2002.)

Leafy Green Vegetables
(eat as much of these as you like)

Arugula	Endive	Parsley
Beet greens	Escarole	Romaine
Chicory greens	Iceberg lettuce	Sorrel
Chives	Kale	Spinach
Collards	Loose leaf lettuce	Swiss chard
Dandelion greens	Mustard greens	Watercress

Nonstarchy Vegetables
(eat as much of these as you like)

Asparagus	Celery/celeriac	Raw sauerkraut
Avocado	Cucumber	Shallots
Bean sprouts	Eggplant	Snow peas
Broccoli	Fennel	Spinach
Brussels sprouts	Garlic	Summer squash
Bok choy	Green beans	Tomatoes/cherry
Chinese cabbage	Mushrooms	tomatoes
Cauliflower	Peppers	Zucchini

Lean protein
(Serving size is 4 ounces, approximately the size of your palm)
Poultry (lean cuts, preferably white meat)

Chicken	Goose	Squab
Duck	Ostrich	Turkey
Eggs	Quail	

Meat

Bison	Nitrate-free bacon,	Venison
Grass-fed beef	sausage, and ham	Wild game
Lamb	Pork	

Seafood and Fish
(no more than once per week due to high mercury levels)

Clams	Mussels	Tilapia
Cod	Orange roughy	Trout
Crab	Oysters	Wild halibut
Flounder	Sardines	Wild Pacific salmon
Lobster	Shrimp	
Haddock	Sole	
Mackerel		

Soy

Miso	Tempeh	Tofu
Soy protein		

Dairy
(serving size varies)

Cheddar and other hard cheeses (1 ounce)	Goat's cheese (1 ounce)	Provolone (1 ounce)
Cottage cheese (1 cup)	Greek style yogurt (1 cup)	Ricotta (1 ounce)
Feta (1 inch)	Mozzarella (1 ounce)	Unsweetened plain
	Plain yogurt (1 cup)	Kefir (1 cup)

Nuts and Seeds
(serving size is approximate, 1-2 ounces of nuts,
about a handful; 1-2 tablespoons of nut butter)

Acorns	Hickory nuts	Pumpkin seeds
Almonds	Macadamia	Sesame
Brazil nuts	Peanut	Sunflower
Cashews	Pecans	Walnuts
Coconut (fresh, shredded)	Pine nuts	
Hazelnuts	Pistachio	

Beans/Legumes
(16 gram carbohydrate portion, cooked)

Adzuki (¼ cup)	Great northern (⅓ cup)	Mung (⅓ cup)
Black beans (½ cup)	Hominy (½ cup)	Navy (⅓ cup)
Fava beans (½ cup)	Kidney (⅓ cup)	Pinto (⅓ cup)
French beans (⅓ cup)	Lentil (⅓ cup)	Split peas (⅓ cup)
Garbanzo (chickpeas)	Lima (⅓ cup)	Yellow beans
(⅓ cup)		(⅓ cup)

Starchy Vegetables
(16-gram carbohydrate portion, cooked)

Acorn squash (½ squash)	Green peas (½ cup)	Potato
Artichoke (1)	Jerusalem artichokes (½ cup)	(½ medium (baked)
Beets (1 cup)	Jicama (⅔ cup)	Rutabaga (1 cup)
Butternut squash (⅔ cup)	Leeks (1 cup)	Sweet potato or
Carrots (1 cup)	Okra (1 cup)	yam (½ medium)
Corn (½ cup)	Parsnip (⅔ cup)	Pumpkin (1 cup)
		Turnip (1 cup)
		Winter squash (½ cup)

Fruit
(from lowest sugar loads to highest)
(16-gram carbohydrate portion)

Blackberries (¾ cup)	Cherries (1 handful)	Peach (1 medium)
Blueberries (½ cup)	Honeydew (1 2-inch wedge)	Pear (½)
Boysenberries (¾ cup)	Kiwi (1)	Pineapple (raw)
Grapefruit (½ cup)	Lemons (3)	(¾ cup)
Raspberries (1 cup)	Limes (2)	Plums (2)
Strawberries (1 ¼ cups)	Mango (½)	Pomegranate (½ fruit)
Apple (1 small)	Nectarine (1)	Rhubarb (8 stalks)
Apricots (2)	Orange (1 small)	Tangerines (2 small)
Cantaloupe (1 2-inch wedge)	Papaya (1 cup)	Banana (½ small)

Whole Grains and Cereals
(16-gram carbohydrate portion, cooked)

Barley (⅓ cup)
Brown rice (⅓ cup)
Buckwheat (whole) (⅓ cup)
Bulgur (⅓ cup)
Corn grits (½ cup)
Brown rice pasta (½ cup)

Couscous (⅓ cup)
Kasha (⅓ cup)
Millet (⅓ cup)
Oats (⅔ cup)
Polenta (⅓ cup)
Quinoa (⅓ cup)

Rye (¼ cup)
Wheat Bran (dry)
  (½ cup)
Wheat germ (dry)
  (⅓ cup)
Wild rice/black rice
  (½ cup)

Sweet Treats

As I've said, the fastest, easiest way to start shedding those toxic pounds is to eliminate all baked goods—including bread, junk food, cookies, cakes, pastries, scones, waffles, popovers, pizza dough, and so on—and all extra sugar and gluten from your diet. If you are gluten-sensitive, eating products containing gluten (which includes most conventional baked goods) can start a vicious cycle of cravings. However, life being what it is, I know you will be tempted to indulge every once in a while. It's okay to be tempted! Acknowledge the craving, accept it, and then ask yourself if something else will do. (For hints on calming specific cravings without giving in to them, see page 74.)

In Chinese medicine, a craving for sugar and sweetness is a need for mothering energy—no wonder we turn to it for comfort. So you can wean yourself off sugar by learning how to mother yourself and others in healthier ways. In the meantime, if you simply must have a sweet treat, here are a couple of acceptable choices. Try to keep these indulgences down to twice a week for the next 14 days. And if you know you can't stop once you start, don't even go there. Go directly to the Core Imbalance Quiz on page 93, and we'll figure out what is making you eat compulsively.

- One small slice of fresh fruit pie with unsweetened whipped cream

- Two ounces of bittersweet dark chocolate (above 65 percent cacao)

When Craving Strikes

My Essential Eating Plan is designed to keep your metabolism humming and your belly filled, but if you find you are really hungry, make a big pot of potassium broth or miso soup (recipe, page 269) and sip throughout the day to your heart's content. Or, if you're constantly craving certain foods, try these craving busters.

If you're craving...	Try...
Sweet and creamy	Avocado guacamole (page 263) or a spoonful of healthy nut butter
Sugar	400 milligrams of chromium before meals
Salty foods	Licorice tea with ginseng
Alcohol	Adding 1000 milligrams of L-glutamine to your daily supplements and/or drinking kudzu tea
Coffee	Drinking a cup of hot water, lemon juice, and a sprinkle of cayenne pepper, or a cup of miso soup

Fill Up on Fiber

Try drinking this shake in the morning before breakfast or instead of your afternoon snack every other day—it will do wonders for your hunger pangs and help cleanse your colon.

The Core Balance Fiber-Full Shake

1 scoop powdered psyllium husks, gluten-free
⅓ cup full-fat plain yogurt (I like Greek-style Fage yogurt), or 2 percent if you are
   watching your saturated fat intake because of high cholesterol and/or high triglycerides
3 tablespoons orange or pomegranate juice
6 ounces cold water
4 ice cubes

Optional: sweeten with a pinch of stevia or ⅛ teaspoon of honey, or add 1 scoop of whey or rice protein powder.

Place all ingredients in a blender. Blend on high for 5 seconds or until smooth.

* Recipes start on page 259.

Essential Menu
DAY ONE

BREAKFAST

Tomato and Asparagus
Frittata*
½ cup blueberries

MORNING SNACK

Tropical Prosciutto Rolls*

LUNCH

Sweet Chicken Salad*
½ cup strawberries

AFTERNOON SNACK

Olive Tapenade* with ½ cup
sliced vegetables

DINNER

Creamy Cilantro Chicken*
Crunchy Snow Peas*
⅓ cup wild rice

Essential Menu
DAY TWO

BREAKFAST

2 eggs, any style
Zucchini Cakes*
⅓ cup blueberries

MORNING SNACK

1 small apple, sliced and
spread with 1 tablespoon
cashew butter

LUNCH

Not Your Mom's Chicken Salad*
on 1 cup mixed salad greens

AFTERNOON SNACK

2 Cheese Balls with Parsley*
1 unsweetened rice cake
or 4 rice crackers

DINNER

Pork Chop Medley*
⅓ cup wild rice

Essential Menu
DAY THREE

BREAKFAST

Cheeseless Artichoke Omelet*
½ cup raspberries

MORNING SNACK

Avocado and Pear Dip*
with ½ cup sliced cucumber
or zucchini

LUNCH

Best Ever Egg Drop Soup*
1 cup mixed salad greens
with 1 teaspoon olive oil
and juice of ½ lemon

AFTERNOON SNACK

½ nectarine stuffed with
2 tablespoons ricotta cheese
and sprinkled with cinnamon
or nutmeg

DINNER

baked or broiled chicken
breast, salt and pepper to taste
Asparagus with a Zing*
½ sweet potato with
½ tablespoon butter, sprinkled
with cinnamon if desired

Essential Menu
DAY FOUR

BREAKFAST

2 Salmon Cakes*
½ cup sliced strawberries

MORNING SNACK

½ cup cantaloupe
1 ounce sliced cheese

LUNCH

Curried Chicken Salad* on
1 cup mixed salad greens

AFTERNOON SNACK

2 stalks celery, each stuffed
with 1 tablespoon Lemony
Hummus*

DINNER

Creole Fish*
¼ cup wild rice
1 cup mixed salad greens
with 1 teaspoon olive oil
and balsamic vinegar

Essential Menu
DAY FIVE

BREAKFAST

Creamy Cheesy Scramble*
2 slices nitrate-free bacon
½ cup blueberries

MORNING SNACK

Olive Tapenade* with ½ cup
sliced vegetables

LUNCH

2 leftover Salmon Cakes*
1 cup mixed salad greens
with 1 teaspoon olive oil
and juice of ½ lemon
Cheesy Cauliflower Bake*

AFTERNOON SNACK

Minty Cantaloupe Balls*
2 tablespoons almonds

DINNER

Rosemary Lamb*
Crunchy Green Beans*
¼ cup wild rice

Essential Menu
DAY SIX

BREAKFAST

Creamy Salmon Omelet*
½ cup raspberries

MORNING SNACK

1 small baked apple sprinkled
with cinnamon and
2 tablespoons crushed pecans

LUNCH

Curried Chicken Salad* on
1 cup mixed salad greens
½ gluten-free roll

AFTERNOON SNACK

Avocado and Pear Dip*
with ½ cup sliced cucumber
or zucchini

DINNER

grilled or broiled steak
Asparagus Soup*
½ sweet potato with
½ tablespoon butter, sprinkled
with cinnamon if desired
2 cups steamed spinach

Essential Menu
DAY SEVEN

BREAKFAST

Spicy Fiesta Eggs*
¼ cup blueberries with
1 tablespoon heavy cream,
sweeten with stevia to taste

MORNING SNACK

½ cup sliced strawberries
1 tablespoon pecans

LUNCH

leftover grilled or broiled steak
over 1 cup mixed salad greens
Asparagus Soup*
½ gluten-free roll

AFTERNOON SNACK

Olive Tapenade* with ½ cup
sliced vegetables

DINNER

Fillet of Fish Amandine*
Edamame Mix*
¼ cup wild rice
1 cup mixed salad greens
with 1 teaspoon olive oil
and balsamic vinegar

Essential Menu
DAY EIGHT

BREAKFAST

½ cup cottage cheese
2 Homemade Turkey Patties*
½ cup blueberries

MORNING SNACK

½ baked pear sprinkled with
cinnamon or nutmeg and
1 tablespoon crushed pecans

LUNCH

Spinach Salad*

AFTERNOON SNACK

2 Cheese Balls with Parsley*
1 unsweetened rice cake
or 4 rice crackers

DINNER

Chicken Cacciatore*
⅓ cup brown rice
1 cup mixed salad greens
with 1 teaspoon olive oil
and balsamic vinegar

Essential Menu
DAY NINE

BREAKFAST

Ricotta and Leek Frittata*
¼ cup blueberries

MORNING SNACK

1 small apple, sliced and
spread with 1 tablespoon
cashew butter

LUNCH

leftover Fillet of
Fish Amandine*
½ cup steamed spinach
¼ cup wild rice

AFTERNOON SNACK

Tropical Prosciutto Rolls*

DINNER

Greek Stuffed Chicken Breasts*
½ cup steamed broccoli
¼ cup wild rice

Essential Menu
DAY TEN

BREAKFAST

Crab and Swiss Pie*
⅓ cup raspberries

MORNING SNACK

2 Cheese Balls with Parsley*
1 unsweetened rice cake
or 4 rice crackers

LUNCH

leftover Greek Stuffed Chicken
Breasts* on 2 cups raw
spinach with 1 tablespoon
sliced almonds
½ cup sliced strawberries

AFTERNOON SNACK

2 stalks celery, each stuffed
with 1 tablespoon Lemony
Hummus*

DINNER

Sweet Salsa Smothered Steak*
½ cup steamed broccoli
¼ cup brown rice

Essential Menu
DAY ELEVEN

BREAKFAST

2 eggs, any style
Zucchini Cakes*

MORNING SNACK

1 ounce string cheese
1 tablespoon almonds

LUNCH

2 cups Romaine lettuce topped
with leftover Sweet Salsa
Smothered Steak*

AFTERNOON SNACK

1 small baked apple sprinkled
with cinnamon and
2 tablespoons crushed pecans

DINNER

Glazed Lamb Chops*
Zucchini Ribbons*
¼ cup wild rice

Essential Menu
DAY TWELVE

BREAKFAST

1 Salmon Cake*
½ cup unsweetened full-fat
or 2% yogurt
½ cup blueberries

MORNING SNACK

2 Cheese Balls with Parsley*
1 unsweetened rice cake
or 4 rice crackers

LUNCH

Not Your Everyday Egg Salad*
on 1 cup mixed salad greens

AFTERNOON SNACK

Avocado and Pear Dip*
with ½ cup sliced cucumber
or zucchini

DINNER

Stuffed Red Peppers*
1 cup mixed salad greens
with 1 teaspoon olive oil
and juice of ½ lemon

Essential Menu
DAY THIRTEEN

BREAKFAST

Delicious Crustless
Seafood Quiche*
½ cup raspberries

MORNING SNACK

Lemony Hummus* with ½ cup
sliced vegetables

LUNCH

leftover Stuffed Red Peppers*
½ cup strawberries with
1 tablespoon heavy cream,
sweetened with stevia to taste

AFTERNOON SNACK

½ nectarine stuffed with
2 tablespoons ricotta cheese
and sprinkled with cinnamon
or nutmeg

DINNER

baked or broiled chicken
breast, salt and pepper
to taste
Tasty Tomatoes*
⅓ cup wild rice

Essential Menu
DAY FOURTEEN

BREAKFAST

Spinach Scramble*
½ cup strawberries with
1 tablespoon heavy cream,
sweetened with stevia to taste

MORNING SNACK

1 small apple, sliced and
spread with 1 tablespoon
cashew butter

LUNCH

Gazpacho*
Easy Chicken Florentine*
½ cup cantaloupe

AFTERNOON SNACK

2 Cheese Balls with Parsley*
1 unsweetened rice cake
or 4 rice crackers

DINNER

grilled or broiled hamburger
Vegetable Confetti*
¼ cup wild rice

chapter six

THE CORE BALANCE
ESSENTIAL ACTION PLAN

Food is medicine, and the Core Balance Essential Eating Plan that you've just read about is a crucial component of the healing you'll be doing in these first 14 days. But eating well is only one part of cultivating a healthy Core Balance. Your actions count, too. Remember, everything you do becomes a voice that participates in your internal conversation and contributes to change. Part of your Essential Plan is to shift your daily routine so that it synergizes with your changes in diet and becomes as supportive a participant as possible. Habits (which we now know can be defined as the way you've conditioned your cells) can be very hard to change—that's why most conventional medical practitioners steer away from counseling patients about their lifestyles. But lifestyle changes are extremely effective in making sure that your weight loss becomes permanent and not just a blip on your scale's timeline. It's all about small steps leading to big shifts. Don't take on too many changes at once. Make a commitment, do what you can, and reward yourself with lots of praise and self-care when you succeed. And keep in mind that once you do something regularly for about two to three weeks, it becomes a habit!

Marcelle's Prescription for
CORE PHYSICAL WELLNESS

1. Begin a moderate exercise program, three to four times a week, if you are new to exercise.

2. If you already have an exercise routine, incorporate high-intensity "bursting" and weight resistance training into half of your exercise sessions.

3. Set a bedtime for yourself that allows you seven to nine hours of sleep a night, and stick to it for the next month.

4. Breathe!

5. Go out and play.

6. Make a self-care ritual part of your daily routine; make it loving and mindful, and make time for it each day.

Why Exercise?

As a species, we are meant to be active. Our ancestors had to walk, run, dig, and till for their food. Today, food comes much easier to most of us in the industrial world—so we must find some other reason to move around.

As we get older, we lose lean muscle tissue, and our metabolic rate naturally begins to slow down. Lean muscle is more metabolically active than fat and stores fewer toxins, so the more we have, the better off we are. And the best way to combat a stalling metabolism and loss of lean tissue? Exercise. This doesn't mean you have to become a fanatic, but you do have to incorporate physical activity into your daily routine. The right amount and type will, like everything else in the Core Balance program, depend on your individual circumstances and metabolic profile.

Here's how exercise works, in brief. Your body stores energy in two ways: as long-term fat reserves and as a shorter-term glycogen supply. Glycogen is glucose stored in the muscles—about 12 hours' worth as a ready supply. Regular exercise, both aerobic and anaerobic, depletes these stores at a faster rate while you are exercising and for hours afterward, forcing the body to dip into fat reserves. On a calorie-restricted diet, you may well drop five or ten pounds right away, but it will be primarily glycogen loss (that is, muscle), not fat. Once you resume eating regularly, those pounds will reappear as quickly as they went away. A diet high in simple carbohydrates means that your body always has a ready supply of glucose and rarely has to resort to burning fat. A balanced diet that includes more protein, fat, and fiber encourages the body to burn fat and build muscle. You may not see the quick, drastic weight loss that results from losing muscle and stressing your metabolism with deprivation, but neither will you have the immediate bounceback on the scale. Instead, you will slowly, steadily lose pounds as you make more lean muscle and ensure that your metabolism is properly stoked and accessing energy from the right place—those pesky fat reserves!

Muscle strength depends on good bone health and nutrient absorption—including an often-overlooked nutrient, oxygen, which we take in both in air and in water—as well as a healthy demand for work. Cardiovascular or aerobic exercise (the kind that gets your heart pumping) increases the rate of oxygen absorption, stimulates the breakdown of fat, and helps your body eliminate toxins through sweat and urine. Anaerobic exercise (the kind that occurs in the absence of oxygen, when you are lifting weights or working out intensely) helps build stronger muscle tissue and encourages the body to withstand the buildup of toxins in muscles, and it also improves the body's ability to rid itself of these toxins—an important ally in losing toxic weight. So while you are on my program, it's important to do both kinds of exercise. Weight resistance training is particularly important for women over 40 as a way to fight bone loss and osteoporosis. Bones react to stress by becoming thicker, and lifting weights is a safe way to "stress" your bones. But, again, you don't have to go crazy—too much exercise is its own form of stress. So use the following guidelines and experiment to find what suits you best.

If You're Just Beginning to Exercise

Try to walk 10,000 steps a day, five or more days a week. Wear a pedometer to count your steps. This is easier than you think! Or you can order a "burst" machine (see page 344), a simple step machine that will quickly help you improve your fitness level if you use it just eight minutes a day. It's compact and easy to use, so you can take it anywhere.

If You're an Easygoing Exerciser

Continue walking—30 to 40 minutes a day, three or four days a week—or use a burst machine. Now, add two 20-minute weight-lifting sessions a week. If you're not sure how to get started, call a neighborhood gym or your local Y and ask about personal training. Many gyms now offer free consultations that can get you going. Or buy a DVD or record

If you are increasing your activity level while you're on the program, and you find that you are ravenous or exhausted on the Essential Plan, you can add up to five grams of carbs per meal for every step you move up the exercise scale. If you are still ravenous, it may be that you need some extra healthy fat. Try adding a serving of avocado, feta cheese, or more olive oil to each meal.

a TV exercise show, buy your own free weights, and follow along.

If You're Becoming a More Active Exerciser

Exchange two days of walking for another aerobic activity, such as biking, swimming, running, basketball, in-line skating, hiking, rowing, soccer, or tennis. Keep up the weight training twice a week, adding weight and repetitions as you get stronger.

If You're Already an Active Exerciser

Incorporate "bursting" into your aerobic routine, either by using the burst machine or by cranking up your effort in any activity for a short period, then slowing down. For example, if you are walking, try jogging or running for one minute, then walking for three, then jogging again, and so on. If you are on an exercise machine such as a stair climber, turn up the intensity for two minutes every five minutes. Continue your weight training twice a week. On one of your days "off," add a stretch class such as yoga, Pilates, or body rolling. You should be active five to six days a week.

Why Sleep?

Getting a good night's sleep is underrated in our go-go culture, but if you are struggling with toxic weight it is an absolute must. There is a causal link between disrupted or short sleep time and obesity, and it seems to be more prevalent in women than in men. There are many factors that contribute to this connection, but the primary one, in my opinion, is the fact that sleep is when the body does its maintenance work. When we are awake and active, the body must be primed to react to whatever we put in its path. During sleep, our cells can take the time to heal and detoxify, refueling and recharging for the day ahead.

Melatonin, the body's natural sedative, rises in the evening as the sun goes down and we prepare for bed. The hypothalamus sends a signal to increase the level of the hormone glucagon, which helps in the uptake of glucose from cells into the bloodstream. This keeps our blood sugar stable through the night and ensures that our cells have a good supply of energy to do their maintenance work without triggering our hunger hormones. As morning nears, and the hypothalamus registers light, melatonin and glucagon ebb and cortisol and adrenaline rise slightly. We wake up refreshed—and hungry.

This is a natural biochemical rhythm that promotes a healthy metabolism while you are awake and while you sleep. In fact, a good night's sleep is probably the best thing you can do to help yourself get rid of toxic weight—and it's easy and pleasurable! However, we do tend to make things difficult these days, with all our electronics and artificial lights. If you are having trouble getting a full seven to nine hours of sleep, try practicing a better sleep routine by creating a strict prebedtime schedule and doing the same things at the same time each evening. Disconnect a couple of hours before bed. Turn off the TV, the computer, and the radio, and dim the lights; or turn off the lights and just use candles (but be sure to blow them out before you fall asleep). Keep your room cool and your nightclothes comfortable and loose. Keep your room dark—if you live in the city, buy blackout shades to block light. Let your brain know that evening is upon you and it's time to begin the hormonal cascade triggered by nightfall and a lack of light that ultimately leads to a good night's sleep.

One other important part of a good sleep routine: set a bedtime and stick to it. Some women find that reading is too stimulating. If this sounds like you, put your book or newspaper down an hour before bed and take a hot bath or breathe or simply be still and calm instead.

Why Breathe?

A surprising number of my patients show irregularly high levels of carbon dioxide in their blood even when all the other tests of the blood are fine. In fact, I probably see more abnormal results for carbon dioxide than on standard glucose, kidney, or liver tests. While this is not life-threatening, it does tell me that my patient is not breathing deeply; she's not inhaling enough oxygen or exhaling enough carbon dioxide. I often note on a patient's chart "needs to breathe." Not the shallow chest breathing many of us default to, but deep, meaningful breaths, or "belly breathing."

Deep breathing is the fastest way to send a calming message to your hypothalamus and to trigger your parasympathetic nervous system, through what some practitioners call the relaxation response. The sympathetic nervous system, which is stimulated in times of stress and anxiety, controls your fight-or-flight response, including spikes in cortisol and adrenaline that can be damaging when they persist too long. When you are excited, scared, or nervous, your breath is rapid and shallow. Your muscles constrict and your chest and lungs feel tight. When you are calm and relaxed, your diaphragm softens and you can breathe slowly and deeply.

Breathing serves as the pump for the lymphatic system, just as the heart serves the circulatory system. To thrive, cells rely on a complex exchange between the circulatory system and the lymphatic system. Blood flow carries nutrients and ample amounts of oxygen into the capillaries, while a healthy lymphatic system carries away destructive toxins. Proper breathing is the moderator of this exchange. But unlike your circulatory system, your lymph system does not have a built-in pump. It relies on the act of breathing and bodily movement to move all that waste fluid around. The expansion and contraction of the diaphragm actually stimulate your lymphatic system and massage your internal organs, helping the body rid itself of toxins and leaving more room in the cells for an optimal exchange of oxygen.

Deep breathing also delivers many of the benefits of exercise, including facilitating weight loss. Though not a substitute for exercise, it's a great first step for women just beginning an exercise plan, and deep breathing enhances the benefits of any form of exercise. One basic measure of fitness is cardiovascular capacity—how much oxygen our heart and lungs can deliver to our cells. When muscle cells spring into action, they must have energy to burn and they need the waste products of that metabolism removed. The good news is that deep breathing itself helps raise cardiovascular capacity.

To help you get the benefits of breath, try these exercises.

Simple Deep Breathing

The most basic thing to remember is that your breath begins with a full exhalation. I know this seems counterintuitive, but it's true. You can't inhale fully until you empty your lungs completely.

Now try this: sit in a comfortable position with your hands on your knees. Relax your shoulders. Close your eyes. On your next exhalation, breathe out slowly through your nose, counting to five. Tense your abdominal muscles, drawing in your diaphragm to help your lungs deflate. At the bottom of your breath, pause for two counts, then inhale slowly to the count of five. Expand your belly as you breathe in. Now repeat five to ten times. Think of your diaphragm as the pump and your breath as the power.

If you find that your mind wanders during this exercise, don't worry. Just refocus on your counting. Some of my patients find it helpful to think of a word to focus on. In Buddhist meditation, this word is called a mantra. I find the Sanskrit mantra *Ham Sa* ("I am that") to be very helpful in focusing my breath. Breathe in on the word *Ham* and out on the word *Sa*. As your awareness increases, you'll find that it becomes easier to breathe deeply without so much attention.

The Bellows, or Fire Breath

Many forms of yoga begin with breathing techniques, or *pranayama*. *Prana* means "breath" or "life force" in Sanskrit. The bellows breath is a yogic exercise that stimulates energy when you need it, toning the abdomen and massaging the internal organs and lymph system. Though it's not deep breathing, the bellows does activate the lungs, neck, chest, and abdomen so that deeper breathing comes more naturally.

Again, sit in a comfortable position. With your mouth closed, breathe in and out through your nose as fast as possible. Think of pumping up a balloon or water toy. Try to keep the in and out breaths equal. Continue for ten seconds, no more at first. As you become more accustomed to this technique you can extend the exercise to one full minute.

The Breath of Life

Try this whenever you are feeling groggy or lethargic—it will reinvigorate and refresh you. Stand with your feet hip width apart, arms hanging by your sides. Take a quick breath in through your nose as you lift your arms up over your head (in a "touchdown" pose). Without stopping or exhaling, breathe in more and throw your arms open; then without exhaling, breathe in more and raise your arms over your head. Exhale loudly through your mouth as you bow down and let your hands touch the floor. Do this quickly, three to five times in succession.

Why Play?

Joy is an underrated but very powerful healing mechanism. When you engage in an active, pleasurable activity, you trigger life-enhancing biochemicals, such as serotonin (the "happy" neurotransmitter) and DHEA (dehydroepiandrosterone), also called the joy hormone, which is a natural steroid and precursor hormone to your sex hormones. When you play outside in the sunshine, you make vitamin D, a valuable nutrient that supports the immune system, among various other functions. These feel-good chemicals can become part of a self-sustaining cycle if you activate them on a regular basis (the body is always learning!). But just as important to your long-term health is the connection playing makes with your younger, less encumbered self and the things you used to like to do. Whether it's strapping on some ice skates, taking a walk, giggling with a friend, playing tag with your kids, or learning something new, make sure you incorporate some play time into each week. What are the requirements of play? It doesn't feel like something you have to do—but something you want to do! Go ahead. Let yourself go.

Why Adopt a Self-Care Ritual?

The Core Balance Essential Plan is your first step in beginning to take care of your whole self: body, intellect, instinct, and emotions. As you go through the next month, you may find that in addition to ridding your body of physical toxins, you also notice some emotional "garbage" swimming to the surface. It may take the form of mind-chatter —the negative script that plays in your head, which we will address at length in Stage IV. Taking 30 minutes every day to calm down and nourish a peaceful, loving mind is just as important to getting rid of toxic weight as everything else I'm talking about.

Now, every woman will have a different perspective on what she considers a nurturing self-care ritual—one of my patients likes to groom her cat—but here are a few ideas:

- Journaling
- Lighting candles
- Meditating
- Making tea and drinking it slowly and quietly
- Bathing or massaging with essential oils
- Deep breathing
- A slow, calming walk
- Prayer or worship

Do your ritual activity at the same time every day. For me, doing it upon waking works best. Set aside time to devote to it, and do it to the exclusion of everything else— no TV, radio, iPod, conversation, or other distracting or extraneous stimulation. And don't share this activity with anyone else. Instead, keep it private and personal.

A Day in the Life of the
Core Balance Essential Plan

Time	Activity
6:00-7:00 A.M.	Wake up. Stretch. Drink a full glass of water.
7:00-7:30	Self-care ritual.
7:30-8:00	Bathe, dress. Set a positive intention for the day, such as "Today, I will try to take things slowly."
8:00-8:30	Breakfast, take supplements. Eat breakfast outside, if you can. Drink more water.
9:00	Work, household chores, take care of obligations.
10:30	Snack. Take a 15-minute walk if you can. Drink more water or herbal tea.
12:00 P.M.	Lunch.
2:00	Snack. Drink water.
3:00	Tea break. Breathe!
5:00	Walk home or other physical activity. (If you prefer to exercise in the morning, set your alarm accordingly but go to bed earlier!)
6:30	Dinner.
7:00	Play, journal, listen to music. Socialize with supportive friends or partners.
8:30	If you are taking a separate calcium and magnesium supplement, take now. It can be very helpful with sleep.
9:00	Relax, practice deep breathing, meditate, or journal—whatever helps you let go of the day.
9:30	Bedtime.

There! You're ready to begin your journey.

Check in with yourself often over the next two weeks and notice how you are feeling. What's different? What's changed? Try not to judge yourself, just notice. Remember, this is the first phase, where you and your unadulterated biochemistry are getting to know each other again. The reunion might be fantastic, or it might have its bumps and letdowns. My patient Marlene almost quit after the first week because she felt so tired and didn't want to spend so much time cooking. She called me up and I asked her to give it another 24 hours. I got a call from her the following afternoon and she was over the moon. For the first time in over two years, she had slept through the entire night and woken up feeling like she could outrun her teenage son. By the end of two weeks, she had begun to steadily lose weight. Results are as unique as the individuals who experience them. So don't hold yourself to some unrealistic standard. Do the best you can and don't be too hard on yourself. Treat yourself as you would your best friend.

If by the end of the first two weeks you are feeling great and shedding those toxic pounds, feel free to go back and continue on the Essential Plan until you've lost the weight you set out to lose. If you aren't sensing a shift or would like to see quicker results, continue to Stage III, take my Core Balance Quiz, and we'll dig a little deeper into what's holding you back.

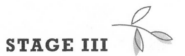

STAGE III

The Next 14 Days:
The Core Balance
Custom Plan

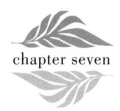

chapter seven

THE CORE BALANCE QUIZ

I'm hopeful that those of you who are reading this have found the past two weeks helpful. You may not be shedding the toxic pounds as quickly as you would like, but if all is going well you should be feeling a shift in how you feel and look—for the better! I also hope that you feel encouraged and empowered from the changes you've been able to make, changes that are shoring up your health and creating a foundation of wellness as we speak. As I've said many times in these pages, true weight loss begins with wellness. If you are dealing with toxic weight, you must restore balance and health in your body first before your body feels safe enough to let go of that weight for good.

If you feel better after the previous two weeks but not great, or if you haven't felt a positive shift yet, chances are that you are experiencing an entrenched core imbalance (or more than one) that is making it more difficult to get your body into the safety zone. But I hope that over the past two weeks you've learned how powerful your day-to-day choices can be when it comes to how you feel. Now you are going to refine those choices even more. First, we need to do a little sleuthing.

Because every system in the body overlaps and each one of us has a unique physiology, identifying and treating a core imbalance isn't always straightforward. It helps if you are working closely with a trusted medical professional who knows your history. But the truth is, most of us aren't, which makes it that much harder to get better. I've created this quiz as a place to start. After years of listening to and caring for so many women with serious weight-loss resistance, I found that their symptoms pointed to six major core imbalances that influence metabolism and toxic weight gain. These imbalances deal with large, overarching systems; healing one often led to the healing of another—or made it possible to identify other issues. We need to figure out which core imbalance is affecting you most right now. Then I will explain how to heal it.

Take a few minutes to answer the questions in this quiz. This is a very important step—please don't skip it. Just get a pencil and circle the answers that feel right; don't think too hard. When you get to the end of each section, add up your score in the place provided. At the end of the quiz, look at each score. The section with the highest number reflects the area that needs your attention.

You may have overlapping issues that need to be addressed simultaneously. In this case, I suggest you read all of the appropriate chapters and adopt as many of the actions as you can. (The different plans call for some of the same actions, so this is easier than it sounds!) It will be easiest to tell which of your core imbalances needs your attention most if you take this quiz after successfully following the Core Balance Essential Plan for two weeks.

Once you've identified the core imbalance you will start with, you can turn to the appropriate chapter to learn more about what's going on in your body and start the customized eating and action plan I've designed to support and heal this imbalance. In each of these chapters, you'll find guidelines similar to those you followed in the Essential Plan: foods to eat in abundance, foods to avoid, supplements to ensure your body gets the active nutrients it needs, as well as "Marcelle's Prescription" highlighting the major points of the plan and a sample "Day in the Life" to help you know what to expect. You'll also find recommendations for diagnostic tests you can arrange for through your practitioner to give you a greater understanding of the issues affecting you. The results will help you fine-tune your Core Balance Custom Plan even more.

The key to this quiz is:

1. Strongly disagree
2. Mostly disagree
3. Mostly agree
4. Strongly agree

Digestive Sensitivities

		1	2	3	4
1.	After eating a meal, I often feel bloated and gassy.	○	○	○	○
2.	I am constipated or have diarrhea more often than not.	○	○	○	○
3.	I have foul-smelling gas and/or stools.	○	○	○	○
4.	I often feel foggy and lethargic and lack focus after I eat.	○	○	○	○
5.	I crave certain foods and beverages and/or often eat the same things.	○	○	○	○
6.	I often feel nauseous after eating or after taking a supplement.	○	○	○	○
7.	I use over-the-counter pain relievers regularly.	○	○	○	○
8.	I tend to crave alcohol, sugar, bread, and other "yeasty" foods.	○	○	○	○
9.	I often (2-3 times a week) have headaches, intestinal pain, and/or joint pain.	○	○	○	○
10.	I feel ill when it is muggy or damp or in specific environments (e.g., my office, my basement).	○	○	○	○
11.	I regularly (two or three times a week) eat out at restaurants or get takeout.	○	○	○	○
12.	I am prone to flushing, pimples, and/or acne breakouts.	○	○	○	○

Score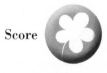

Hormonal Imbalance

		1	2	3	4
1.	Lately, my periods are more irregular and can be very heavy.	○	○	○	○
2.	I am having trouble falling asleep and/or staying asleep at night.	○	○	○	○
3.	I have intense mood swings and cravings before I get my period.	○	○	○	○
4.	Lately I cry at everything, even cheesy TV commercials.	○	○	○	○
5.	My hair and skin feel dry and coarse.	○	○	○	○
6.	I am experiencing heart palpitations, hot flashes, and/or night sweats.	○	○	○	○
7.	I feel much calmer after my period starts.	○	○	○	○
8.	I have little interest in sex, and even when I do have interest, my vagina stays dry.	○	○	○	○
9.	I've lost a lot of muscle recently or I can't make muscle, no matter how much I exercise.	○	○	○	○
10.	I tend to store my extra weight around my hips and thighs.	○	○	○	○
11.	Lately, my breasts are more tender and/or painful.	○	○	○	○
12.	I have a history of PMS, postpartum depression, and/or abnormal periods or irregular bleeding.	○	○	○	○

Score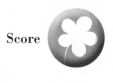

Adrenal Imbalance

		1	2	3	4
1.	I feel as if I am always on the go and am known for getting things done.	○	○	○	○
2.	I am exhausted and irritable a lot of the time—I have a short fuse.	○	○	○	○
3.	When I'm not exhausted, I feel restless and agitated. I can't relax.	○	○	○	○
4.	Usually, I crash in the afternoon, only to get a second wind in the evening.	○	○	○	○
5.	I often crave salty foods, or I crave sugar and can't stop eating it.	○	○	○	○
6.	I am light-headed and queasy in the mornings, or when I get up too fast.	○	○	○	○
7.	I find it difficult to wake up and/or get out of bed—I can't live without coffee!	○	○	○	○
8.	I often feel anxious and have no idea why.	○	○	○	○
9.	Sex is about the last thing on my mind these days.	○	○	○	○
10.	When I want something done right, I have to do it myself.	○	○	○	○
11.	If I sit or lie down for a minute in a warm spot, I tend to fall asleep.	○	○	○	○
12.	I usually need a sugar or caffeine jolt in the afternoon.	○	○	○	○

Score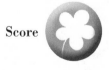

Neurotransmitter Imbalance   *1*   *2*   *3*   *4*

		1	2	3	4
1.	I binge-eat regularly, especially on carbohydrates.	○	○	○	○
2.	I don't get much pleasure out of most of my activities.	○	○	○	○
3.	I'm drinking more alcohol than I used to.	○	○	○	○
4.	I crave comfort food.	○	○	○	○
5.	I feel tense, guilty, and anxious much of the time.	○	○	○	○
6.	I feel flat, unfocused, and empty much of the time.	○	○	○	○
7.	Lately I've been sleeping a lot more/less than usual.	○	○	○	○
8.	I've been told that I'm moody.	○	○	○	○
9.	Sometimes, I just want to scream at everybody.	○	○	○	○
10.	Eating makes me feel better.	○	○	○	○
11.	I worry a lot.	○	○	○	○
12.	I feel stuck and my self-esteem is pretty low.	○	○	○	○

Score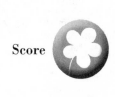

Inflammatory Issues

		1	2	3	4
1.	Most of my weight gain is around my belly.	○	○	○	○
2.	I have a BMI over 28 and/or I am more than 30 pounds overweight.	○	○	○	○
3.	I'm prone to acne and skin rashes like eczema and psoriasis.	○	○	○	○
4.	I have high blood pressure and/or high cholesterol.	○	○	○	○
5.	I've been diagnosed with irritable bowel syndrome, or I often have diarrhea and/or intestinal pain.	○	○	○	○
6.	I suffer from chronic pain, multiple joint/ arthritic pain, and/or chronic headaches and migraine.	○	○	○	○
7.	I'm under so much stress!	○	○	○	○
8.	I smoke.	○	○	○	○
9.	When I get injured, it takes a long time to heal.	○	○	○	○
10.	I catch every bug that goes around, without fail.	○	○	○	○
11.	Since taking certain medications or a combination of medications, I've gained more weight.	○	○	○	○
12.	I've been diagnosed with asthma, chronic allergies, Type II diabetes, fibromyalgia, heart disease, hypertension, or metabolic syndrome.	○	○	○	○

Score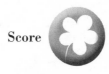

Detoxification Issues

		1	2	3	4
1.	I'm very sensitive to medications; I usually only take a half dose.	O	O	O	O
2.	I have a stuffy nose/congestion, and/or postnasal drip often.	O	O	O	O
3.	I consume caffeine and/or alcohol on a daily basis.	O	O	O	O
4.	I use recreational drugs on a regular basis, including nicotine and/or marijuana.	O	O	O	O
5.	I'm often constipated (two to three times a week).	O	O	O	O
6.	I think I eat too much junk food and candy.	O	O	O	O
7.	I am gaining weight, even though I'm not overeating.	O	O	O	O
8.	I have problem skin and/or rosacea.	O	O	O	O
9.	I have five or more metal alloy fillings.	O	O	O	O
10.	I used to tolerate caffeine and alcohol much better than I do now.	O	O	O	O
11.	I'm very sensitive to chemical/environmental odors and perfumes; I get headaches when I go into certain stores or offices.	O	O	O	O
12.	I was once exposed to a high level of toxic chemicals, or I've been exposed to small amounts of toxic substances and/or heavy metals over an extended period of time.	O	O	O	O

Score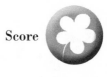

Tally your scores here:

Digestive Sensitivities   _____

Hormonal Imbalance   _____

Adrenal Imbalance   _____

Neurotransmitter Imbalance   _____

Inflammatory Issues   _____

Detoxification Issues   _____

Take a look at your scores and compare them. Generally speaking, if you scored 12 to 20 points on an imbalance, it is not an area that needs your immediate attention. A score of 20 to 30 means the imbalance may be contributing to your weight gain but may not be the primary cause. Scoring 30 to 48 in an area means this imbalance needs your attention, now. If there is a score that is significantly higher than the others, turn directly to the appropriate Custom Plan chapter. This is the imbalance you will be working on for the next 14 days. If, however, you have a tie between scores, you are probably dealing with overlapping imbalances—a very common occurrence. The good news is that if you heal one imbalance, the others often follow suit, since every system in the body is inter-connected. I believe that the digestive system is the doorway to vital health, so if you are in a tie but one of your high scores is Digestive Sensitivities, I suggest you begin there. If digestive issues are not one of your high scores, you can use your intuition to discern which imbalance is impacting you most, or you can stick with the Core Balance Essential Plan for two more weeks and then take the quiz again. If imbalances are entrenched, it can take a little longer to quiet the "noise" and really hear your symptoms.

A Note on Diagnostic Testing

In each of these customized plans I recommend a series of appropriate diagnostic tests. My list is by no means comprehensive; however, the tests I recommend are fundamental and will give you a better idea of underlying problems. I have included a detailed description of each test in the Appendices, as well as the results I like to see and a list of clinical labs where the tests can be ordered. Many conventional practitioners do not offer these tests, so you may have to schedule an appointment with an integrative or alternative practitioner to receive them (see Referrals and Resources for help finding one in your area). That's a good thing! The more people you have on your team, the better. The more precise you can be about your health picture, the easier it will be to prescribe the right supplements and healing agents to restore your core balance.

chapter eight

THE DIGESTIVE
IMBALANCE CUSTOM PLAN

If you scored highest on Digestive Sensitivities in my Core Balance Quiz, there's a good chance that something is off-kilter in your digestive system. This is extremely common and it happens to many of us from time to time. The majority of my patients rank bloating, gas, and gastrointestinal (GI) distress high on their list of symptoms. Many of them can't remember a time when they didn't have discomfort after eating!

In fact, it's a rare Westernized human who does not have some digestive imbalance. Often we don't notice it because we're just used to the symptoms. There's speculation that perhaps 90 percent of the population has food sensitivities that are genetic. Most of these sensitivities lie hidden or dormant until other stress burdens trigger a response. Many GI problems stem from such undiagnosed food sensitivities, which put your immune system on alert and your body into protective mode. Imbalances can also result from low stomach acidity; a deficiency in digestive enzymes; yeast overgrowth; overly acidic pH in the intestines; or an infestation of parasites or overpopulation of unwelcome bacteria in the intestinal tract that leads to a condition called dysbiosis.

Chronic digestive imbalances that aren't dealt with can seriously undermine your health, your metabolism, and your ability to get rid of "defensive" weight. That's because your digestive system is your body's powerhouse. Its two major functions are to break down food into usable nutrients and to control toxicity by getting rid of the unusable portions, and it has to work efficiently if you want to avoid overburdening your body. Unfortunately, years of yo-yo dieting, eating too much of the same foods, overusing antibiotics and antifungal medications, chemical exposure, and emotional stress can gum up the works and overburden not only the digestive system, but the immune system and the central nervous system, too—and you know what that eventually leads to: toxic weight.

Conventional practitioners can be skeptical when it comes to the degenerative effects of GI issues, but I've seen women transform their health by healing their guts. My patient of many years, Carla, suffered with constipation for most of her adult life—she had a bowel movement once a week, and she thought that was normal, because for her at that point in her life, it was. After we began treating her digestive imbalance with the protocol I'll lay out for you in this chapter, she began to go every day like clockwork— a simple thing, but one that brought her an immense amount of relief. "It was amazing," she reported. "I had no idea how much I was suffering from holding in all those toxins. Releasing them was a fantastic feeling. Now I don't know what I'd do if I had to go back to the way I was before."

Sometimes a digestive imbalance is at the root of seemingly unrelated symptoms, so it can be hard to spot. I think it's a smart idea to check out digestive health if you are experiencing any chronic problem—I've seen too many women suffer for too long with unnecessary complications of a GI imbalance, including stubborn weight, not to believe that the first line of defense for everyone is a healthy digestive tract. Take my patient Natasha for an example of someone with a more extreme digestive imbalance. She first came to see me when she was 42 years old and suffering from chronic urinary tract infections and yeast infections. During that time, she'd dutifully trekked to one OB-GYN after another and taken scores of antibiotics, and nothing had worked. Along the way, she'd accumulated more than ten pounds of stubborn excess weight gain that she couldn't lose no matter how many calories she cut out or how much exercise she did. She was under tremendous stress and had very little energy. "All I want is to feel better," she said on that first visit, "but nothing I do makes any difference."

I was suspicious of a yeast overgrowth in her GI tract, so I ordered all the appropriate tests. We did a stool test and an adrenal test (because of her low energy). When the tests came back, it was clear that Natasha was not absorbing nutrients sufficiently due to an overgrowth of bacteria, systemic yeast, and low digestive enzymes. It was as if the furnace in her house hadn't been cleaned in years and was reduced to working on the lowest possible setting. Our first step was to rid Natasha's system of the bacteria and yeast that were interfering with her proper digestion. I treated her with Diflucan (an antifungal) and Candex (a supplement to support the reduction of yeast in the GI tract). She followed the Digestive Imbalance Custom Plan and took a medical food and a probiotic. Within six weeks, Natasha felt so much better—it was obvious from the minute she entered my office. No more yeast infections or urinary tract infections. She began to lose the extra weight that was bothering her and felt energetic enough to begin exercising regularly.

The Digestive Imbalance Custom Plan loosely follows the classic "4R" plan first introduced by my mentor, friend, and fellow functional healer Dr. Jeff Bland. Over the next two weeks we will rebalance your diet and your habits; remove the allergens most offensive to your GI tract; replace lost and poorly utilized enzymes and nutrients; and finally reinoculate your gut with probiotics, those helpful, beneficial bacteria.

First, though, we'll take a look at where we're going.

A Fast Trip Through the GI Tract

The GI tract is an amazing piece of organic machinery: a 25- to 30-foot tube inside your skeleton that works automatically to maximize nutrition and minimize exposure to harmful substances. If you were a tree, your gut would be your taproot—your life source.

Digestion begins in the mouth, where the teeth break up food and mix it with saliva. Then the stomach mechanically churns food, hydrochloric acid (HCl) breaks up and emulsifies fat, and food molecules are exposed to multiple enzymes and pancreatic juices. If HCl levels are insufficient in your stomach, a condition called low gastric acidity results and you cannot adequately break down your food. This leads to indigestion and, ironically, heartburn as the stomach wall churns out more and more acid to compensate for the low acidity. It can also contribute to acid reflux and, in more severe cases, putrefaction of undigested food in the GI tract. For patients who have this problem, I sometimes prescribe a digestive aid, betaine HCl, made up of hydrochloric acid and the vitamin-like substance betaine. Its high acid content can irritate the stomach, so it should be taken only in the middle of a meal. Because it can significantly change pH in the stomach, I recommend that betaine HCl be used under the guidance of an experienced practitioner. (For more information, see the Appendices.)

It takes about four hours for food to be processed in the stomach. The resulting semiliquid mass, called chyme, is passed from the stomach to the small intestine, where it is

Symptoms of Low Gastric Acidity

- Bloating, burning, belching, and/or gas after meals

- Sensation of fullness after eating

- Diarrhea or constipation

- Indigestion, gas, or pain in upper digestive tract

- Food allergies

- Nausea after taking supplements

- Rectal itching

- Weak, peeling fingernails

- Broken capillaries on cheeks and nose

- Acne

- Iron deficiency

- Chronic intestinal parasites

- Undigested food in stool

- Chronic yeast infections

- Foul, smelly stools or gas

further emulsified with the aid of bile from the liver. Bile, an alkaline, soapy substance, helps neutralize the acidic contents coming out of the stomach to prepare them for the more alkaline environment of the intestines. It also increases the water-solubility of certain fats and encourages enzymatic activity in the small intestine. Bile is stored in the gallbladder, a small but precious organ. If your gallbladder is overtaxed—a result of a diet heavy in sugar and unhealthy fats—you will often feel nauseous after meals.

The small intestine has hundreds of folds along its membranous wall, called villi and microvilli, which act like bouncers at the doorway to your bloodstream: they allow useful nutrients to pass, but turn away substances that are useless or harmful. In many cases, digestive imbalance is caused by a certain confusion on the part of these bouncers. A poor diet, undiagnosed food sensitivities, overuse of medications, and chronic stress can all create an abnormal environment in which the villi can no longer discern what should be turned away; they begin to let larger proteins and foreign substances through, triggering an immune response. When your intestine becomes too permeable, you may have a condition known as leaky gut syndrome, with many uncomfortable symptoms, including chronic inflammation, indigestion, and weight gain.

The gut flora that live in your small intestine and help keep you healthy have evolved in tandem with our digestive systems over thousands of years. Depending on where you live and what you eat, different strains either perish or thrive. (Travelers who come home with a bout of Montezuma's revenge haven't bred the right kind of gut flora to fight off an invasion of foreign bacteria—that's why tourists get sick and the locals don't.) When your intestines contain the right balance of good and bad bacteria, they are described as being in a state of symbiosis. When the balance is upset, it's called dysbiosis, a condition that impairs the GI tract's ability to absorb nutrients. Dysbiosis is a very common little thief that steals your body's most valuable resource.

This is where probiotics come in—foods or supplements that help us fortify or rebuild our own supply of beneficial gut flora to digest and absorb our food, shore up our immune systems, neutralize toxins, and aid in the production of essential vitamins. Probiotics are active in most fermented foods, such as yogurt, kefir, sauerkraut, beer, kimchi, miso, and tempeh, but you would have to eat a lot of these foods to get enough bacteria to repopulate a damaged gut. That's why I recommend taking a probiotic supplement every day you're on the Core Balance program.

The Trouble with Yeast

One of the biggest bugaboos when it comes to digestive imbalance is an over-abundance of yeast in the GI tract, a condition also called candidiasis after *Candida albicans,* a type of yeast organism that normally helps us digest carbohydrates. Think of weeds in a garden: once yeast is out of control, it's hard to keep the other flora healthy. An overgrowth of yeast in the GI tract interferes with nutrient absorption, stressing the immune system and causing weight gain. Symptoms of candidiasis include fatigue, foggy thinking, insomnia, chronic vaginitis, vaginal yeast infection, rectal itching, low blood sugar, sensitivity to damp and mold, PMS, depression, and ringing in the ears—to name just a few. What's more, when yeast microorganisms die, they release a lot of putrefying gas that causes bloating, smelly flatulence, and nausea.

There is still a lot of resistance in Western medicine to the concept of yeast over-growth, but I've seen too many women walk through my door with candidiasis to pooh-pooh it. Once it is diagnosed, it's easy to fix, and women feel so much better! The basic treatment is to wipe out existing yeast colonies by depriving them of their favorite foods—refined sugar and grains; fermented foods like beer, wine, and vinegar; yeasted breads; and dried fruit—and to repopulate the gut with good bacteria by taking a potent probiotic supplement. If necessary, you can also use a natural antimicrobial supplement such as Candex or, in more severe cases, a prescription antifungal medication such as Diflucan or Nystatin.

Another major player in the process of digestion is the almighty and all-important liver. The liver breaks down fat and fat-soluble nutrients with the help of bile and filters digested food of alcohol, drugs, extra hormones, and other extraneous material for absorption into the bloodstream. Whatever remains is either stored or broken down for elimination. The liver makes and breaks down cholesterol and hormones, including estrogen, progesterone, and testosterone. If it is not operating properly, your body cannot detoxify—so one of the goals of the Digestive Sensitivities plan is to reduce the burden on the liver.

When the liver and small intestine have made the most of your food, the remaining water, bacteria, and fibrous waste is passed into your large intestine. Your large intestine has beneficial flora of its own that produce an array of essential vitamins, including A, B, and K, and ferment dietary fiber, which wards off colon disease. Here, the remnants of the digestive process are turned into stool and evacuated. The whole digestive process takes anywhere from 6 to 24 hours to complete, depending on the food and amount of water you've consumed, how robust your stomach acids and pancreatic enzymes are, the population of your gut flora, and the action of your immune system.

Food Allergies

Food allergies are an immune response triggered by a kind of lymph tissue called gut-associated lymph tissue, or GALT, which is woven throughout the gut and serves as a backup defense against invading pathogens. If a potential offender has survived the digestive process thus far, GALT samples it and, if it doesn't like what it tastes, launches a full-blown attack. A severe GALT-initiated response can cause sweating, flushing, increased mucus production, diarrhea, nausea, and vomiting—so you know something doesn't agree with you. But the same response can be triggered on a much less severe scale by foods

Take a look at your poop! A healthy stool is a warm brown color that exits (without strain) in the shape of a banana. If you are eating enough fiber, it will float. If your stool is hard, pebbly, overly smelly, yellow, green, shreddy, or poorly formed—or if it sinks like a stone—there's a good chance your GI tract needs some TLC. A healthy stool moves one to three times a day; if yours moves less, it's another sign that something is awry.

that you've become sensitized to over the years. Many of us have become so used to feeling slightly sick that we don't know how good we can feel until a particular food is removed.

Ironically, the foods that don't work for us are usually the very foods we crave all the time. Practitioners call this allergic addiction.[1] Allergies and sensitivities often lead to nutrient deprivation, which can trigger cravings for the allergen that creates the deficiency in the first place. For instance, if you are sensitive to strawberries, you may have a reaction to vitamin C, which means your body is not absorbing vitamin C properly. Since the body needs vitamin C, you end up craving all foods that contain vitamin C—the ultimate vicious cycle. In fact, if there are certain foods you crave all the time (even healthy foods like bananas), you may want to remove them from your diet while you're on this plan, in addition to eating the foods I recommend. Many of my patients have been living with low-grade food sensitivities and allergies for years and need a bigger supplemental boost to help heal digestive imbalances; in such cases, I use a medical food designed to manage this condition. If you are not seeing the results you would like after two weeks of following the Digestive Imbalance Custom Plan, talk to your practitioner about this option or call my clinic for more information. I've also included a basic formula of supplements to provide the equivalent of a medical food that supports digestive healing in the Appendices.

The Role of Emotions

Emotional stress, too, plays a part in the biochemical reaction to digestive sensitivities. Stress triggers the central nervous system, which shuts down digestion in favor of more urgent physical responses. When you are stressed and in fight-or-flight mode, adrenaline and the stress hormone cortisol skyrocket. This switch into high gear ratchets up the acids in your blood just when your digestive and elimination processes are being told to slow down. This can lead to a pH imbalance, making your internal environment overly acidic. Some enzymes and beneficial gut flora work best in an alkaline environment, so if the internal environment is overly acidic, they can't do their jobs. Over time, an overly acidic environment will lead to dysbiosis.

That Time of the Month

Why are women more prone than men to GI distress? In Western cultures, women are two to three times more likely to seek medical help for digestive disorders. There is still a lot of research to be done on this topic, but preliminary data suggest that ovarian hormones (estrogen and progesterone) influence digestion.[2]

Most of us know the bloated feeling that may occur around our periods. This is partly because the stomach and intestines empty more slowly during the last two weeks of the menstrual cycle, when progesterone levels are higher, than in the first two weeks. I've witnessed a marked rise in digestive symptoms in many of my patients right before a period starts. Post-menopausal women often feel a similar slowing.

As you can see, the digestive process is a long and winding road. If at any point there's a diversion or detour, it can have a lasting detrimental effect on your health and your weight. Moreover, an entrenched digestive imbalance can ultimately contribute to illnesses such as cancer, Alzheimer's disease, cardiovascular disease, Crohn's disease, psoriasis, autoimmune disorders, and even some psychiatric conditions. So be kind to your digestive system. Take the next two weeks to give it what it needs. It may be difficult at first—this is one of the more stringent plans—but if you just see it through for three or four days, I think you'll find yourself feeling so energized and fabulous that you'll know it's worth it.

The Digestive Sensitivities Eating and Action Plan

Over the next two weeks, your biggest challenge will be to keep an open mind. You're going to be on a hypoallergenic food plan that removes the most common allergens from your diet: dairy, gluten, corn, and soy. These are the most frequent offenders when it comes to food sensitivities, so they're a great place to start figuring out what is at the root of your GI issues. You are going to cook with grains that may be unfamiliar—but trust me, they're very tasty. This is not a calorie-restricted plan; still, you don't want to overeat, as that stresses the digestive system. So I urge you to eat slowly and chew your food well. That way your mouth will help your stomach get a jump on digesting its contents and your brain will have time to receive the signal that you're full.

By now, you've been following the Core Balance Essential Plan for two weeks, which should make the adaptations here easier. All of the Core Balance Essential guidelines and suggestions still apply; we're just going to build on them to remove the substances that may be causing you problems and rebalance your diet. At the same time, if you take your supplements as directed, you'll replace the nutrients you're lacking and reinoculate your gut with beneficial bacteria. And it's only for two more weeks!

A bit earlier we talked about reducing the burden on your liver. You can make this easier by avoiding stimulants, chemicals, additives, and alcohol for the next two weeks. Give your liver a vacation! Keep some activated charcoal tablets on hand so that if you do slip up and ingest something less than beneficial, the charcoal can absorb additional toxins in your stomach before they have a chance to pass through.

Remember, too, to check in with yourself every day to gauge how you're feeling. This is important throughout the Core Balance program, and especially when you're focusing on digestive issues. You may feel a little worse in the short run, but don't let that discourage you. It's a natural, temporary response as your body releases fat and the toxins that have been stored there. If you feel worse for more than a week or ten days, it's a red flag that something needs medical attention, so call your practitioner.

As you make these dietary changes, it's important to pay attention to the way you're feeling emotionally, too. As I mentioned a short while ago, stress can play a significant role in the biochemistry of your digestion. What's more, we tend to hold fear and worry in our guts, which adds to problems of indigestion, heartburn, and acid reflux—all symptoms of digestive imbalance. The GI tract has over 30 hormones that influence the digestive processes but also act as neurotransmitters, like serotonin, and it is in constant communication with other organs, including your brain. Remember my patient Carla, who thought it was normal to move her bowels once a week? Her digestive sensitivities were exacerbated by feelings she had kept bottled up for decades about her mother and her family life. Carla had structured her life so that she was always helping others and never had much time to attend to her own needs—either nutritionally or emotionally. When Carla's digestive symptoms began to settle down and she had more energy, she found herself able to look at the other pieces of her puzzle. "I felt I had awoken a sleeping giant," she recalled. "I learned that the body is a living organism and when you treat it intelligently, with respect and mindfulness, it can teach you an awful lot."

So the next two weeks are about healing your gut, but they are also about healing the fear you hold there. We'll look more closely at what this means and how to do it in Stage IV.

Marcelle's Prescription for
DIGESTIVE SENSITIVITIES

1. Follow the menu plan beginning on page 116.
2. Sit down when you eat, take your time, and chew properly.
3. At meals, sip your drink. Too much liquid may dilute your digestive juices.
4. Take your supplements at the prescribed times.
5. Set a bedtime that allows you seven to nine hours of sleep per night and stick to it.
6. When you wake up in the morning, lie quietly for a moment and set your intention for the day.
7. Add a mindful, restorative exercise class to your weekly regimen—one that focuses on calming the central nervous system, such as yoga or tai chi.
8. Cancel any obligations, such as meals out, that might sabotage your efforts to heal your GI tract.
9. Schedule at least one massage in the next two weeks.
10. Read Stage IV and think about whether you tend to "swallow" your feelings.
11. Schedule diagnostic tests if you aren't seeing any progress at the end of two weeks.

Diagnostic Testing for Digestive Sensitivities

- ALCAT (a test designed to determine food and chemical sensitivities) and intestinal permeability test for food sensitivities and allergies
- Comprehensive Digestive Stool Analysis (CDSA) to test digestion and absorption and bacterial balance
- Comprehensive Parasitology 2 (CP x 2) to identify abnormal intestinal microflora
- Breath test for small-intestine bacterial overgrowth
- H. pylori: An antigen test for bacteria correlated with peptic and duodenal ulcers
- Celiac Profile to test for gluten sensitivity/allergy
- Urine Toxic Metals to test for heavy metals

Foods to Include for Digestive Sensitivities

- Vegetables (all kinds!)
- Nongluten grains—brown rice, oats, millet, quinoa, amaranth, teff, tapioca, buckwheat, potato flour, rice pastas
- Animal protein—fresh or water-packed fish, wild game, lamb, duck, organic chicken and turkey
- Nuts and seeds
- Fruits
- Sweeteners—brown rice syrup, agave nectar, stevia, molasses
- Lemons and lemon juice
- Herbs—basil, garlic, cinnamon, carob, cumin, dill, ginger, mustard, oregano, parsley, pepper, rosemary, tarragon, thyme, turmeric
- Celtic or other sea salt

Foods to Avoid for Digestive Sensitivities

- Caffeine

- Alcohol

- Dairy products

- Carbonated beverages (except carbonated spring water)

- Whipped products

- Oranges and orange juice

- Gluten and grains—wheat, barley, spelt, kamut, rye, triticale

- Soybeans and soy products

- Peanuts and peanut butter

- Refined sugars, honey

- Sauces and condiments—chocolate, ketchup, relish, chutney, soy sauce, barbecue sauce, teriyaki sauce

Supplements for Digestive Sensitivities

Basic:

- High-potency multivitamin with additional calcium and magnesium

- Essential Fatty Acid (EFA)

- Probiotic (take 5 to 15 minutes before each meal with water)

- L-glutamine (1000 mgs with each meal)

- Digestive enzyme full-spectrum tablet (take with each meal) or betaine HCl (mid-meal, for bloating: start with one tablet, increase to two as needed)

- Charcoal tablets to neutralize any digestive toxins; take as needed as soon as you ingest a potential offender

Additional (for use under medical guidance and/or with diagnostic testing):

- Medical foods to soothe symptoms caused by food allergies/sensitivities (morning and afternoon)

Digestive Enzymes

Digestive enzymes turn big food molecules into smaller ones and allow us to absorb vital nutrients. Because certain enzymes should not be used by people with a history of certain digestive disorders, such as peptic ulcers, I recommend you work with a practitioner to find the best solution for your situation. But there are a few exceptions—enzymes that are safe to take on your own:

- alpha-galactosidase
- amylase
- bromelain
- cellulase
- glucoamylase
- hemicellulase
- invertase (sucrase)
- lactase
- lipase
- maltase
- papain
- peptidase
- protease
- phytase

Multi-enzyme products contain a spectrum of enzymatic ingredients, some of which work in the stomach and some of which function further down the digestive tract.

A Day in the Life of the
Digestive Imbalance Custom Plan

Time	Activity
7:00 A.M.	Drink glass of warm water with lemon, dash of cayenne optional.
7:00-7:30	Self-care ritual.
7:30-8:00	Shower and dress. Take probiotic with water.
8:00-8:30	Breakfast. Take supplements. Brush teeth and floss.
8:30-9:00	Walk to work, light housework, correspondence—gentle busyness.
10:30	Snack with water.
12:00 P.M.	Lunch, supplements, followed by 15-20 minute walk.
1:00	Herbal tea break. Deep breathing.
4:00	Snack with water.
5:00	Walk home, exercise, get outdoors if possible.
6:00	Dinner.
6:30	After-dinner stroll.
7:00	Recreational activities, chores.
8:00	Time to wind down: turn off electronics, lower lights.
8:30	Journal day's triumphs and challenges; read.
9:00	Take calcium and magnesium supplement if having trouble sleeping. Brush teeth and floss.
9:30-10:00	Lights out.

The Core Balance Menu Plan for Digestive Imbalance

Snack Ideas:

- Rice cakes or apple slices with almond or cashew butter
- Celery sticks, carrot sticks, or pepper slices with hummus
- One piece of fresh fruit
- A handful of nuts or seeds
- Half a serving of the previous evening's dinner entrée

* Recipes start on page 259. If you have a sensitivity to eggs, you can substitute a fiber and rice or whey protein smoothie for breakfast (page 74) for breakfast.

Digestive Sensitivities Menu
DAY ONE

BREAKFAST	LUNCH	DINNER
2 eggs, any style	Not Your Mom's Chicken Salad*	Cashew Chicken*
Zucchini Cakes*	on 1 cup mixed salad greens	½ cup steamed broccoli
	(½ cup cantaloupe optional)	¼ cup brown rice

MORNING SNACK
Avocado and Pear Dip*
with ½ cup sliced cucumber
or zucchini

AFTERNOON SNACK
1 small baked apple sprinkled
with cinnamon and
2 tablespoons crushed pecans

Digestive Sensitivities Menu
DAY TWO

BREAKFAST	LUNCH	DINNER
Cheeseless Artichoke Omelet*	Turkey Frittata*	Ginger Salmon*
½ cup raspberries	2 cups mixed salad greens	Crunchy Snow Peas*
	with 1 teaspoon olive oil	½ cup wild rice
	and juice of ½ lemon	
	(½ cup raspberries optional)	

MORNING SNACK
2 stalks celery, each stuffed
with 1 tablespoon Lemony
Hummus*
(½ cup cantaloupe optional)

AFTERNOON SNACK
½ pear spread with
1 tablespoon cashew butter

Digestive Sensitivities Menu
DAY THREE

BREAKFAST

Confetti Scramble*
½ cup blueberries

MORNING SNACK

2 unsweetened rice cakes or
8 rice crackers spread with
1 tablespoon cashew butter

LUNCH

Sweet Arugula Salad
with Chicken*

AFTERNOON SNACK

½ cup sliced strawberries
2 tablespoons pecans

DINNER

Fillet of Fish Amandine*
⅓ cup wild rice
½ cup steamed broccoli

Digestive Sensitivities Menu
DAY FOUR

BREAKFAST

2 Salmon Cakes*
½ cup cantaloupe

MORNING SNACK

1 small baked apple sprinkled
with cinnamon and
2 tablespoons crushed pecans

LUNCH

Eggs Florentine*
2 cups mixed salad greens
with 1 teaspoon olive oil
and juice of ½ lemon
(¼ cup blueberries optional)

AFTERNOON SNACK

2 unsweetened rice cakes or
8 rice crackers spread with
1 tablespoon cashew butter

DINNER

Rosemary Lamb*
Zucchini Ribbons*
½ sweet potato with
½ tablespoon butter, sprinkled
with cinnamon if desired

Digestive Sensitivities Menu
DAY FIVE

BREAKFAST

Spinach Scramble*
¼ cup raspberries

MORNING SNACK

Lemony Hummus* with ½ cup
sliced vegetables

LUNCH

Turkey Tarragon Salad*
½ millet roll

AFTERNOON SNACK

½ cup cantaloupe
2 tablespoons almonds

DINNER

Chicken and Asparagus Sauté*
2 cups mixed salad greens
with 1 teaspoon olive oil
and juice of ½ lemon
½ millet roll

117

Digestive Sensitivities Menu
DAY SIX

BREAKFAST

2 eggs, any style
2 slices nitrate-free bacon
(½ cup sliced strawberries
optional)

MORNING SNACK

Olive Tapenade* with ½ cup
sliced vegetables

LUNCH

leftover Chicken and
Asparagus Sauté*
(½ cup cantaloupe optional)

AFTERNOON SNACK

1 small apple, sliced and
spread with 1 tablespoon
almond butter

DINNER

Garlic Poached Haddock*
Crunchy Green Beans*
¼ cup brown rice

Digestive Sensitivities Menu
DAY SEVEN

BREAKFAST

Turkey Hash*
½ cup cantaloupe

MORNING SNACK

2 unsweetened rice cakes or
8 rice crackers spread with
1 tablespoon almond butter

LUNCH

Mushroom Scramble*
2 cups mixed salad greens
with 1 teaspoon olive oil
and juice of ½ lemon
(¼ cup blueberries optional)

AFTERNOON SNACK

Olive Tapenade* with ½ cup
sliced vegetables

DINNER

Sherry Chicken*
½ cup steamed broccoli
¼ cup brown rice

Digestive Sensitivities Menu
DAY EIGHT

BREAKFAST

Cheeseless Artichoke Omelet*
½ cup blueberries

MORNING SNACK

Avocado and Pear Dip*
with ½ cup sliced cucumber
or zucchini

LUNCH

baked or broiled
chicken breast,
salt and pepper to taste
Gazpacho*
½ millet roll

AFTERNOON SNACK

½ cup raspberries
2 tablespoons almonds

DINNER

Cinnamon Lamb Chops*
Spinach with Lemon
and Garlic*
¼ cup wild rice

Digestive Sensitivities Menu
DAY NINE

BREAKFAST

Turkey Frittata*
½ cup sliced strawberries

MORNING SNACK

2 unsweetened rice cakes or
8 rice crackers spread with
1 tablespoon cashew butter

LUNCH

leftover Cinnamon Lamb Chops*
¼ cup wild rice
1 cup mixed salad greens
with 1 teaspoon olive oil
and juice of ½ lemon

AFTERNOON SNACK

1 small baked apple sprinkled
with cinnamon and
2 tablespoons crushed pecans

DINNER

Dilled Salmon*
Rosemary Green Beans*
¼ cup wild rice

Digestive Sensitivities Menu
DAY TEN

BREAKFAST

2 eggs, any style
Zucchini Cakes*

MORNING SNACK

Lemony Hummus* with ½ cup
sliced vegetables

LUNCH

leftover Dilled Salmon*
2 cups mixed salad greens
with 1 teaspoon olive oil
and juice of ½ lemon

AFTERNOON SNACK

½ pear spread with 1
tablespoon cashew butter

DINNER

Summertime Grilled Chicken*
½ cup brown rice

Digestive Sensitivities Menu
DAY ELEVEN

BREAKFAST

Onion Tomato Scramble*
½ cup raspberries

MORNING SNACK

Olive Tapenade* with ½ cup
sliced vegetables

LUNCH

Spinach Salad*
½ millet roll

AFTERNOON SNACK

2 unsweetened rice cakes or
8 rice crackers spread with
1 tablespoon cashew butter

DINNER

Simple Sautéed Fish*
Stir Fry Broccoli with Ginger*
¼ cup wild rice

Digestive Sensitivities Menu
DAY TWELVE

BREAKFAST

2 Salmon Cakes*
(½ cup blueberries optional)

MORNING SNACK

Guacamole* with ½ cup sliced
vegetables

LUNCH

Sweet Chicken Salad*
½ gluten-free roll

AFTERNOON SNACK

Avocado and Pear Dip*
with ½ cup sliced cucumber
or zucchini

DINNER

Cheeseless Artichoke Omelet*
2 cups mixed salad greens
with 1 teaspoon olive oil
and juice of ½ lemon

Digestive Sensitivities Menu
DAY THIRTEEN

BREAKFAST

Spinach Scramble*
½ cup raspberries

MORNING SNACK

2 unsweetened rice cakes or
8 rice crackers spread with
1 tablespoon cashew butter

LUNCH

Turkey Hash*
2 cups mixed salad greens
with 1 teaspoon olive oil and
juice of ½ lemon

AFTERNOON SNACK

2 stalks celery, each stuffed
with 1 tablespoon
Lemony Hummus*

DINNER

Tarragon Chicken*
Asparagus with a Zing*
½ cup wild rice

Digestive Sensitivities Menu
DAY FOURTEEN

BREAKFAST

Cheeseless Artichoke Omelet*
½ cup cantaloupe

MORNING SNACK

1 small baked apple sprinkled
with cinnamon and
2 tablespoons crushed pecans

LUNCH

leftover Tarragon Chicken*
½ cup steamed broccoli
¼ cup wild rice

AFTERNOON SNACK

2 unsweetened rice cakes or
8 rice crackers spread with
1 tablespoon cashew butter

DINNER

Red and Green Turkey
Stir Fry*
¼ cup brown rice
2 cups mixed salad greens
with 1 teaspoon olive oil
and juice of ½ lemon

Digestive Sensitivities FAQ

What happens if my digestive symptoms get worse?

Continue with the Custom Plan for a week and see if your symptoms begin to resolve. Sometimes women feel worse before they feel better. If you continue to feel terrible, or if your symptoms worsen, call your practitioner and schedule your tests. You may be dealing with an underlying issue, like low gastric acidity or systemic yeast, that needs additional attention. It's also possible that you are more sensitive than you thought and other allergens (such as dander, mold, or food additives) are making themselves known in the absence of an overriding dietary offender.

How quickly will I see changes?

You should notice changes within five to seven days. If you had bloating and GI distress, 80 to 85 percent of it should resolve in that time. If you do not feel any improvement in 14 days, go back to the Core Balance quiz and look at your scores. Another of the high-scoring imbalances may be holding you back! You may also be one of the many women who need a medical food to support their recovery.

If I go off the plan for a day, will I undo all the work I've done?

No. Going off the program for a day may make you uncomfortable, but it will not set you back permanently. Resume the plan as soon as you can and don't get down on yourself. If you need to, break things down into steps that are easier to manage. You don't have to give up everything at once; just remember that working by degrees may make your progress slower. Note how you feel when you reintroduce a food (even if it's by mistake) and keep a list of the foods that make you feel sick.

chapter nine

THE HORMONAL
IMBALANCE CUSTOM PLAN

If you scored highest on Hormonal Imbalance in my quiz, I suspect that you are experiencing an imbalance in the ratio of your androgen, or sex, hormones—estrogen, progesterone, and testosterone—that's being exacerbated by environmental factors, toxic weight, and life stress. When you consider that such an imbalance also contributes to toxic weight—and the added stress you may feel from that alone—you'll see that this is a cycle you would do well to break!

Female sex hormones orchestrate, among other functions, sex development, fertility, pregnancy, lactation, bone and muscle growth, libido, and your monthly cycle. When one is off-kilter, it undermines the action of the other two (and of other hormones). And when your sex hormone ratio is thrown off, your body lets you know with a raft of uncomfortable symptoms. In older women, these symptoms are often associated with perimenopause—the years leading up to menopause—and menopause, such as hot flashes, rapid heartbeat, irritability, and loss of libido. Younger women may experience irregular menses and worsening symptoms of PMS, such as bloating, cravings, breast tenderness, and mood swings. And of course, the common denominator in most of us with a hormone imbalance is weight gain!

It's very common for women to experience a slight thickening waist, and/or a shift in fat distribution, as they get older, but a ballooning waistline is a different matter. (And keep in mind that it's also quite possible for younger women to experience hormonal weight gain.) More than a few women have stood in my office grabbing at their extra inches and asking, "Where did this come from?" Not only is it upsetting and frustrating, it's a health risk: Excess belly fat at any age is linked with a host of degenerative issues that contribute to accelerated aging and chronic disease, such as inflammation, cardiovascular disease, and insulin resistance—so it's imperative that you begin to whittle it away.[1] But take heart! Though hormonal weight gain is stubborn, it does not have to be permanent. By now you know better than to be afraid of this weight. By now you can call this weight what it really is—toxic—and recognize it as a symptom that can be healed with the right support.[2]

Hormones In and Out of Balance

Hormonal imbalance is very common, and often complicated, simply because we have so many hormones in our bodies—and more are being discovered all the time. (You'll find a list of known hormones in the Appendices.) We use a lot of metaphors to describe the endocrine system, but the best one I've heard is that if your body were a business, your hormones would be all the e-mails being sent back and forth between offices relating relevant information to get work done—and your hypothalamus would be your server. If the flow of information gets blocked or misdirected in any way—or if the server breaks down—work deteriorates or stops altogether and the business starts to fall apart. Because hormones are extremely agile and adaptive, however, they don't just stop working; they often find other ways of working as the body tries to compensate, and the changes cause symptoms that can alert you to a problem long before any permanent damage occurs. So you may just want to revise your thinking about your hormonal symptoms—including toxic weight—and be glad that your body has let you in on its struggle before anything more serious happens.

Estrogen and progesterone are sister hormones that work in sync, providing an important check and balance to each other, with testosterone providing crucial support; the ratio of these hormones to one another is what matters. At any stage of a woman's life this relationship can get stuck, for lack of a better word, in a dysfunctional pattern, but it is far more common as we get older and our hormones start to fluctuate more wildly. The key to restoring hormone balance is to give your body the working materials it needs to manufacture enough hormones and get rid of any extra. Your sex hormones are steroids, meaning they are made from cholesterol (fat) and are fat-soluble (stored in fat cells). Cholesterol is made in your liver from dietary fat. If you don't eat enough fat, which often happens on low-fat diets, your liver is tasked with making up the difference. This means double duty, because the liver is also the organ responsible for clearing and excreting excess hormones from the bloodstream.

There is still much to be discovered about how our myriad hormones interact, but one thing is clear: They all operate in a feedback loop that influences and is influenced

by fat cells. And the amount of fat cells you have is related to your blood sugar levels and your insulin levels. The equation is simple: the higher your glucose levels, the higher your levels of insulin, the more fat cells your body creates to store the extra glucose. Now this wouldn't necessarily be more than an aesthetic problem if fat cells were just inactive lumps of gelatinous tissue—but they are not. Your fat cells, especially the ones around your belly, are metabolically active: They store and secrete fat-soluble hormones, including estrogen, and they hold loads of glucose receptors.[3] Talk about a hard-to-break pattern: an insulin imbalance has caused you to gain weight, and your extra fat is making the hormonal imbalance symptoms worse! What's even more disturbing is that declining levels of estrogen during perimenopause and menopause raise levels of testosterone in women, like a seesaw, and women naturally begin to store weight in more of a "male" pattern (around our bellies) than we did during our reproductive years (when fat went to breasts, arms, thighs, and bottom).

Holding on to some extra weight may actually be good for your body—at menopause. Remember, your fat cells store estrogen; they also manufacture hormonal precursors to estrogen in very small amounts. As ovarian function declines, estrogen levels fluctuate, and your body begins to guard its estrogen reserves with a vengeance (to help impede bone loss, among other essential functions). By holding on to fat cells, your body is taking out insurance for the future—so if you put on some extra weight at this time, no more than five pounds, it should not be considered toxic. Give yourself a break and give your body a year or two to find its post-menopausal equilibrium. The good news is that menopausal weight, particularly around the belly, responds well to exercise. So if you have gained more than is healthy, adding consistent exercise to your Custom Plan will really help.

Insulin Resistance

We all start off in life being "insulin sensitive." Our cells' demand for fuel varies from moment to moment, but the brain needs our blood sugar level to remain stable. So getting the cells the energy they need without changing that level is a critical function—and that's the role that insulin plays. Insulin signals the cells to absorb glucose from the bloodstream. The body monitors blood sugar levels, cell demands, and the food we digest, and it releases insulin in perfectly calibrated amounts. When the feedback between the cells and the insulin release is efficient and healthy, cells are described as insulin sensitive.[4]

In contrast, when we consistently overeat or subsist on a diet high in "empty" calories, refined sugar, and simple carbohydrates, high levels of insulin are required to keep the level of glucose in the bloodstream from spiraling out of control. Cells are simply awash in the stuff, so they quit responding to the signal, just as you would if someone kept ringing your doorbell all the time. At this point, the body is insulin resistant, and this is a precursor to diabetes type II, obesity, inflammation, cardiovascular disease, and the umbrella condition that links all of these: metabolic syndrome.

You can test for insulin resistance by having a fasting glucose/insulin level taken, followed by another glucose/insulin level two hours after eating a high-glucose meal, such as pancakes and syrup. High triglycerides may also point to this problem; if you can multiply your HDL by 4 or 5 and the sum equals your triglyceride levels or higher, you are probably insulin resistant.

Bringing It All into Balance

As important as sex hormones are to your well-being and your weight, they are minor players on the hormonal stage; there are major players—including cortisol, your thyroid (T3, T4, and parathyroid) hormones, and, as we've seen, insulin—to examine as well when we treat hormonal imbalance. You simply must balance the major players before you can balance the minor players. Sally, a life coach we work with at Women to Women, first came to see me as a patient because she had classic symptoms of perimenopause: night sweats, hot flashes, and increasing bouts of severe anxiety. Her tests revealed that she was indeed approaching menopause and her sex hormones needed support, but—very important—they also told me that her cortisol levels were extremely low. (For more information on cortisol and your adrenals, read about the Adrenal Imbalance

Custom Plan in Chapter 10.) Some patients who come in with menopause symptoms actually have overlapping hormonal issues, such as thyroid or insulin issues, and more often than not they have digestive issues on top of everything else.

The point is this: restoring balance to your sex hormones begins by stabilizing other major hormones, like insulin, first. That's because all of your major and minor hormones "dance" together in a complicated pattern dictated by your diet, your lifestyle, and your physiology, including your hypothalamus. In other words, if you have hot flashes and weight gain and you are insulin resistant, the hot flashes and extra weight won't go away until you first heal the insulin resistance. And in my experience, most women approaching menopause are predisposed to insulin resistance. This doesn't have to become a permanent state, but it does mean that if you are experiencing hormonal symptoms, one of the first ways to regain control is to pay more attention to blood sugar.

One good thing about a sex-hormone imbalance is that it often makes itself heard loud and clear, especially as you approach menopause. For many women, it's as if they've been walking along all these years with a silent partner who suddenly starts to yell. This happened to Letitia, one of the many women who come to see me for dysfunctional uterine bleeding and weight gain related to menopause. At 56 years old, Letitia was on HRT (synthetic hormone replacement therapy) and bleeding all the time. She also had about 25 extra pounds that she wanted to be rid of. Letitia told me she had tons of energy and felt great on hormones but she was frustrated: the constant bleeding really hampered her lifestyle. All of her conventional tests were negative, but try as we might, we couldn't regulate Letitia's bleeding while she continued on HRT. Nothing was working. As Letitia's frustration mounted, we decided to wean her off hormones completely (albeit slowly) and see how that affected the bleeding. For the first few weeks, Letitia's menopausal symptoms came back—she called me about night sweats, hot flashes, sleeplessness, the whole shebang. She was bloated and puffy and felt, in her words, "like a stuffed pig!" I prescribed the Hormonal Imbalance Custom Plan and supplements to help her through the transition, which Letitia followed scrupulously, along with a supplemental soy drink containing 80 mgs of soy isoflavones and beneficial herbs, such as red clover, black cohosh, ashwaganda, passionflower, and wild yam (among others). To Letitia's immense credit, she didn't give up on herself or the plan. Soon enough her diligence was rewarded. Her bleeding had stopped; her symptoms were gone; and she had lost 17 pounds! Today, more than a year later, she has not regained any of the weight.

If you suspect that you have a sex-hormone imbalance, it's worth the time and money to discover which of your sex hormones is off-kilter. In some cases, women in perimenopause may have low levels of progesterone in comparison to their estrogen levels. In other cases, women's progesterone levels are fine, but their estrogen levels are too high. And more and more frequently, all three of the key hormones in flux during this time—estrogen, progesterone, and testosterone—are too low. Additionally, your sex hormones may be responding to an underlying imbalance in thyroid hormones or the stress-adaptive hormone cortisol. If you aren't feeling any better on your own, you may want to be evaluated by a medical practitioner conversant in integrative or alternative medicine. Begin the Hormonal Imbalance Custom Plan tomorrow to start restoring balance and clearing away clutter so you can see what's really going on. Once you've followed the plan for two weeks, schedule time to get some diagnostic tests if you are still symptomatic to investigate your hormonal upset and see whether or not your thyroid is involved (there are several scenarios).

In the end, keeping your major hormones well balanced through your life is the key to maintaining a healthy metabolism and a wellspring of vitality. The spectacular thing about this is that many women don't need a lot of pills and potions to help heal their hormonal imbalance—even at menopause! Some do, and that's where those diagnostic tests come in handy. If you decide you want to pursue some form of bioidentical HRT, you'll find information in the Appendices. But first give the next two weeks your best shot and then see how you feel. If you follow this plan diligently, I suspect you'll be feeling so much better—and lighter—in 14 days that your symptoms of hormonal imbalance will follow suit.

The Hormonal Imbalance Eating and Action Plan

Your challenge over the next two weeks will be limiting your carbohydrate intake (and having patience with yourself when you struggle with this). A diet high in sugar and refined carbs—especially with overeating—can lead to a sex hormone imbalance by triggering spikes in insulin levels, which causes insulin sensitivity and a complicated biochemical reaction that alters the level of estrogen in the bloodstream.[5] The Hormonal Imbalance menu is designed to provide optimal nutrition and supplemental support to help your body synthesize adequate sex hormones without jacking up insulin levels.

Most of my patients with hormonal imbalance report a significant improvement in hormonal symptoms and weight loss—especially belly fat—when they completely remove refined carbs from their diets and follow my guidelines for supplements and stress reduction. In my practice we call this addition by subtraction! Don't worry—you are still going to eat lots of delicious food, including lean protein and dairy products and plenty of complex carbohydrates and good fats. Try as hard as you can for the next two weeks to stay away from baked and processed goods, sugary snacks, all junk food, and alcohol, the ultimate sugar buzz, as you have been the past two weeks.

I will also be asking you to avoid, or at least limit, caffeine and other stimulants to help regulate your levels of adrenaline and cortisol, which at higher levels make symptoms of sex-hormone imbalance worse. This means you must find other ways to counteract fatigue and stress. Consider canceling engagements and try to avoid excessive emotional stimulation—you have my permission to give yourself a break! As another way to support yourself emotionally, you may want to explore a creative activity. Estrogen is the seed of our reproductive ability, which can be thought of as our creative potential. If you're in menopause, you may feel the sense of loss some of us experience when our organs no longer have the ability to reproduce; it helps to remember that your creativity doesn't go away, it just moves onto another plane. Trying your hand at an art or a craft can be a fantastic—even transformative—way to channel your creative energy.

Keep in mind that your hormones are always changing and adapting to meet your body's requirements. This makes them very impressionable—susceptible to bad diets and bad habits, but just as eager to respond to a good diet and healthy habits. In fact, women with hormonal imbalance frequently feel better after just a few days on the Hormonal Imbalance Custom Plan; they also tend to see faster weight loss than women with other imbalances. Knowing that your hormones are so quick to take impressions, think about how you've conditioned yourself to react to others (and to yourself) over the years—reactions that trigger the same hormonal response over and over again—and then focus instead on the wealth of possibilities that the future always holds. Wherever you are today, whatever you feel today, is not where you have to be or what you have to feel tomorrow.

Marcelle's Prescription for
HORMONAL IMBALANCE

1. Follow the menu plan beginning on page 136 as strictly as possible.

2. Take your supplements at the prescribed times.

3. Set a bedtime that allows you seven to nine hours of sleep per night and stick to it.

4. When you wake up in the morning, linger in bed for five to ten minutes and set a positive intention for your day.

5. Try to get an hour of physical activity at least five times a week, including resistance training twice weekly.

6. Drink plenty of pure, unfiltered water and noncaffeinated herbal teas.

7. Reduce your "to do" list to bare necessities. Reschedule appointments and engagements if necessary. You are healing!

8. Schedule a relaxing treatment, such as acupuncture, massage, or energy healing, at least once over the next two weeks. For more information on options, see the Appendices.

9. Go outside and play!

10. Read Stage IV and consider ways you can begin to tap into your creative potential.

11. Schedule diagnostic tests (following) if you are not feeling an improvement within two weeks.

Diagnostic Testing for Hormonal Imbalance

Basic:

- If you are premenopausal, hormone saliva testing for estrogen, progesterone, and free and total testosterone, as well as sex hormone binding globulin (SHBG) and DHEA levels.

- If you are menopausal or postmenopausal, hormone panel for serum hormone levels

- Fasting blood sugar (glucose) and insulin, then two-hour postprandial glu-cose/insulin test (for insulin resistance and metabolic syndrome)

- Adrenal Stress Index to test adrenal function

- At-home iodine patch test; if positive, proceed with scheduling an Iodine Urine test

Advanced:

- Thyroid testing: TSH, free T3, free T4, thyroid antibodies

- Blood Lipid Panel to test HDL, LDL, and triglycerides (Note: If you have a high ratio of triglycerides to HDL, I advise getting tested for insulin resis-tance to rule out metabolic syndrome. If you can multiply your HDL by 4 four or 5 five and the sum equals your triglyceride number or higher, you are probably insulin resistant; still, have the test to make sure.)

Foods to Include for Hormonal Imbalance

- Nonstarchy vegetables, especially from the *Brassica* family—broccoli, cab-bage, brussels sprouts

- Leafy greens

- Alfalfa beans and sprouts

- Complex grains

- Lean animal protein

- Soy protein

- Dairy, use 2% or full fat

- Eggs

- Legumes

- Sea kelp

- Nuts and seeds

- Lemons and limes

- Sweeteners—agave nectar, stevia

- Lemons and lemon juice

- Herbs and spices—all, especially basil, cardamom, cinnamon, cumin, fennel, garlic, ginseng, oregano, pepper, and sea salt

- Balancing teas—gingko, ginseng, green, fenugreek, dandelion, red raspberry, dong quai (see page 65)

Foods to Avoid for Hormonal Imbalance

- Caffeine

- Alcohol (including wine and beer)

- Sugar, fructose, high-fructose corn syrup, maltose, dextrose, honey, and maple syrup

- Refined flour, grains, and breads

- Baked goods

- Chocolate and candy

- Crackers, chips, and salty snacks

Supplements for Hormonal Imbalance

Basic:

- High-potency daily multivitamin with additional calcium and magnesium

- Essential fatty acids

- Probiotic (take 5 to 15 minutes before each meal with water)

- Herbal supplement for menopausal symptom relief, preferably one that contains extracts of black cohosh, red clover, ashwaganda, passionflower, kudzu, chasteberry, and wild yam

- Soy—80 mgs isoflavones in powder or shake form

- Calcium d-gluconate to help estrogen metabolism and impede bone loss if you're postmenopausal

Additional:

- Take these supplements if your diagnostic tests show persistent high levels of estrogen compared to progesterone or you suspect you have low progesterone; discontinue use if you experience breast tenderness or unusual bleeding

- Over-the-counter topical USP (United States Pharmacopeia, an official standard) progesterone cream or wild yam cream—½ teaspoon on wrist daily from day 14 of menstrual cycle to beginning of next period

- Indole-3-carbinole (if tests show sustained high levels of estrogen, use with medical supervision) or DIM, an estrogen balancer derived from cruciferous plants, especially if you have a family history of breast cancer or if you have a problem with estrogen metabolism

Food for Your Hormones

Soy

The soybean belongs to the legume or pulse family, whose members include peas, beans, and peanuts. Soybeans are renowned for their phytonutrient content, which includes a high concentration of isoflavones, omega-3s, and protein. Soy has been closely studied and found supportive for a wide range of menopausal and perimenopausal symptoms: improved insulin regulation; weight loss; bone health; improved nail, skin, and hair health; and decrease in menopausal discomforts, particularly vaginal dryness, hot flashes, and night sweats.[6] Studies abound on both the benefits and the detrimental effects of soy, with sometimes conflicting results. From what I've seen, the preponderance of evidence falls clearly on the beneficial side—especially as a safe alternative to conventional HRT-based menopausal treatments. Soy has been helpful for people who have difficulty metabolizing estrogen—80 mgs isoflavones seems to be the key.

Soy works extremely well for some women and moderately well for others, while there are some who do not metabolize it well and a smaller subset who react adversely to it. If you are experiencing menopausal symptoms, try adding whole, non-GMO (not genetically modified) soy foods to your diet, such as edamame, tofu, tempeh, and soy protein powders, and see how they work for you.

Iodine

Iodine is a component of the thyroid hormones thyroxine (T4) and triiodothyronine (T3) and as such is essential for healthy metabolism. An enlarged thyroid gland (goiter) is an early sign of iodine deficiency. Governments solved potential mass iodine deficiencies by iodizing salt to the extent that it prevented goiter but not necessarily to the optimal level for health; however, over the past 25 years we've been cautioned to watch our salt intake. So now fewer of us are getting enough iodine, let alone too much. Plus, certain foods called goitrogenic compounds—cruciferous vegetables like cabbage, cauliflower, broccoli, and kale—may interfere with the absorption of iodine. If you have thyroid deficiencies, you may want to consider decreasing these foods; however, they are very healthy, so get your iodine levels tested before you decrease them.

I've been surprised to see how many of my patients have an iodine deficiency that may be related to their thyroid function and hormonal balance. Because iodized salt is bleached, I recommend that you ingest a gentler source such as natural unbleached sea salt, Celtic sea salt, or kelp salt. The downside of this is that natural salt does not provide enough iodine, so add dried seaweed products to your diet to ensure that you're getting adequate iodine. I do not recommend that anyone take iodine supplements without medical testing and guidance. It can be problematic if your iodine levels are too high, but I seldom see this at my practice.

A Day in the Life of the
Hormonal Imbalance Custom Plan

Time	Activity
6:30-7:00 A.M.	Wake up. Linger in bed for five to ten minutes. Set a positive intention for the day. Transition slowly. Exercise in the morning if this works best for you.
7:15	Drink two to three glasses of water or warm water with lemon, followed by self-care ritual. Take probiotic.
7:30	Breakfast.
8:00	Shower, dress.
8:30	Walk to work or take a 15-minute walk or practice deep breathing if possible.
10:30	Snack with water.
11:30	Tea break.
12:20-1:00 P.M.	Lunch, followed by a walk.
3:00	Snack.
4:30	Drink two to three glasses of water.
5:00	Exercise (if you haven't already done so), go outdoors, or find a playful activity that makes you happy.
6:00	Make dinner and take probiotic.
6:30	Dinner.
7:00	Catch up with family, friends, chores, crafts, correspondence. Stay away from the nightly television news, which can pile on stress.
8:00	Reading, journaling, meditation—begin to wind down.
9:00	Bedtime.

The Core Balance Menu Plan for Hormonal Imbalance

Snack Ideas:

- ¼ cup mixed nuts or soy nuts
- 1 serving of cheese and 1 piece of fruit
- 1 cup 2 percent or full-fat plain yogurt
- 1 hard-boiled egg
- Sliced veggie sticks with hummus or yogurt

* Recipes start on page 259.

Hormone Imbalance Menu
DAY ONE

BREAKFAST
2 eggs, any style
Zucchini Cakes*

MORNING SNACK
1 small baked apple sprinkled
with cinnamon and
2 tablespoons crushed pecans

LUNCH
Curried Chicken Salad* on
1 cup mixed salad greens

AFTERNOON SNACK
Avocado and Pear Dip*
with ½ cup sliced cucumber
or zucchini

DINNER
Fillet of Fish Amandine*
Sautéed Green Beans*
⅓ cup wild rice

Hormone Imbalance Menu
DAY TWO

BREAKFAST
Spinach Quiche*
½ cup raspberries

MORNING SNACK
Tropical Prosciutto Rolls*

LUNCH
leftover Fillet of
Fish Amandine*
½ cup steamed broccoli with
½ tablespoon butter
¼ cup wild rice

AFTERNOON SNACK
Lemony Hummus* with
½ cup sliced vegetables

DINNER
Sumptuous Chicken Stew*
½ gluten-free roll
½ cup steamed broccoli with
½ tablespoon butter

Hormone Imbalance Menu
DAY THREE

BREAKFAST

Spicy Fiesta Eggs*
½ cup sliced strawberries

MORNING SNACK

1 ounce string cheese
2 tablespoons almonds

LUNCH

Sweet Chicken Salad*
½ gluten-free roll

AFTERNOON SNACK

Avocado and Pear Dip*
with ½ cup sliced cucumber
or zucchini

DINNER

Steak with Blockbuster
Bleu Cheese*
Crunchy Snow Peas*
⅓ cup wild rice

Hormone Imbalance Menu
DAY FOUR

BREAKFAST

2 Salmon Cakes*
½ cup unsweetened full-fat
or 2% yogurt
½ cup raspberries

MORNING SNACK

2 hardboiled eggs
½ cup cantaloupe

LUNCH

leftover Spinach Quiche*
1 cup mixed salad greens
with 1 teaspoon olive oil and
balsamic vinegar
¼ cup blueberries

AFTERNOON SNACK

1 small nectarine
1 ounce sliced cheese

DINNER

Sizzling Shrimp Scampi*
½ cup braised kale
¼ cup wild rice

Hormone Imbalance Menu
DAY FIVE

BREAKFAST

Tomato and
Asparagus Frittata*
½ cup blueberries with
1 tablespoon heavy cream,
sweetened with stevia to taste

MORNING SNACK

½ pear spread with
1 tablespoon cashew butter

LUNCH

Not Your Everyday Egg Salad*
on 1 cup mixed salad greens

AFTERNOON SNACK

Lemony Hummus* with ½ cup
sliced vegetables

DINNER

Creamy Cilantro Chicken*
Edamame Mix*
¼ cup wild rice

Hormone Imbalance Menu
DAY SIX

BREAKFAST

2 eggs, any style
Zucchini Cakes*
½ cup cantaloupe

MORNING SNACK

Olive Tapenade* with
½ cup sliced vegetables

LUNCH

baked or broiled chicken
breast, salt and pepper to taste
Tasty Tomatoes*
⅓ cup wild rice

AFTERNOON SNACK

2 unsweetened rice cakes or
8 rice crackers spread with
1 tablespoon almond butter

DINNER

Rosemary Lamb*
Zucchini Ribbons*
½ sweet potato with
½ tablespoon butter, sprinkled
with cinnamon if desired

Hormone Imbalance Menu
DAY SEVEN

BREAKFAST

Cheeseless Artichoke Omelet*
¼ cup blueberries

MORNING SNACK

½ nectarine stuffed with
2 tablespoons ricotta cheese
and sprinkled with cinnamon
or nutmeg

LUNCH

leftover Rosemary Lamb*
2 cups mixed salad greens with
1 teaspoon olive oil and
juice of ½ lemon
½ cup sliced strawberries

AFTERNOON SNACK

½ cup blueberries
1 ounce sliced cheese

DINNER

Mediterranean Scallops*
¼ cup wild rice
Spinach with Lemon
and Garlic*

Hormone Imbalance Menu
DAY EIGHT

BREAKFAST

½ cup cottage cheese
2 Salmon Cakes*
½ cup raspberries

MORNING SNACK

1 small apple, sliced and
spread with 1 tablespoon
cashew butter

LUNCH

leftover Cheeseless
Artichoke Omelet*
1 cup mixed salad greens
with 1 teaspoon olive oil
and balsamic vinegar

AFTERNOON SNACK

1 ounce string cheese
2 tablespoons almonds

DINNER

Chicken Lyonnaise*
¼ cup wild rice
1 cup mixed salad greens
with 1 teaspoon olive oil
and balsamic vinegar
¼ cup blueberries with
1 tablespoon heavy cream,
sweeten with stevia to taste

Hormone Imbalance Menu
DAY NINE

BREAKFAST

Delicious Crustless
Seafood Quiche*
½ cup sliced strawberries

MORNING SNACK

2 Cheese Balls with Parsley*
½ cup sliced strawberries

LUNCH

Easy Chicken Florentine*
½ cup cantaloupe

AFTERNOON SNACK

2 stalks celery, each stuffed
with 1 tablespoon
Lemony Hummus*

DINNER

grilled or broiled hamburger
Brussels Sprouts
with Mushrooms*
¼ cup brown rice

Hormone Imbalance Menu
DAY TEN

BREAKFAST

2 eggs, any style
2 slices nitrate-free bacon
½ cup raspberries with
heavy cream, sweetened
with stevia to taste

MORNING SNACK

1 small baked apple sprinkled
with cinnamon and
2 tablespoons crushed pecans

LUNCH

baked or broiled chicken
breast, salt and pepper to taste
Crunchy Snow Peas*
⅓ cup wild rice

AFTERNOON SNACK

Olive Tapenade* with ½ cup
sliced vegetables

DINNER

Jazzy Cajun Jambalaya*
1 cup mixed salad greens
with 1 teaspoon olive oil
and balsamic vinegar
½ cup sliced strawberries

Hormone Imbalance Menu
DAY ELEVEN

BREAKFAST

½ cup unsweetened full-fat
or 2% yogurt
Zucchini Cakes*
½ cup cantaloupe

MORNING SNACK

1 hardboiled egg
2 tablespoons almonds

LUNCH

leftover Jazzy
Cajun Jambalaya*
1 cup mixed salad greens
with 1 teaspoon olive oil
and balsamic vinegar
½ cup blueberries with
1 tablespoon heavy cream,
sweetened with stevia to taste

AFTERNOON SNACK

½ pear spread with
1 tablespoon cashew butter

DINNER

baked or broiled chicken
breast, salt and
pepper to taste
Mushroom Soup*
½ cup steamed broccoli with
½ tablespoon butter
½ gluten-free roll

Hormone Imbalance Menu
DAY TWELVE

BREAKFAST

Spicy Fiesta Eggs*
½ cup sliced strawberries with
1 tablespoon heavy cream,
sweeten with stevia to taste

MORNING SNACK

1 unsweetened rice cake or
4 rice crackers spread with
1 tablespoon almond butter

LUNCH

Curried Chicken Salad* on
1 cup mixed salad greens
½ cup raspberries

AFTERNOON SNACK

2 Cheese Balls with Parsley*
1 tablespoon almonds

DINNER

Hearty Pork Stew*
1 cup mixed salad greens
with 1 teaspoon olive oil
and balsamic vinegar
¼ cup cantaloupe

Hormone Imbalance Menu
DAY THIRTEEN

BREAKFAST

Creamy Salmon Omelet*
½ cup blueberries

MORNING SNACK

Avocado and Pear Dip*
with ½ cup sliced cucumber
or zucchini

LUNCH

Not Your Everyday Egg Salad*
on 1 cup mixed salad greens

AFTERNOON SNACK

Tropical Prosciutto Rolls*

DINNER

Sweet Salsa Smothered Steak*
Spinach with Lemon
and Garlic*
¼ cup wild rice

Hormone Imbalance Menu
DAY FOURTEEN

BREAKFAST

Tomato and
Asparagus Frittata*
½ cup raspberries with
heavy cream, sweetened with
stevia to taste

MORNING SNACK

1 ounce sliced cheese
2 tablespoons almonds

LUNCH

leftover Sweet Salsa
Smothered Steak* on
1 cup mixed salad greens
½ cup sliced strawberries

AFTERNOON SNACK

Guacamole* with ½ cup
sliced vegetables

DINNER

Quick and Easy Chicken*
1 cup mixed salad greens
with 1 teaspoon olive oil
and balsamic vinegar
½ gluten-free roll

Hormonal Imbalance FAQ

Is it possible to relieve hormonal symptoms naturally at menopause? I don't want to take HRT, but I'm sick of this roller-coaster ride.

Yes! And you are on your way right now just by following this plan. Improving hormonal balance is possible through diet and lifestyle changes and by adding certain supplements and foods to our diet that enhance hormonal stability. And the sooner you intervene the better. For more in-depth information, I encourage you to read the Appendices section on natural HRT and visit www.womentowomen.com, which explores many ways to restore hormone balance safely, effectively, and naturally.

I'm on birth-control pills (or HRT) and I want to go off. Can I just quit?

I don't recommend going off hormone therapy cold turkey. While you are on this plan, talk to your practitioner about slowly reducing the amount of hormones you are currently on. As you regain your core balance, you may find you really don't need hormone therapy, unless you want it for birth control reasons. If you're on the Pill, try to follow this plan for two months and then stop the Pill.

I'm not losing weight on this plan. What should I do?

Have patience with yourself and give it the full two weeks. If you aren't using a medical food, see Appendix for more information, and consider doing so—it really helps! If you still don't notice an improvement, go back to the Core Balance Quiz and look at your other high scores. It may be that your adrenals or your digestive tract need some help, or that you aren't detoxifying well.

chapter ten

THE ADRENAL
IMBALANCE CUSTOM PLAN

If you scored highest on Adrenal Imbalance in my quiz, there's a high likelihood that your adrenals are shouting for help. The adrenals are walnut-sized glands located on top of each kidney, and they are important control centers for many of the body's hormones. The outer layer of the gland, called the adrenal cortex, produces small amounts of steroid hormones including cortisol, DHEA, estrogen, and testosterone. The centers of the glands produce adrenaline, the hormone named after them. (Adrenaline is also called epinephrine; it is made from a similar hormone, norepinephrine.)

Your adrenal glands give a lot of bang for the buck. They ignite the fight-or-flight response when you are under stress, either real or perceived. You probably know what it feels like when you face a physical threat, like a shark attack! (Okay, you may not know what that feels like, but you get the idea.) Your heart pounds, your breathing speeds up, and you feel mentally sharp. The fight-or-flight response creates a tremendous amount of energy in milliseconds to keep you, or someone you're protecting, alive. But unlike your thinking brain, which has evolved to distinguish real threats from perceived ones, this automatic response does not register a difference between, say, a real shark attack and a scene of a shark attacking in a scary movie, or between physical danger and a particularly frustrating traffic jam. All the hypothalamus reads is "Danger!" and it sounds the alarm throughout the central nervous system.

When the adrenals get the signal, they release a barrage of chemicals, specifically adrenaline and norepinephrine for that quick spurt of superhuman energy. This energy requires fuel, so adrenaline also stimulates a breakdown of fats and of glycogen to glucose, which results in a spike in blood sugar and an increase in the level of free fatty acids circulating in the blood.[1] These adrenaline-charged cellular changes trigger the release of cortisol and other hormones that raise insulin levels, which helps channel more glucose to your muscles and brain, so your senses sharpen while secondary functions, including your digestion, slow. If the original stressor was emotional or imagined, your cerebral cortex steps in within moments and you know intellectually that you aren't in physical danger (That's not a real shark! It's only a movie!). But it doesn't matter—your central nervous system is already fired up.

The fight-or-flight response may be your body's most important, most efficient defense mechanism for surviving another day in the jungle, but there's one problem: It wasn't designed to last very long. Long enough to get you to safety, perhaps, but then it was intended to subside and return you to normal with the help of the parasympathetic nervous system, the countering actions in the body related to relaxation. The adrenals were designed to sprint and then rest, not run a cross-country race. But these days, when stress has become a chronic condition, that's precisely what we ask them to do. As a result, our health is showing the strain—and our waists are showing it, too, in the form of toxic weight.

A Short Course in Adrenal Burnout

Remember I explained in the Introduction how toxic weight gain is a symptom of a body under stress? Well, overworked and burnt-out adrenals—and the toxic weight they cause us to pack on—are the result of chronic stress. Unlike our great-great-grandmothers and our ancestors before them, we in our modern life are exposed to unrelenting stress over a long span of years. We're constantly overworked, overwired, overmedicated, undernourished, and exposed to an allergic and chemical cocktail of environmental toxins. We live in a technology- and media-saturated age that keeps us perpetually stimulated. All of this, along with our personal emotional challenges, creates a huge demand on the adrenal glands. This is particularly true of women in their 30s and 40s—years otherwise known as the "crunch" decades—the time of life when they are sandwiched between raising children and taking care of elders, often while holding down a job or doing volunteer work.

Some of us may have the support we need to combat this constant toll, but in my clinical experience, only 10 to 15 percent of the women I test have normal adrenal function. That leaves 85 to 90 percent who are operating with impaired adrenals. A few years ago a woman named Denise came to see me. She had been diagnosed with chronic fatigue, and her doctors had told her that she would just have to live with it, so she did— for 20 years! By the time she came to see me, she couldn't drive a car. She could barely walk up the stairs to my office—her husband practically had to carry her. Her tests proved that her adrenal function was low, and she had to make some major life changes to heal. She began a journey back to health that began with the same plan I'm going to present to you.

How do the adrenals get so burned out? It's complicated, but the short answer is: stress itself—physical, environmental, and emotional. Stress taxes the adrenals, forcing them to make a lot of cortisol. And over time, cortisol in large amounts stresses your body even further. Designed to help you respond to challenges by converting proteins into energy, it stimulates the liver to release glycogen into the bloodstream to quickly fuel the brain, and it counteracts inflammation by suppressing the immune reaction. For a short time that's okay, but at sustained high levels, cortisol gradually tears your body down as it breaks apart larger molecules to release their energy. Over extended periods, it actually destroys healthy muscle and bone, impairs digestion and metabolism, and decreases insulin sensitivity, which can be a step toward putting on unwanted weight. At the same time, when the adrenals strain to maintain high cortisol levels, they lose the ability to produce sufficient amounts of the hormone DHEA, a precursor to estrogen, progesterone, and testosterone and a key player in moderating your body's hormone balance. Insufficient DHEA contributes to fatigue, bone loss, depression, joint pain, decreased sex drive, and impaired immune function, among other concerns.

Adrenal imbalances are so common in my patients that I've almost come to believe they are the price we all may pay at some point for our mile-a-minute lifestyle. When the adrenals are overworked, you feel tired—it's that simple. And by tired, I mean wiped—as if you have nothing left in your tank. The tricky part, of course, is that everyone complains of being tired these days, so women may go for months and years without medical care. I have one patient, Heather, who came to see me last year. She was in her late 30s and wanted an overall checkup and help losing 15 toxic pounds. During our first interview, she told me that she was exhausted all the time. She had an autistic son and an ex-husband who helped as much as he could, but it was getting to the point where she could barely get out of bed in the morning. She was tired all day long, relying on coffee and snacks to keep her going; if she rested for more than a few minutes, overwhelming fatigue washed over her. Heather had always prided herself on being the go-to person, but now she felt as if she could barely hold it together. She admitted to me that her stress levels were very high and she was extremely worried about how to keep up enough energy to care for her son.

Heather's exhaustion immediately made me curious about her adrenal health, so we ordered an Adrenal Stress Index test along with all the other appropriate tests. All of her conventional tests were normal but her ASI showed that her adrenal function was flatlined. I immediately asked Heather to stop exercising and she started the Adrenal Imbalance Core Diet Plan the next day, including nutritional supplements for adrenal support, such as ginseng, rhodiola, licorice, and the Chinese mushroom extract *Cordyseps sinensis*. Heather promised to make it a priority to try to engage some extra help with her son and she began to get strict with her own bedtimes. It took her four months, but by the end of that time she felt and looked like a different woman. Not only had she changed her lifestyle so that she had more support with her son, she had learned how to support her body with the right nutrition and her adrenals were back on track—and, happily, her extra weight fell off in the process.

Interestingly, with an adrenal imbalance, your own body may be trying to cope with either too much or too little cortisol. At one end of the spectrum, women with poor adrenal function leading to low cortisol levels may be diagnosed with the very rare Addison's disease; at the other end, women with Cushing's syndrome may have overproductive adrenals that release too much cortisol. Most of you will fall somewhere in between, slowly moving from excessive cortisol production in your 30s and 40s to insufficient production in your 50s and 60s. It's important to know whether you are experiencing high cortisol levels or low; however, women often go to their healthcare practitioners with their symptoms only to find out that the standard tests come back negative or "normal." In my opinion, conventional adrenal testing (the ACTH challenge) leaves a far too generous margin for "normal," So I prefer to use the Adrenal Stress Index (ASI) for diagnosis. This is a saliva test taken at different times of the day (read more in the Appendices). Whatever your test says, no woman should feel a big drop in energy for more than a few days at a time. Chronic fatigue is not normal—it's another symptom, just like toxic weight. If your energy levels are low, or sinking fast, and more rest does not help, you need to have your adrenals tested with the ASI and your thyroid tested as well. The thyroid and the adrenals are intimately connected through the HPA (hypothalamus-pituitary-adrenal) axis, and adrenal imbalance can mask symptoms of an underlying thyroid problem, which can make you feel worse once your adrenals heal; testing will let you know if you are dealing with both.

Is Your Cortisol High or Low?

Symptoms of too much cortisol include feeling tired and wired, hyper, hungry, forgetful, and depressed. You may find yourself bingeing on food or having intense cravings even when you're not really hungry (that's what stress eating is all about). You may crave sleep, only to lie down at night and toss and turn. Or you may go to sleep easily but wake up a few hours later unable to go back to sleep. You may even be eating well and exercising without losing weight, but feeling terribly fatigued the whole time.

Symptoms of low cortisol and adrenal burnout include extreme fatigue, even upon waking; feeling light-headed and queasy when you stand up; falling asleep whenever you sit down; foggy thinking; inability to lose weight; falling asleep only to wake up and feel exhausted; and relying on caffeine and sugar jolts to make it through the day.

The Stress Response and Your Weight

It's commonplace that we eat when we're stressed—and stress is the most commonly reported trigger for binge eating—but how does that make sense in the context of the adrenal response? Think about it: If you were running away from an attacker, would you stop to eat a sandwich? The fight-or-flight response is designed to turn hunger signals down and divert energy away from digestion to the pressing business of survival—that's why leptin, the satiety hormone, rises with cortisol levels.[2] But as with many things in the body, what works in the short term isn't so healthy in the long term. Like a slow leak in your house, persistently high levels of cortisol damage the foundations of the HPA axis. The biochemistry is extremely complex, but the idea is that chronic stress simply drowns out normal signaling and hijacks HPA axis processing, keeping these glands overstimulated and all the hormones they produce ever-present. (This is one reason why chronic stress leads to insulin resistance and leptin resistance: because constantly high levels of these hormones signal so relentlessly—stimulating the HPA axis over and over, in a manner of speaking—that the brain stops responding to the signal.[3] And leptin resistance means your brain never gets the signal that you're full.) The stress response has a shutoff switch built in—when cortisol reaches the brain, it tells the hypothalamus to stop signaling for its production—but research has found that chronic stress drowns out normal signaling. So while stress continues, so does cortisol production, sending you on the hunt for cheap and easy comfort foods that will bring the most quick energy and fat for the effort—like candy bars, donuts, and, of course, caffeine-laden mocha frappuccinos.[4]

Many women with impaired adrenals try to power through their fatigue in just this way, relying on caffeine (which stimulates adrenaline in your system) or eating more to try to sustain their energy levels (and usually resorting to junk food and refined sugar for the quick jolt). Others try to boost their energy by increasing their exercise, which gives them the temporary energy surge that accompanies the release of endorphins. But what goes up must come down, and this energy roller coaster just makes adrenal imbalance worse! Cortisol and insulin levels are intertwined: when cortisol rises, so does insulin, and leptin, and a whole related cascade of hormones that we are just beginning to understand. In this way, excessive stimulation of the HPA axis and cortisol production can artificially keep insulin levels high, inducing resistance and stubborn weight gain. Once cells are conditioned to be insulin- or leptin-resistant, it takes a big shift to restore metabolic balance.[5] If you'd like to know more about insulin resistance, please read Chapter 9 about the Hormonal Imbalance Custom Plan. It's not uncommon for adrenal imbalance and hormonal imbalance to go hand in hand.

There are many metabolic hormones that regulate hunger and fat accumulation (see the Appendices). Remember that all of your hormones work together in a feedback loop that influences all of your body's functions. We've talked about the high adrenaline–high cortisol–high insulin–high leptin loop. Conversely, some hormones and functions are suppressed when cortisol levels are high: thyroid hormones, immune function, sex hormones, and other steroid hormones, such as DHEA and human growth hormone. That's why adrenal fatigue can be a factor in many related conditions, including fibromyalgia, hypothyroidism, dysmenorrhea, chronic fatigue syndrome, insomnia, depression, arthritis, and others. It may also produce a host of other unpleasant symptoms, from acne to anxiety to hair loss. And it can lead to problems after menopause, when the adrenals are tasked with making small amounts of estrogen and other hormones once produced by the ovaries; if they're not up to the job, they won't contribute their share, which will interfere with your biochemistry and make all the symptoms of menopause worse. But many of my patients first tune in to their adrenal fatigue because they suddenly have huge difficulty losing weight—especially around their abdomens. A ballooning waistline is a good indicator that your body is in serious defense mode and it's time to pay attention.

The good news here is that the adrenals are like the rest of your physiology: they're fairly easy to heal with the right support, once you know you need to, and the next 14 days will put you well on your way. In order to keep your adrenals in good shape, you'll simply need to learn what your stressors are—physical and emotional—then eliminate them where you can and learn how to cope better with the stress where you can't. We call any event that sets off your stress response a "trigger," including the stress of childhood trauma that's retrieved when you experience a triggering event. Go back to Chapter 1 and look at my list of common stressors; you'll see that I include experiences in your past. When it comes to stress and stubborn weight gain, such subconscious triggers are just as powerful as those we're aware of—and they are usually buried deep in our emotional and instinctive brains. We'll talk about this at greater length in Stage IV, where you can explore ways of taking further action to really get to the bottom of what stresses you and why. In my experience, this, more than anything else, will help you keep the weight off for life.

The Adrenal Imbalance Eating and Action Plan

The biggest challenge for those of you dealing with an adrenal imbalance is restructuring your mind-set so that you stop multitasking and allow a healthy balance between rest and activity—and this means putting yourself first! Adrenal imbalance types tend to be always on the go; if you're one, you may think you thrive on stress, going and going until you run out of gas or get sick. Maybe you're just stuck in a relentless cycle of caretaking and work that feels impossible to break. Meals are taken on the run, sleep is fitful and brief, and you may be dieting, bingeing, and then either overexercising or starving yourself to make up for it. If you feel like you are burning the candle at both ends—you probably are! It's time to stop.

Your plan for the next 14 days emphasizes protein and fiber in the morning and afternoon to keep you satiated and your energy levels up without an afternoon dip. As you begin to wind down for the evening, it uses the right amount of complex carbs to help you relax and get a restful sleep. What it doesn't contain is wheat or other gluten products. In my experience, symptoms of adrenal imbalance are immensely complicated by sensitivity to gluten, a main component in all wheat (and some other grains). Celiac disease is an allergy to gluten; if you have this condition you probably already know, since the symptoms can be quite severe. However, a much larger portion of our society is gluten-sensitive, and this sensitivity becomes increasingly common with age. Over time it wears on the body, but you may not have any noticeable symptoms beyond feeling less than well for a long time. Eliminating gluten from the diet is a shortcut to healing many other core imbalances, including digestive and inflammatory issues.

The menu and supplements here should have you feeling more refreshed, energized, and able to cope with the demands of your life. You should also begin to lose some of the weight your stressed-out body is holding on to. Then you can look to see if there are underlying reasons why you keep yourself busy all the time. Are there things you don't want to take the time to deal with? Ask yourself what you are running away from, and read Stage IV to get more insight and support. And remember, regardless of what our go-go culture tells you, it is not natural or healthy to be on the run all the time. Look around you at the natural world—all living things need rest and activity in equal measure to thrive. So take the next 14 days to cultivate balance in all things and let your adrenals heal.

Marcelle's Prescription for
ADRENAL IMBALANCE

1. Follow the menu plan beginning on page 157.

2. Take your supplements at the prescribed times.

3. If you are currently exercising, reduce the intensity by half for the next two weeks. Do not let your heart rate get above 90 until your adrenals are healed.

4. If you are not currently exercising, make it a goal to walk for 15 minutes after each meal, preferably outdoors.

5. Set a strict bedtime that allows you eight to nine hours of sleep per night and stick to it. If you are having trouble sleeping, please read more on pages 84–85.

6. Listen to your body's needs—allow yourself time to nap on the weekends.

7. Cancel any obligations that are not strictly necessary for the next two weeks.

8. Try to avoid activities and contacts that fire up your central nervous system. This includes dramatic TV shows and evening news, as well as vigorous exercise, confrontations, and so on. Give your stress response a holiday.

9. If you haven't already done so, reduce your caffeine intake or wean yourself off it completely (see page 155). Removing artificial stimulants, like caffeine, is important for women with adrenal issues.

10. Have a massage or another form of therapeutic bodywork at least once during this time. For more information on options, see the Appendices.

11. Unplug at least two hours before bed: no TV, no radio, no computer, no cell phone. Dim the lights, take a bath, or simply do nothing. You are healing!

12. Schedule diagnostic tests if you are not feeling an improvement within two weeks.

Diagnostic Testing for Adrenal Imbalance

Basic:

- Adrenal Stress Index (ASI) to check cortisol levels at different times throughout day

- Complete Blood Count (CBC with differential) to test for anemia, infection, or other blood disorders

- Standard Comprehensive Metabolic Profile (CMP) to test electrolytes, blood sugar, blood protein, pH level, and liver and kidney function

- Blood thyroid panel—TSH levels, free T4 and T3, and thyroid antibodies

- Celiac profile to test for gluten sensitivity/allergy

Additional (if other tests are normal):

- Epstein-Barr/Lyme disease/Mono test (to rule out Epstein-Barr virus, mononucleosis, and Lyme disease)

- ACTH challenge, if desired

- At-home Iodine patch test; if positive, proceed with Urine Iodine test

Please note that many Western practitioners are still skeptical about the role of adrenal health. You may need to see a functional or integrative practitioner for these tests; see Referrals and Resources for information. It's my belief that Western medicine will fully embrace the reality of adrenal fatigue within the next 10 years—you have the chance to get the jump on your own health in the meantime!

Foods to Include for Adrenal Imbalance

- Asparagus
- Avocados
- Cabbage
- Celery
- Cucumbers
- Fruits
- Garlic
- Ginger

- Lean protein
- Sunflower and sesame seeds
- Salt, especially if your adrenal function is low

Foods to Avoid for Adrenal Imbalance

- Alcohol

- Caffeine

- Gluten and grains—wheat, barley, spelt, kamut, rye, triticale, oats if not gluten-free

- Refined and processed sugars, including corn syrup

- Packaged, processed, and junk foods

- Overly spicy foods

Supplements for Adrenal Imbalance

Basic:

- High-potency daily multivitamin with additional calcium and magnesium
- Essential fatty acids
- Probiotic (take 5 to 15 minutes before each meal with water)

Additional—if your cortisol levels are high:

- Astralagus

- Kelp

- A good B complex with B6 if your multivitamin does not offer this

- Melatonin (half a tablet—1 to 3 mgs—half an hour before bed) or 500 mgs Phosphatidyl serine supplement to purge excess cortisol

- Supportive herbs: ginseng, rhodiola, Cordyseps sinensis extract (as directed on package)

Additional—if your cortisol levels are too low:

- Astralagus
- Ashwaganda,
- DHEA (25 mgs)
- Licorice extract or, if you have high blood pressure, deglycerized licorice
- If you are having trouble sleeping, melatonin (half a tablet—1 to 3 mgs— half an hour before bed)
- Supportive herbs: ginseng, rhodiola, Cordyseps sinensis extract

Are You Addicted to Caffeine?

- Do you use caffeine to facilitate a physical activity (waking up, exercising, concentrating, having a bowel movement)?

- Do you have to have caffeine in the morning?

- Do you crash or have caffeine/sugar cravings in the afternoon or early evening?

- Do you grow irritable, have headaches, or feel disembodied if you miss your caffeine fix?

- Do you have difficulty falling asleep at night and waking feeling refreshed?

- Do you need caffeine to heighten the effects of other substances— nicotine, alcohol, sugar?

- Do you feel your social routines would suffer without caffeine use?

- Does the idea of going without caffeine almost bring you to tears?

If you answered yes to two or more of these questions, the time may be ripe to examine your attachment to caffeine. Follow the advice below for weaning yourself off caffeine—if you haven't already begun doing so on the Core Balance Essential Plan—and read more about it in the Appendices.

First, switch to half caf/half decaf for all the coffee you drink. Make sure your coffee is decaffeinated without chemicals (e.g., Swiss water-processed). Next, substitute a decaf variety for one cup of coffee or tea during the day. If you are drinking caffeine throughout the day, alternate with water. Each day, remove more caffeine, weaning yourself slowly to lessen any withdrawal symptoms. After two weeks, you should be drinking decaffeinated beverages exclusively. Then keep going—decaf can have up to one-third the caffeine of the "high-test." If you love the ritual of a warm beverage, don't forget to try interspersing coffee with herbal teas!

A Day in the Life of the
Adrenal Imbalance Custom Plan

Time	Activity
6:30-7:00 A.M.	Rise slowly. Linger in bed for five to ten minutes and set a positive intention for the day. If you feel queasy when you get up, keep a glass of water by your bedside, sit on your bed, and sip it slowly. Do some easy stretches and your self-care ritual.
7:00	Take probiotic with full glass of water. Make breakfast.
7:15-7:45	Eat breakfast slowly. Don't read the paper. Focus on one thing at a time. Take your supplements.
8:00	Bathe and dress.
8:30	Walk to work or leave time for a gentle 15-minute stroll outside.
10:00	Snack.
12:00 P.M.	Lunch. Go somewhere peaceful to eat—not your desk. Take supplements and another 15-minute walk, if possible.
2:00	Snack.
4:00	Tea or water break. Do some deep breathing exercises.
5:00	Walk home or do some gentle exercise, outside if possible, such as gardening or playing with the kids or your pets. Have some fun—a little joy is very relaxing!
6:00	Dinner.
7:00	Self-care ritual.
7:30	Resist the urge to turn on your electronics. Journal, write letters, read, take a bath, or listen to soft music instead. Dim lights and move slowly. Think about powering down.
8:30	Drink a cup of sleep-inducing tea. After, lie down with an eye pillow or towel across your eyes. This stimulates the vagus nerve, which helps trigger the relaxation response.
9:00	Lights out.

The Core Balance Menu Plan for Adrenal Imbalance

* Recipes start on page 259.

Adrenal Imbalance Menu
DAY ONE

BREAKFAST

Spinach Quiche*
⅓ cup blueberries

MORNING SNACK

1 small nectarine
1 ounce sliced cheese

LUNCH

Not Your Everyday Egg Salad*
on 1 cup mixed salad greens

AFTERNOON SNACK

Olive Tapenade* with ½ cup
sliced vegetables

DINNER

Sumptuous Chicken Stew*
2 cups mixed salad greens
with 1 teaspoon olive oil
and juice of ½ lemon
½ gluten-free roll

Adrenal Imbalance Menu
DAY TWO

BREAKFAST

2 scrambled eggs
2 Homemade Turkey Patties*

MORNING SNACK

1 small baked apple sprinkled
with cinnamon and
2 tablespoons crushed pecans

LUNCH

leftover Spinach Quiche*
2 cups mixed salad greens
with 1 teaspoon olive oil
and juice of ½ lemon

AFTERNOON SNACK

Avocado and Pear Dip*
with ½ cup sliced cucumber
or zucchini

DINNER

grilled or broiled steak
½ sweet potato with
½ tablespoon butter, sprinkled
with cinnamon if desired
Brussels Sprouts with
Mushrooms*

Adrenal Imbalance Menu
DAY THREE

BREAKFAST

Creamy Cheesy Scramble*
½ cup sliced strawberries

MORNING SNACK

½ pear spread with
1 tablespoon cashew butter

LUNCH

leftover Sumptuous
Chicken Stew*
½ gluten-free roll

AFTERNOON SNACK

Guacamole* with ½ cup
sliced vegetables

DINNER

Mediterranean Scallops*
2 cups mixed salad greens
with 1 teaspoon olive oil
and juice of ½ lemon
¼ cup blueberries with
1 tablespoon heavy cream,
sweeten with stevia to taste

Adrenal Imbalance Menu
DAY FOUR

BREAKFAST

leftover Creamy Cheesy
Scramble*
Zucchini Cakes*

MORNING SNACK

Lemony Hummus* with ½ cup
sliced vegetables

LUNCH

½ cup diced baked or broiled
chicken with 1 ounce Feta
cheese on 2 cups mixed salad
greens with 1 teaspoon olive
oil and juice of ½ lemon
½ cup sliced strawberries with
1 tablespoon heavy cream,
sweeten with stevia to taste

AFTERNOON SNACK

Tropical Prosciutto Rolls*

DINNER

Rosemary Lamb*
Zucchini Ribbons*
½ sweet potato with
½ tablespoon butter, sprinkled
with cinnamon if desired

Adrenal Imbalance Menu
DAY FIVE

BREAKFAST

Cheeseless Artichoke Omelet*
½ cup cantaloupe

MORNING SNACK

1 small apple, sliced and
spread with 1 tablespoon
cashew butter

LUNCH

Best Ever Egg Drop Soup*
1 cup mixed salad greens with
½ cup sliced vegetables,
1 teaspoon olive oil,
and juice of ½ lemon
½ cup cantaloupe
½ cup unsweetened full-fat or
2% yogurt

AFTERNOON SNACK

2 Cheese Balls with Parsley*
½ cup sliced vegetables

DINNER

Salmon with Fresh Thyme*
½ cup braised kale
½ gluten-free roll

Adrenal Imbalance Menu
DAY SIX

BREAKFAST

2 scrambled eggs
2 slices nitrate-free bacon
½ cup sliced strawberries

MORNING SNACK

1 ounce string cheese
1 tablespoon almonds

LUNCH

Curried Chicken Salad* on
1 cup mixed salad greens

AFTERNOON SNACK

Avocado and Pear Dip*
with ½ cup sliced cucumber
or zucchini

DINNER

Stuffed Red Peppers*
1 cup steamed spinach
¼ cup blueberries with
1 tablespoon heavy cream,
sweeten with stevia to taste

Adrenal Imbalance Menu
DAY SEVEN

BREAKFAST

Spicy Fiesta Eggs*
½ cup sliced strawberries

MORNING SNACK

2 stalks celery, each topped
with ½ ounce cream cheese
and 2 sliced Kalamata olives

LUNCH

leftover Stuffed Red Peppers*
1 cup mixed salad greens
with 1 teaspoon olive oil
and juice of ½ lemon

AFTERNOON SNACK

Olive Tapenade* with ½ cup
sliced vegetables

DINNER

Greek Stuffed Chicken Breasts*
Spinach with Lemon
and Garlic*
¼ cup wild rice

Adrenal Imbalance Menu
DAY EIGHT

BREAKFAST

2 Salmon Cakes*
¼ cup blueberries

MORNING SNACK

1 hardboiled egg
½ cup cantaloupe

LUNCH

Curried Chicken Salad* on
1 cup mixed salad greens

AFTERNOON SNACK

2 Cheese Balls with Parsley*
½ cup sliced strawberries

DINNER

Caribbean Jerk Pork*
⅓ cup wild rice
2 cups mixed salad greens
with 1 teaspoon olive oil
and juice of ½ lemon

Adrenal Imbalance Menu
DAY NINE

BREAKFAST

½ cup cottage cheese
2 Homemade Turkey Patties*
½ cup blueberries

MORNING SNACK

½ cup cantaloupe
1 ounce string cheese

LUNCH

leftover Caribbean Jerk Pork*
⅓ cup wild rice

AFTERNOON SNACK

1 small apple, sliced and
spread with 1 tablespoon
cashew butter

DINNER

Marinated Sicilian Steak*
⅓ cup wild rice
Sautéed Green Beans*

Adrenal Imbalance Menu
DAY TEN

BREAKFAST

Ricotta and Leek Frittata*
½ cup cantaloupe

MORNING SNACK

½ baked pear sprinkled with
cinnamon or nutmeg and
1 tablespoon crushed pecans

LUNCH

leftover Marinated Sicilian
Steak* on 2 cups mixed
salad greens
½ cup sliced strawberries

AFTERNOON SNACK

2 stalks celery, each stuffed
with 1 tablespoon Lemony
Hummus*

DINNER

Lemon Chicken*
⅓ cup wild rice
½ cup steamed broccoli with
½ tablespoon butter

Adrenal Imbalance Menu
DAY ELEVEN

BREAKFAST

Crab and Swiss Pie*
½ cup blueberries

MORNING SNACK

2 Cheese Balls with Parsley*
1 unsweetened rice cake or
4 rice crackers

LUNCH

leftover Lemon Chicken*
Asparagus with a Zing*
⅓ cup wild rice

AFTERNOON SNACK

1 ounce string cheese
1 tablespoon pecans

DINNER

Sizzling Shrimp Scampi*
¼ cup wild rice
1 cup mixed salad greens
with 1 teaspoon olive oil and
balsamic vinegar
½ cup sliced strawberries

Adrenal Imbalance Menu
DAY TWELVE

BREAKFAST

2 eggs, any style
½ cup cantaloupe
2 Homemade Turkey Patties*

MORNING SNACK

½ nectarine stuffed with
2 tablespoons ricotta cheese
and sprinkled with cinnamon
or nutmeg

LUNCH

2 cups Romaine lettuce with
Creamy Parmesan Dressing*
topped with
grilled or broiled steak
½ cup sliced strawberries

AFTERNOON SNACK

Avocado and Pear Dip*
with ½ cup sliced cucumber
or zucchini

DINNER

Orange Chicken Stir Fry*
½ cup steamed broccoli
¼ cup wild rice

Adrenal Imbalance Menu
DAY THIRTEEN

BREAKFAST

2 eggs, any style
Zucchini Cakes*
⅓ cup blueberries

MORNING SNACK

2 unsweetened rice cakes or 8
rice crackers spread with
1 tablespoon cashew butter

LUNCH

2 cups mixed salad greens
with Creamy Parmesan
Dressing* topped with baked
or broiled chicken and 1 ounce
shredded cheddar cheese
½ cup sliced strawberries

AFTERNOON SNACK

Tropical Prosciutto Rolls*

DINNER

Salmon with Dilled Butter*
½ cup steamed green beans
½ sweet potato with
½ tablespoon butter, sprinkled
with cinnamon if desired

Adrenal Imbalance Menu
DAY FOURTEEN

BREAKFAST

Pepper and Onion
Breakfast Omelet*
⅓ cup cantaloupe

MORNING SNACK

Avocado and Pear Dip*
with ½ cup sliced cucumber
or zucchini

LUNCH

Not Your Mom's Chicken
Salad* on 1 cup mixed
salad greens

AFTERNOON SNACK

1 unsweetened rice cake or 4
rice crackers spread with
1 tablespoon almond butter

DINNER

Spicy Crunchy Chicken*
Spinach with Lemon
and Garlic*

Adrenal Imbalance FAQ

I know you say take it easy–but I'm busy!
Who's going to do what needs to get done?

For the next two weeks, think of yourself as a patient and heal yourself. If you had the flu, you'd rearrange whatever you could to allow yourself time to recover, wouldn't you? Well, adrenal fatigue should be no different. You need to quiet both the outer and inner—as well as your past and present—stressors and take the time to figure out what's eating you. Learn to say no. This is the only real way to break the cycle of stress that's keeping your body on defense so you can't lose weight. If you don't decide to take this time to heal your adrenals, they may do the deciding for you later on. It's time to really shift gears and recoup your losses—that way you'll have abundant health and energy for the rest of your life.

I've never heard about the adrenals–and my healthcare
practitioner doesn't think they're that important.

Western medicine is taking its time recognizing the importance of adrenal health—but Eastern cultures have always given the adrenals their due. Here, the standard adrenal function test, the ACTH challenge, shows only the most acute adrenal-related conditions—Addison's disease and Cushing's syndrome—which are not exceedingly common. However, more sensitive testing will show a trend toward one end of the spectrum that, though not an illness, may point to a vulnerability. My goal is to have you intervene with diet, supplements, and good habits before things get more serious.

I'm not losing weight as quickly as I would like on this plan.

Continue diligently for the full two weeks and really try to rest as much as you can. If you aren't feeling a shift in weight but you have more energy, know that the plan is working; it's just taking more time! You should also be sure to have your thyroid levels checked—many women need to heal both the thyroid and the adrenals simultaneously. Alternatively, go back to the Core Balance Quiz and look at your other scores. You may be dealing with overlapping issues. Consider getting adrenal testing for more precise results.

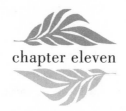

chapter eleven

THE NEUROTRANSMITTER IMBALANCE CUSTOM PLAN

If you scored highest on Neurotransmitter Imbalance in my quiz, there's a good chance that your brain chemistry is making it hard for you to lose weight. Neurotransmitters are brain chemicals that affect our appetite and how we think and feel, but they impact—and are impacted by—so much more. Like hormones, they operate throughout the body and are interconnected with other physiological systems via the hypothalamus. (Neurotransmitters are hormones by another name, in other words: chemical messengers, only they operate between neurons in your nervous system.) So the systems activated by your hormones are also impacted by neurotransmitter levels—including appetite, immunity, digestion, and elimination—and vice versa. Healing a neurotransmitter imbalance restores health to the mind and the body at once.

A User's Guide to Brain Chemistry

Neurotransmitters are chemical messengers made from amino acids that travel the central nervous system and carry impulses between nerve cells. These impulses orchestrate many functions, including but not limited to mood, sleep, appetite, cognitive processes, and responses to hot, cold, and pain—in fact, almost everything that influences your behavior. Neurotransmitters have either an "excitatory" effect or an "inhibitory" effect on the organs of the central nervous system (most important, the brain!) and dance together in a give-and-take that tries to keep your nervous system stable.

If you are feeling agitated, shaky, and hyperalert, as though your nerves are frayed, that's a symptom of a neurotransmitter balance tipped toward the "excitatory" end of the scale. Normally, this agitation will trigger the release of an inhibitory neurotransmitter that will calm you down. If your body can't access enough of the calming agent internally, you'll often find yourself on a hunt for an outside source—such as a glass of wine. In this way, the state of your neurotransmitters impacts how you feel and what you do minute by minute—an important connection to make when you're trying to lose weight. Many natural and synthetic chemicals in our diet facilitate, block, and/or mimic the action of neurotransmitters in the body (like sugar, nicotine, and MSG), making the state of your neurotransmitters extremely vulnerable to nutrition and lifestyle choices.

The Weight-Loss Transmitters

We know of more than 50 chemical compounds that function as neurotransmitters, including peptides, nitrous oxide, and cytokines. Their interplay is vastly complex and very individual. But in my experience, most women struggling with a neurotransmitter imbalance and stubborn weight are dealing with the following neurotransmitters:

- Serotonin: The "up with life" neurotransmitter. It makes you feel good; it's also the chemical targeted by most antidepressants. Serotonin rises and dips with blood sugar levels.

- Dopamine: Another "up" neurotransmitter involved in attention, anxiety, pleasure seeking, and reward. Imbalances are linked with ADHD (attention deficit hyperactivity disorder) and addictions. Caffeine stimulates the release of dopamine.

- GABA (gamma-aminobutyric acid): The anesthetizing neurotransmitter—a major brain inhibitor. It slows locomotion and reflexes and dulls inhibition and pain. Drinking alcohol raises GABA levels.

- Glutamate: An excitatory neurotransmitter connected with memory, learning, pain perception, and pain amplification. It has been linked with mood swings, mania, anxiety, chronic pain, and depression. Heavy metal toxicity (specifically mercury), recreational drugs (such as Ecstasy and PCP), and overuse of MSG impact glutamate production. Chronic overstimulation of glutamate may raise your risk of stroke.

- Norepinephrine: A neurotransmitter triggered by the release of adrenaline in the fight-or-flight response. It suppresses appetite and immunity to free up more energy for the fray.

These neurotransmitters all communicate with your hunger hormones via the hypothalamus. When balanced, they go a long way in maintaining regular appetite and helping your body feel safe enough to let go of stubborn weight.

Neurotransmitters are synthesized in the body from amino acids and nutrients found in food from an age-old recipe dictated by your DNA. Some women may have inherited a wrench in the works (called a genetic polymorphism) that makes it difficult for them to synthesize or metabolize enough of a certain neurotransmitter. This is why certain mood disorders, like clinical depression, are believed to run in families. However, as I've said before, DNA is not destiny. And nowhere does this seem to be more true than in the production and supply of neurotransmitters: we synthesize more of them each day, depending on what we eat and how we act. In fact, neurotransmitters are controlled by what we eat and how we process feelings and associations. One good example of this is the "happy" neurotransmitter serotonin, which rises when we experience joy. It is also influenced by something I call the "carb effect."

Carbohydrates, generally speaking, contain a good amount of the amino acid L-tryptophan, which is a precursor to serotonin. When we eat foods high in tryptophan, it increases serotonin and makes us feel calm, sleepy, and content—briefly. (Turkey is high in tryptophan, which is why you feel drowsy after a Thanksgiving turkey feast.) And this effect is doubled if we wash everything down with a glass of wine or beer. After the initial sugar rush, the alcohol initiates higher levels of GABA, which acts as a sedative. High-protein foods (those that don't contain a lot of tryptophan like turkey) promote the production of dopamine and norepinephrine, which have the opposite, stimulating effect. Weight-loss drugs and stimulants operate on this mechanism: They raise levels of the neurotransmitters involved in the fight-or-flight response (adrenaline, dopamine, and norepinephrine), resulting in a loss of appetite—for as long as you take the pills. The soothing, happy-making effect of eating carbohydrates is one of the reasons it is so difficult to sustain a high-protein, low-carb diet for a long time—it tends to make us crabby!

Food and Feelings

When you feel stressed, physically or emotionally, your body releases the hormone cortisol, which is the major hormone responsible for a neurotransmitter imbalance. A surge in cortisol is always accompanied by some degree of the fight-or-flight stress response, followed by a surge in serotonin and the hormone insulin—and then a drop in both a few hours later.[1] Women with neurotransmitter imbalance who suffer from

165

fatigue and cravings for carbohydrates in the late afternoon are probably on the high-cortisol-low-serotonin roller coaster: low serotonin causes food cravings, especially in the late afternoon, which precipitates a carb binge, which leads to an evening crash. I often hear these women say that they can be "good" all day when it comes to eating well, only to come home and lose control—they just can't stop eating carbs. In effect, they are trying to self-modulate their neurotransmitter imbalances with an excess of simple carbs. Now, eating a ton of carbs in the evening is not a reason to punish yourself (remember, neurotransmitters are also influenced by thoughts!), but it is keeping you from shedding toxic weight and rebalancing your core.

When your neurotransmitters are balanced, your brain and your belly—and your fat cells—are communicating well: you feel energetic, content, and stable. When they're not, you're in for this kind of roller-coaster ride, with surges of "highs" followed by precipitous crashes, marked by mood dips and intense food cravings. This is the same mechanism on which recreational drugs work—so if you feel as if you are addicted to carbs or caffeine, you may not be far from the truth! Because your hypothalamus is part of your limbic brain, the part that stores memory and triggers emotional reactions, hunger is intricately woven into the fabric of your emotions with the help of neurotransmitters.

One important—but often overlooked—factor in neurotransmitter balance is the effect of personal, family, and social pressures on what, when, and how we eat. These factors can create a powerful emotional eating pattern that is imbalanced on its own. Partly because of this, many of us come to our plates with deep-seated emotional attachments to food that have little to do with what our bodies actually need to thrive. Consciously or unconsciously, these emotions influence what we eat and thereby influence the nutrients available to manufacture neurotransmitters. This can very quickly become a vicious cycle.

For instance, let's say you are given a sweet treat whenever you fall and hurt yourself or have a bad day. Your brain begins to associate pain with a sugar hit. As you get older, whenever you feel pain, you crave the sugar hit and the chain of biochemical reactions sparked by consuming it—even if those biochemical reactions are abnormal and unhealthy. As you feed your pain with sugar, often to the exclusion of other, more nutritious foods, your body becomes nutritionally stressed and begins to compensate by putting on weight. The extra weight makes you feel bad about yourself, which creates more pain and more stress. What a rut! And let's not forget about deprivation, which is often at work in anorexia nervosa. Depriving yourself can be a powerful motivator, too (and of course starvation comes with its own set of biochemical reactions that can become addicting). Self-deprivation is a great way to feel as if you have control and to exert control over other people. For some women, depriving themselves of food feels very virtuous while it lasts, but often ends in binge eating.

In my experience, most women who struggle with emotional eating actually "hunger" for a deeper sustenance. They fill that psychological yearning with food. At my practice I call this your emotional black box; other practitioners call it your soul-shaped hole. Recognizing that you have one and that no amount of food will fill it is a great first step to dealing with your emotions and food. But it's important to remember that emotional and compulsive eating often has undiagnosed physical underpinnings that need to be healed before you can tackle the emotional work.[2] Hormonal and neurotransmitter imbalances can spark insatiable cravings that contribute to overeating. Food allergies are sometimes the root of food addiction: we crave the food we are allergic to because we've grown used to the abnormal biochemical state that the food produces or we crave the food to fill a deficiency. In my clinical experience, women with a neurotransmitter imbalance have psychological symptoms, to be sure, such as depression and anxiety, but they also have definite physical symptoms—namely, insatiable cravings, inflammation, violent mood and energy swings, food addictions, and, of course, toxic weight gain. For most women, once we clear up the neurotransmitter imbalance, these symptoms start to diminish and maintaining an optimal weight becomes so much easier.

Take my patient Julie, for example. She's a busy physician and a 46-year-old mother of two small children who first came in complaining of anxiety, PMS, and significant depression. She was also struggling unsuccessfully to lose about 15 pounds left over from her pregnancies. Julie had a demanding job and admitted to me that her life "was not going well." All of her conventional tests were normal, so we had Julie take a neurotransmitter test and found that her serotonin was severely depleted and her dopamine was elevated. We also discovered that her adrenals were suffering and needed support. Our first step was to start Julie on the Core Balance Neurotransmitter Custom Plan; we helped her body begin to heal by removing caffeine, sugar, gluten, and wheat from her diet; and we added a few targeted nutrients to support Julie's body's ability to replenish her neurotransmitters and hormones naturally.

On the lifestyle front, Julie vowed to start putting more limits on her practice and to take more time for herself. I also recommended more exercise, at least three times per week, intense enough to break a sweat and get her endorphins going. Julie entered psychotherapy and carved out time to exercise regularly. She was strict with herself about meals and sleep, and she reduced some of her work demands. Within a month, Julie reported a huge shift in her mood and energy levels and began losing weight. She felt inspired to stay with her clean diet and lifestyle changes and continued on neurotransmitter supplemental support. Now, six months later, she feels that her life is back on track. She's lost all the weight, her mood is great, and she has all the resilience and energy she needs to take care of her kids and her medical practice. But best of all, Julie is back in control and happy with her life.

Julie's depression and neurotransmitter imbalance was on the low end of the scale. If you have a diagnosed clinical biochemical imbalance—such as clinical depression or post-traumatic stress disorder—it may take more work (with help from a team of trusted health-care practitioners and therapists, I hope). However, following my Neurotransmitter Imbalance Plan is a great place to begin.

Are You Depressed?

Depression includes a range of normal negative emotions and often manifests physically in symptoms that won't respond to treatment, including but not limited to weight gain, chronic pain, and digestion disorders. But clinical depression differs significantly from minor or situational depression or mood disorders, even though the symptoms can be the same. How can you tell which you have?

The difference is that in mild depression the symptoms ebb and flow and eventually lift, while in major depression they spiral down into a full-blown mental health crisis. Patients often describe the sense that they are on the edge of, or slipping into, a deep, dark hole. If you've been feeling any of the following symptoms consistently for over a month, you should immediately seek medical advice, preferably from a trained psychiatrist, psychologist, or social worker.

- Overwhelming, persistent feelings of grief, anxiety, guilt, or despair
- A sense of numbness or hollowness
- Feelings of hopelessness
- A loss of interest or pleasure in activities that you once enjoyed, including sex
- Dullness
- Decreased energy
- Difficulty concentrating or making decisions
- Disrupted sleep patterns
- Loss of appetite
- Suicidal thoughts or attempts and obsessing about death—these are serious warning signs that need to be addressed immediately

If this sounds like you, please don't worry. You can get better. Depression is a physical and mental condition that responds very well to treatment, both conventional and integrative. The most important thing is to get some help.

Having a steady and reliable supply of neurotransmitters is so important to your long-term psychological and physical well-being that the body is naturally inclined to make more quite easily—given the right nutritional support. Women with neurotransmitter imbalance often see significant improvement after just a few days of following this plan. As you move through the next two weeks, you'll find that you are sleeping better, feeling more grounded and content, losing weight, and—more important—feeling more resourceful. You may also find that lesser imbalances will begin to heal once you get your biochemistry back on the right track. So let's not wait a minute more!

The Neurotransmitter Imbalance Eating and Action Plan

The biggest challenge for those with a neurotransmitter imbalance is going to be managing your carbohydrates so that you eat enough, but not too much, which could destabilize your blood sugar. The following menu is geared to deliver you the perfect combination of nutrients, designed to help smooth out the highs and lows of a neurotransmitter imbalance while boosting the availability of important precursors and nutrients of certain neurotransmitters, namely serotonin, dopamine, and GABA. Many women who struggle with this imbalance tend to be slightly addicted to carbohydrates, which makes going without them even for a meal a very stressful proposition. If this sounds familiar, take heart. You will be eating plenty of complex carbohydrates, especially toward the end of the day. This will encourage your body to synthesize more serotonin while you sleep.

One cardinal rule of this eating plan is that you must eat a high-protein breakfast, lunch, and snacks. This will keep you from bingeing and stabilize your energies throughout the afternoon. It will also help if you try to skip the morning caffeine jolt, as caffeine really takes your neurotransmitters on a joy ride—and then straight into a burnout. Continue to exercise as you have been the past couple of weeks, going outside in daylight as much as possible. If you have ever suffered from SAD (Seasonal Affective Disorder) you know that sunlight is directly connected to mood (scientists believe it relates to the body's melatonin production), and exercise triggers the release of bliss-inducing endorphins.

It's important not to skip meals or supplements on this plan. Remember that neurotransmitters are synthesized from nutrients and controlled by them, so make it your job to have plenty available. Another important task is to get a full night's sleep each and every night. Your body makes neurotransmitters at night while you sleep, so give it plenty of time and rest. Think of your neurotransmitters as water from a well—over the next two weeks you will learn how to keep the level high enough to fill as many buckets as your emotional and physical well-being require.

Marcelle's Prescription for
NEUROTRANSMITTER IMBALANCE

If you are currently under acute emotional stress, be kind to yourself. Go slowly!

1. Follow the menu plan beginning on page 174.

2. Take your supplements as directed.

3. Schedule an appointment for talk therapy, if warranted.

4. Sleep eight hours per night.

5. Eat breakfast within 90 minutes of waking.

6. Do not eat after 7 p.m.

7. Make a list of your top ten favorite things to do and clear at least half an hour a day to do one.

8. Get outside in the sunshine as often as you can.

9. If you are currently exercising, continue with a goal of at least 30 to 60 minutes of physical activity five times a week. Or walk at least 30 minutes every day if you aren't currently exercising. More vigorous exercise is better—break a sweat and get those endorphins pumping!

10. Drink plenty of water and herbal tea between meals, especially if you feel a craving. Often our hunger and thirst controls can become confused.

11. Tune in to your hunger levels (see page 172). Are you eating because you are hungry or because your "black box" is calling to you? Read Stage IV and begin to practice some of my tips for emotional freedom.

12. If following the menu causes you too much stress or anxiety, back off for a few days and simply try to take your supplements, read Stage IV, and get plenty of rest. You can try again when you feel calmer.

13. Schedule diagnostic tests if you are not feeling an improvement within two weeks.

Diagnostic Testing for Neurotransmitter Imbalance

- ALCAT test for food sensitivities and allergies

- Adrenal Stress Index to measure cortisol levels throughout the day

- Complete Blood Count (CBC with differential) to test for anemia, infection, or other blood disorders

- Comprehensive Digestive Stool Analysis (CDSA) to test digestion and absorption and bacterial balance

- Comprehensive Metabolic Profile (CMP) to test for amino acid deficiency

- Comprehensive Parasitology 2 (CP x 2) to identify abnormal intestinal microflora

- Neurotransmitter test (this is unconventional, but can give a good overview)

- Epstein Barr/Lyme disease test (to rule out Epstein-Barr virus and Lyme disease)

- Thyroid tests: TSH, free T3, T4, and thyroid antibodies

- Vitamin D level (very important!)

Foods to Include for Neurotransmitter Imbalance

- Dairy (unless you're allergic or sensitive to it), full fat or 2%
- Lean protein
- Leafy greens, rich in vitamin Bs
- Nuts
- Fruits
- Sweet potatoes (especially at night)
- Gluten-free whole grains (especially at night)

Foods to Avoid for Neurotransmitter Imbalance

- Alcohol
- Caffeine
- Chocolate and candy
- Diet soda
- Gluten and grains—wheat, barley, spelt, kamut, rye, triticale
- Sugars, syrups, honeys
- All artificial sweeteners, additives, preservatives, and colorings
- Refined grains
- Junk food and fast food
- MSG

Supplements for Neurotransmitter Imbalance

Basic:

- High-potency daily multivitamin with additional calcium and magnesium

- Essential fatty acids

- Probiotic (take 5 to 15 minutes before each meal with water)

- 5-HTP (a natural precursor to serotonin), from 100 to 400 mgs; if you are on an antidepressant, start with lowest dose and increase with caution

- A daily amino acid support supplement

Additional (if feelings of anxiety, depression, compulsiveness, or irritability persist):

- Tyrosine for GABA support (as directed by a health-care practitioner)
- Specific amino acid support as warranted by neurotransmitter tests

The powerful herb St. John's wort works as a serotonin uptake inhibitor antidepressant, which can really help a serotonin imbalance. However, if you are already on an antidepressant, you need to talk to your health-care provider about using any additional herbs and supplements. Depending on your medication, certain substances may be contraindicated. St John's wort is counterindicated if you are on an antidepressant.[3] 5-HTP can be used if you are on an antidepressant, but check first with a functional medical practitioner.

The Hunger Scale

Why do we eat when we aren't really hungry? Much of it comes down to cell conditioning—we simply get used to eating at certain times (like when we're watching TV). We also eat to fill our black box, even if what we are truly hungry for isn't food. For the next two weeks, use the following scale to rate your hunger and try to eat only when you're in the 3 to 4 range. Eat slowly and stop when you're around 6.

1. Absolutely ravenous, about to faint
2. Politely starving (you would let someone ahead of you in the buffet line)
3. Stomach is rumbling, haven't eaten in 3 hours
4. Hungry but not starving
5. Peckish
6. Content
7. Getting full
8. Full
9. Waistline feels tight
10. Absolutely stuffed—have to unbuckle your belt!

A Day in the Life of the
Neurotransmitter Imbalance Custom Plan

Time	Activity
6:30-7:00 A.M.	Wake up slowly. Breathe into your belly deeply. Don't get out of bed until you feel fully awake and calm. Stand by the window (if possible) and drink in the light. This will signal your hypothalamus to increase production of cortisol and adrenaline to get you on your way. Exercise early if it works best for you.
7:00-7:30	Self-care ritual. Drink water.
7:30	Take probiotic, make breakfast. Sit down to eat and chew slowly. Don't read while you eat, but focus on each mouthful.
8:00	Bathe, dress, pamper yourself and your body by thinking positively. Set a kind intention toward yourself today.
9:00	Work, household chores, duties, and so on. Try not to multitask.
10:00	Snack.
12:00 P.M.	Lunch. Walk 20 minutes if possible.
2:00	Tea break.
3:00	Snack.
5:00	Walk or exercise vigorously if you haven't done so previously. Lift weights. My optimal recommendation is five times per week. Make it fun. Go out and play!
6:00	Make and eat dinner. Light candles, listen to music that you like. Invite relaxation and joy to supper.
7:00	Connect with loved ones. Keep electronics and stimulation to a minimum. Journal your day's triumphs and refer back to your intention. Were you loving to yourself today?
9:00	Practice deep breathing. Drink a cup of sleep-inducing herbal tea, such as chamomile or lemon balm. Dim lights.
9:30	Sleep.

The Core Balance Menu Plan for Neurotransmitter Imbalance

* Recipes start on page 259.

Neurotransmitter Imbalance Menu

DAY ONE

BREAKFAST

Cheeseless Artichoke Omelet*
½ cup sliced strawberries

MORNING SNACK

Tropical Prosciutto Rolls*

LUNCH

baked or broiled chicken
breast, salt and pepper to taste
Green Beans with
Walnuts and Garlic*
½ cup blueberries with 1
tablespoon heavy cream,
sweetened with stevia to taste

AFTERNOON SNACK

½ pear spread with
1 tablespoon cashew butter

DINNER

Cashew Cilantro Chicken*
½ cup steamed broccoli
½ cup wild rice
½ cup raspberries

Neurotransmitter Imbalance Menu

DAY TWO

BREAKFAST

½ cup cottage cheese
Zucchini Cakes*
⅓ cup blueberries

MORNING SNACK

½ nectarine stuffed with
2 tablespoons ricotta cheese
and sprinkled with cinnamon
or nutmeg

LUNCH

Not Your Everyday Egg Salad*
on 1 cup mixed salad greens
½ cup cantaloupe

AFTERNOON SNACK

Avocado and Pear Dip*
with ½ cup sliced cucumber
or zucchini

DINNER

Stuffed Red Peppers*
Spinach with Lemon
and Garlic*
¼ cup raspberries with
1 tablespoon heavy cream,
sweeten with stevia to taste

Neurotransmitter Imbalance Menu

DAY THREE

BREAKFAST

2 scrambled eggs
2 Homemade Turkey Patties*
½ cup blueberries

MORNING SNACK

1 ounce string cheese
1 tablespoon almonds

LUNCH

leftover Stuffed Red Peppers*
½ cup raspberries

AFTERNOON SNACK

½ pear spread with
1 tablespoon cashew butter

DINNER

grilled or broiled steak
Vegetable Confetti*
½ sweet potato with
½ tablespoon butter, sprinkled
with cinnamon if desired

Neurotransmitter Imbalance Menu

DAY FOUR

BREAKFAST

2 Salmon Cakes*
½ cup sliced strawberries

MORNING SNACK

Tropical Prosciutto Rolls*

LUNCH

Curried Chicken Salad* on
1 cup mixed salad greens
½ cup raspberries

AFTERNOON SNACK

Lemony Hummus* with ½ cup
sliced vegetables

DINNER

Orange Chicken Stir Fry*
½ cup steamed green beans
½ cup brown rice

Neurotransmitter Imbalance Menu

DAY FIVE

BREAKFAST

Spicy Fiesta Eggs*
1 Zucchini Cake*
½ cup blueberries with
1 tablespoon heavy cream,
sweeten with stevia to taste

MORNING SNACK

Olive Tapenade* with ½ cup
sliced vegetables

LUNCH

grilled or broiled hamburger
Asparagus Soup*
½ gluten-free roll
½ cup cantaloupe

AFTERNOON SNACK

2 unsweetened rice cakes or
8 rice crackers spread with
1 tablespoon almond butter

DINNER

Creole Fish*
½ cup steamed broccoli
½ cup brown rice
½ cup raspberries

Neurotransmitter Imbalance Menu
DAY SIX

BREAKFAST

½ cup unsweetened full-fat or
2% yogurt
Zucchini Cakes*
½ cup raspberries

MORNING SNACK

½ nectarine stuffed with
2 tablespoons ricotta cheese
and sprinkled with cinnamon
or nutmeg

LUNCH

Spinach Salad*
½ millet roll

AFTERNOON SNACK

¾ cup blueberries
1 ounce string cheese

DINNER

Pork Chop Medley*
½ cup wild rice
½ cup sliced strawberries

Neurotransmitter Imbalance Menu
DAY SEVEN

BREAKFAST

Spinach Quiche*
½ cup cantaloupe

MORNING SNACK

½ cup cantaloupe
1 ounce string cheese

LUNCH

2 Salmon Cakes*
2 cups mixed salad greens
with 1 teaspoon olive oil
and juice of ½ lemon
½ cup blueberries

AFTERNOON SNACK

1 small apple
1 unsweetened rice cake or 4
rice crackers spread with
1 tablespoon cashew butter

DINNER

baked or broiled chicken breast
topped with Festive
Black Bean Salsa*
½ cup wild rice

Neurotransmitter Imbalance Menu
DAY EIGHT

BREAKFAST

½ cup cottage cheese
1 small apple
1 unsweetened rice cake or
4 rice crackers spread with
1 tablespoon cashew butter

MORNING SNACK

Avocado and Pear Dip*
with ½ cup sliced cucumber
or zucchini

LUNCH

leftover baked or broiled
chicken and Festive
Black Bean Salsa*
½ cup cantaloupe

AFTERNOON SNACK

2 stalks celery, each stuffed
with 1 tablespoon Lemony
Hummus*

DINNER

Snappy One Skillet
Turkey Dinner*
¼ cup wild rice
½ cup sliced strawberries

Neurotransmitter Imbalance Menu
DAY NINE

BREAKFAST
2 eggs, any style
2 Homemade Turkey Patties*
½ cup blueberries

MORNING SNACK
Tropical Prosciutto Rolls*

LUNCH
leftover Snappy One Skillet
Turkey Dinner*
¼ cup wild rice

AFTERNOON SNACK
½ pear spread with
1 tablespoon cashew butter

DINNER
Chicken Cacciatore*
½ cup brown rice
½ cup raspberries

Neurotransmitter Imbalance Menu
DAY TEN

BREAKFAST
Crab and Swiss Pie*
½ cup sliced strawberries

MORNING SNACK
Guacamole* with ½ cup sliced
vegetables

LUNCH
2 cups Romaine lettuce with
Creamy Parmesan Dressing*
topped with grilled or
broiled steak
½ cup cantaloupe

AFTERNOON SNACK
1 small baked apple sprinkled
with cinnamon and
2 tablespoons crushed pecans
1 rice cake or 4 rice crackers

DINNER
Glazed Lamb Chops*
¼ cup wild rice
Spinach with Lemon
and Garlic*
¼ cup blueberries with
1 tablespoon heavy cream,
sweeten with stevia to taste

Neurotransmitter Imbalance Menu
DAY ELEVEN

BREAKFAST
½ cup unsweetened full-fat
or 2% yogurt
2 Homemade Turkey Patties*
½ cup blueberries

MORNING SNACK
1 ounce string cheese
1 tablespoon almonds

LUNCH
leftover Crab and Swiss Pie*
2 cups mixed salad greens
with 1 teaspoon olive oil
and juice of ½ lemon

AFTERNOON SNACK
Avocado and Pear Dip*
with ½ cup sliced cucumber
or zucchini

DINNER
Mediterranean Scallops*
¼ cup wild rice
Spinach with Lemon
and Garlic*
½ cup cantaloupe

Neurotransmitter Imbalance Menu
DAY TWELVE

BREAKFAST

Spinach Scramble*
2 slices nitrate-free bacon

MORNING SNACK

½ nectarine stuffed with
2 tablespoons ricotta cheese
and sprinkled with cinnamon
or nutmeg

LUNCH

Asparagus Soup*
½ gluten-free roll
⅓ cup unsweetened full-fat
or 2% yogurt
¼ cup raspberries

AFTERNOON SNACK

Lemony Hummus* with
½ cup sliced vegetables
1 rice cake or 4 rice crackers

DINNER

Salmon with Fresh Thyme*
Zucchini Ribbons*
½ sweet potato with
½ tablespoon butter, sprinkled
with cinnamon if desired
½ cup sliced strawberries

Neurotransmitter Imbalance Menu
DAY THIRTEEN

BREAKFAST

½ cup cottage cheese
2 Homemade Turkey Patties*
¼ cup blueberries

MORNING SNACK

Olive Tapenade* with ½ cup
sliced vegetables

LUNCH

Curried Chicken Salad* on
1 cup mixed salad greens
½ cup sliced strawberries

AFTERNOON SNACK

2 Cheese Balls with Parsley*
2 unsweetened rice cakes or
8 rice crackers

DINNER

Sweet Salsa Smothered Steak*
½ cup wild rice
½ cup steamed broccoli with
½ tablespoon butter

Neurotransmitter Imbalance Menu
DAY FOURTEEN

BREAKFAST

2 eggs, any style
2 slices nitrate-free bacon
½ cup blueberries with
1 tablespoon heavy cream,
sweetened with stevia to taste

MORNING SNACK

Guacamole* with ½ cup
sliced vegetables

LUNCH

leftover Sweet Salsa
Smothered Steak* on
1 cup mixed salad greens
½ cup sliced strawberries

AFTERNOON SNACK

½ nectarine stuffed with
2 tablespoons ricotta cheese
and sprinkled with cinnamon
or nutmeg

DINNER

Fillet of Fish Amandine*
⅓ cup wild rice
½ cup steamed green beans
with ½ tablespoon butter

Neurotransmitter Imbalance FAQ

I'm on antidepressant medication. Can I still do this plan?

Yes, but talk to your practitioner. Certain antidepressants may be contraindicated for use with herbs and serotonin precursor supplements. Begin the eating and action plan immediately and take your essential vitamins and probiotic. When you have your diagnostic tests done, discuss the use of other recommended supplements and emotional help, such as talk therapy. It's my hope that this plan will help you feel so much better over time that you no longer need antidepressants, or need only a reduced dose.

I think I'm addicted to carbs—will this plan break my addiction?

If you love carbohydrates, stop beating yourself up! It's only natural. Carbohydrates are brain fuel and they make us feel calm, full, and content. Who wouldn't like that? Instead of thinking you need to break your addiction, think about changing the kind of carbohydrates you eat—from simple to complex. This plan will certainly teach you how to incorporate plenty of good carbs into your diet—no cold turkey here. However, after two weeks of eating complex carbohydrates at the right time, you should be able to get off the craving-binge-crash cycle so common with neurotransmitter imbalance. This will put you—not the cookie jar—back in control. You may also have a sensitivity to gluten that is sabotaging your best efforts.

I'm not losing weight on this plan. What should I do?

Restoring balance takes time! Don't get discouraged if you aren't seeing significant weight loss this month, as long as you are feeling a shift for the better. Continue for the full two weeks as diligently as possible. If you haven't lost a lot of weight, but feel better, the plan is working. Continue for another two weeks, starting the menu again. If you don't feel significantly better, go back to the Core Balance Quiz and look at your scores again. You may be dealing with overlapping issues. Many women with neurotransmitter imbalance actually have undiagnosed food sensitivities or GI concerns, so be sure to follow up with your practitioner about your diagnostic tests.

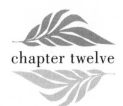

chapter twelve

THE INFLAMMATORY IMBALANCE CUSTOM PLAN

If you scored highest on Inflammatory Issues in my quiz, I'm fairly certain you are dealing with stubborn weight gain caused by inflammation that stems from an imbalanced or overtaxed immune system. And if you have inflammation and weight gain, chances are you are already insulin-resistant or well on your way.[1] (You can read more about insulin resistance on page 126, in the chapter on hormonal imbalance, if you haven't already.)

An inflammatory imbalance is like a fire in a hearth that hasn't been watched and is starting to burn down the house. It roars past its original boundaries in the body and, if we don't intervene, starts to fry all our major systems, including the endocrine, digestive, cardiovascular, respiratory, lymph, and central nervous systems. In time it can contribute to a whole host of conditions, some serious, from heart attack to ulcers to multiple sclerosis to cancer—as well as the accumulation of toxic weight. And it all starts with an overburdened immune system that's just trying to do its job.

The immune system is vastly complex—we don't have room to explain it fully here—but it is intricately connected with your body's ability to age well and maintain a well-functioning metabolism. In fact, it depends on it; your immunity is fueled by your metabolism and your metabolism is protected by your immunity. When it comes to chronic disease, where there's smoke, there's going to be fire: chronic inflammation is the beginning of a downward spiral that can lead to serious metabolic breakdown, with wide and deep ramifications for your long-term health. By healing your inflammation now, you're helping to ensure that you age with vitality and strength—and, of course, with a lean, fit body.

Inflammation in Action

Your immune system has one overarching goal: your survival. To this end, your body synthesizes compounds to moderate your immune response, either pro-inflammatory or anti-inflammatory, from the fatty acids in your blood. Over millennia, the immune system evolved to fight foreign invaders (called pathogens), to neutralize them, and to heal any damage incurred in the process. Pathogens run the gamut from dangerous viruses, bacteria, parasites, and lethal toxins to less harmful forms of bacteria, chemicals, and allergens.

A healthy immune system will spring into action and wipe out any threat. Once it has bested its opponent, it produces specific antibodies that will neutralize that same opponent if it ever comes near you again. (If your immune system didn't remember past skirmishes, your body would always be fighting the same battles over and over.) One of the ways we test for food allergies and sensitivities is to test for certain protein antibodies (called IgE and IgG, among others) that indicate that you have had an immune reaction to a particular food. You are constantly adding to your immune system's memory log, and your immune system is constantly comparing new proteins it encounters to data in that memory log. If you stumble across one that feels threatening, you'll have an inflammatory response.

You're probably familiar with the external signs that appear when inflammation is acute: an injured area gets red, swollen, and painful or itchy, and has you reaching for the ice bag. When the immune system is at work, it produces pro-inflammatory compounds, which create inflammation: prostaglandins, histamines, and proteins called cytokines. (One of these compounds, a cytokine secreted by the liver called C-reactive protein [CRP], is a valuable marker for inflammation; a highly sensitive blood test for CRP measures a patient's level of inflammation and risk of heart attack.[2] Scientists are in the process of discovering a relationship between "bad" or

Inflammation-Related Conditions
(To Name a Few)

- Abdominal obesity
- Arthritis/rheumatoid arthritis
- Asthma
- Physical injury
- Infections
- Allergies
- Autoimmune disorders
- Pulmonary disease
- Bronchitis
- Hypertension
- Cardiovascular disease
- Atherosclerosis
- Cancer
- Alzheimer's disease
- Acne
- Gout
- Eczema/psoriasis/dermatitis
- Gingivitis/periodontitis
- Conjunctivitis
- Gastritis
- Ulcers
- IBS
- Crohn's disease
- Colitis
- Diverticulitis
- Multiple sclerosis
- General obesity
- Diabetes

high LDL cholesterol and chronic inflammation. While the mechanism remains unclear, it's possible that excess LDL feeds inflamed arteries, coating the walls and hardening into plaque. Or it may be that inflammation is exacerbated by preexisting blockages. Either way, inflammation of the arterial wall creates high levels of CRP. Inflamed plaques are highly unstable and prone to rupture, which can then cause a blood clot and heart attack or stroke.

At the site of injury, pro-inflammatory compounds call for your white blood cells to come and clear out infection and damaged tissue. These agents are matched by closely related, equally powerful anti-inflammatory compounds, which move in once the threat is neutralized to soothe the area and begin the healing process. This kind of sporadic, short-lived inflammation balanced by healing is a great signal that your immune system is functioning well.

But when the immune system is out of balance and tipped to the pro-inflammatory side (which is often the case when you have inflammatory issues), you end up with chronic inflammation in the body. It's characterized by a host of physical symptoms, ranging from chronic head and joint pain to acne, arthritis, anxiety attacks, elevated cholesterol levels, high blood pressure—and, of course, the single most common symptom of chronic inflammation: weight gain, particularly the kind that seems to cement around the belly.[3] The link between belly fat and inflammation—which can put you at serious risk for cardiovascular disease—is so clear that if there is a difference of less than ten inches between your waist and your hips, you may want to get tested for an inflammatory condition called metabolic syndrome.

Metabolic Syndrome

Metabolic syndrome, also known as "syndrome X," is the term for a cluster of health-sapping conditions that are strongly associated with insulin resistance and weight gain. These conditions are abdominal obesity, high blood pressure, and elevated cholesterol. Metabolic syndrome is now considered to be a huge red flag for coronary heart disease and type II (adult onset) diabetes. It's also an inflammatory condition.

Fat, by its nature, is inflammatory. Fat cells produce their own pro-inflammatory message-carrying compounds, called adipocytokines, that, in excessive quantities, can seriously disrupt metabolic function.[4] The more fat cells you have, the more adipocytokines you have. And in most cases, the higher your levels of insulin, the more fat cells you accumulate. In this way, inflammation and excess insulin are like the chicken and the egg when it comes to making you vulnerable to metabolic syndrome. Which comes first? Do insulin resistance and obesity cause inflammation or the other way around? There's research to support both views. Time will tell, and it may come down to individual biochemistry. What we do know is that the best way to heal metabolic syndrome is to control insulin levels and cool down inflammation.

What causes chronic inflammation? Everyone has their own triggers, depending on individual biochemistry, but anything we consume or absorb, combined with emotional stress, has the capacity to ignite little flames throughout our bodies that overwork the immune system, occupying it on so many fronts that larger threats may go unnoticed until it's too late. Moreover, we tend to produce more pro-inflammatory compounds naturally as we age, which helps tip the balance. Pro- and anti-inflammatory compounds are synthesized from fatty acids in our blood, respectively, linoleic acid (which comes from omega-6 fats) and alpha-linoleic acid (which comes from omega-3s and omega-9s). We need both of these fatty acids to maintain balance, but our Western diet is too heavy on the pro-inflammatory side. It's also too heavy in animal protein, which raises levels of the pro-inflammatory compound homocysteine. Up to 25 percent of the population has a genetic polymorphism that results in an enzyme deficiency and may disable an individual's ability to convert folate to folic acid, even if she supplements.[5] This condition can lead to elevated homocysteine levels and predispose us to inflammatory issues, such as heart disease. For this reason, if you are having many inflammation-related symptoms that don't improve after a month on this Custom Plan, schedule your diagnostic tests. You may be one of these individuals.

Fuel to the Fire

Generally speaking, chronic inflammation—and the weight gain that goes with it—is fueled by all kinds of stress, internal and external.[6] I recently saw a patient, Maria, who first came to see me about three years ago, when she was 45 years old and 100 pounds overweight. I can tell you now that back then her health was a mess. She suffered chronic menstrual cramps, dysfunctional uterine bleeding, and high blood pressure, as well as many obesity-related ailments. The bleeding was making her miserable, so we decided to start there. But it was difficult to get her bleeding under control, and eventually, Maria agreed to have a hysterectomy. She followed up the surgery with hormone therapy, and we all waited for her to start feeling better. But she didn't. Her bleeding had stopped, but now she was experiencing chronic back pain, bloating, and joint pain, and her weight wasn't budging—all symptoms of underlying inflammation. We ran a number of tests, including the CDSA x 2, CP x 2, and a heavy metal test, and found an overgrowth of numerous strains of bacteria in her GI, including yeast. She also tested positive for parasites and heavy metals. The sum of all this stress had impaired Maria's immune system and she was highly inflamed, which can often be the case with obese patients.

I immediately recommended the Core Balance Inflammation Imbalance diet plan and added a medical food to support Maria's body's healing process. We wanted her to cool her inflammation and lose the weight, but we had to be careful not to mobilize too many toxins for her overburdened system to handle. This is where the medical food really helped bolster her defenses. We also treated Maria's parasites and dealt with the yeast overgrowth. When Maria was feeling well enough, we cleared her heavy metal toxicity with the help of a medical food to support detox, as well as a visit to a biodentist. (For more on biodentistry, see the Appendices.) It took us eight months to get rid of Maria's symptoms, but Maria was a champ—and in the meantime she lost all 100 pounds. Today, you would not recognize her as the same woman I saw three years ago. Back then she was almost bedridden, her skin was terrible, and she showed every inch of the misery she was feeling. Today she looks terrific and has renewed energy and a new attitude. And all that weight? It's been gone for a long time now and she's determined not to let it come back.

Figuring out what your triggers are can take some detective work, just like Maria's, but the best place to start is with your diet and the health of your GI tract. That's because your diet can be either pro-inflammatory (like the typical Western menu of lots of refined grains, sugar, animal protein, and saturated animal fat) or anti-inflammatory (rich in anti-oxidants, lean protein, and healthy fats). The GI tract is the gateway for many pathogens;

we ingest them along with our food. In many cases, certain foods are minor allergens—we just don't know it. The immune system permeates the gut by way of gut-associated lymph tissue, or GALT, creating a kind of weblike filter with the ability to sense even the smallest amount of a foreign substance and send out the alarm. (You can read more about GALT and digestive sensitivities in Chapter 8, if you haven't already.) People with core digestive imbalances such as undiagnosed food sensitivities, IBS, systemic yeast, parasites, dysbiosis, and leaky gut syndrome often suffer from chronic inflammation, as do women who have overly processed diets and difficulty detoxifying.

But let's not forget another inflammatory trigger: your emotions. With inflammation, painful emotional baggage can be as fiery as physical stress. The body can't differentiate between physical stress and psychological stress; it responds equally to both via the HPA axis with the release of cortisol. Cortisol tamps down your immune system, giving inflammation the upper hand; therefore, coping with persistent stress takes a steady toll on your immune system and puts your body on perpetual defense. Thoughts and feelings are very powerful, and they manifest themselves physically all the time with symptoms of inflammation: stress makes your skin break out or your intestines revolt during a painful breakup. Remember that some of your emotional responses may be programmed by early childhood experiences; we'll talk more about exploring these factors in Stage IV. The good news is that your feelings can—and should—be enlisted as your allies in the healing process.

The Inflammatory Issues Eating and Action Plan

The great news for those of you with inflammatory issues is that once you know your weight gain is linked to chronic inflammation, you can take real steps to cool everything down. Just like your sisters with digestive issues and hormonal imbalances, on this plan you'll focus on removing offensive substances, stabilizing glucose levels, and restoring support. In addition, you also need to be vigilant about taking your essential fatty acid supplements. Essential fatty acids help balance out the levels of pro- and anti-inflammatory fatty acids in your blood by upping levels of omega-3s. I also encourage you to schedule the diagnostic tests I recommend below. Because inflammation is linked to so many damaging health conditions, it would be very useful to know if you are dealing with a food sensitivity and/or insulin resistance as well. These overlapping issues can be challenging, but you will get off to a great start by following this plan for the next two weeks. I won't mislead you—this plan is quite restrictive, but trust me, it will make such a difference, so do your best to stick to it.

Many women with inflammatory issues tend to be easily agitated for one reason or another, and many feel emotionally stuck in patterns of anxiety and anger—the classic hair trigger. The challenge for you over the next two weeks will be keeping calm in the face of giving up certain foods and habits that feel comforting but aren't healthy. Don't worry—you will be able to experiment with all of these favorite foods again and instantly feel which ones don't work for you. (You'll read more on this when you've completed these two weeks.) It's my hope that you will learn when it's worth eating the wrong things and feeling bad and when it's not—a thought process that can only empower you and support your weight loss. So take a deep breath and know that you are in control of your choices and that they can change your life!

Marcelle's Prescription for
INFLAMMATORY ISSUES

1. Follow the menu starting on page 193.

2. Take supplements as directed.

3. Drink plenty of filtered water.

4. Floss daily after each meal. Inflammation of the gums has been linked to body-wide inflammation. Your mouth is the first entry point for many inflammatory bacteria.

5. Eat organic. Thoroughly wash all fruits and vegetables. Go through your cabinets and throw out processed food and don't buy any more! This includes products that contain sugar, refined flour, trans fats, artificial preservatives, colors, and sweeteners—all highly inflammatory.

6. Consider adding a gluten-free daily fiber supplement, such as psyllium husks, to your diet.

7. Walk whenever you can and consider inviting more exercise into your life. Exercising at least 30 to 60 minutes per day up to six times a week is optimal to help improve insulin levels and lower blood sugar.

8. Go out and play! Bring more joy and peace into your life. If you live with chronic stress, read Stage IV and consider exploring further stress-reduction techniques.

9. Get plenty of rest. You need to sleep between seven and nine hours a night to give your body time to heal from the previous day's demands. Schedule a regular bedtime and take plenty of naps.

10. Schedule diagnostic tests if you don't feel an improvement within two weeks.

Diagnostic Testing for Inflammatory Issues

- Ultra-sensitive C-reactive protein test and test for elevated levels of the irritating blood acid homocysteine

- ALCAT for food allergies and sensitivities

- Comprehensive Digestive Stool Analysis (CDSA) to test digestion and absorption and bacterial balance

- Standard Comprehensive Metabolic Profile (CMP) to test electrolytes, blood sugar, blood protein, pH level, and liver and kidney function

- Comprehensive Metabolic Profile to test for amino acid deficiency

- Comprehensive Parasitology 2 (CP x 2) to identify abnormal intestinal microflora

- Fasting blood sugar/fasting insulin and two-hour postprandial glucose/insulin to test for metabolic syndrome

- *H. pylori*: An antigen test for bacteria correlated with peptic and duodenal ulcers

- Vitamin D levels

- Thyroid tests: TSH, free T3, T4, and thyroid antibodies

- Celiac test for gluten sensitivity/allergy

- Blood lipid panel to measure HDL, LDL, and triglycerides

- Comprehensive genetic profile to test for genetic SNP leading to methylfolate metabolism defect

Foods to Include for Inflammatory Issues

- Alfalfa sprouts

- Apples/pears

- Avocado

- Beans and lentils, including peas

- Blueberries

- Cherries

- Cinnamon

- Cruciferous vegetables (bok choy, broccoli, cauliflower, cabbage, brussels sprouts, kale)

- Chile peppers

- Flax and sesame seeds

- Garlic

- Green leafy vegetables,

- Oats (gluten-free)

- Pomegranate

- Healthy oils: canola, olive, flaxseed, sesame, safflower, coconut, and nut oils

- Wild Alaskan salmon

- Yogurt/kefir (but no other dairy), full-fat or 2%

Foods to Avoid for Inflammatory Issues

- Alcohol

- Caffeine

- Dairy (except yogurt/kefir)

- Fried foods/fast food

- Gluten and grains—wheat, barley, spelt, kamut, rye, triticale

- Nightshades (tomatoes, potatoes, eggplant, onions)

- Red meat, unless grass-fed

- Refined sugar and grains

- Saturated fats

- Trans fats

- Artificial preservatives, dyes, additives

Supplements for Inflammatory Issues

Basic:

- High-potency multivitamin with additional calcium and magnesium

- Essential fatty acids

- Probiotic (take 5 to 15 minutes before meal with water)

- Glutamine (1000-mg tablets with each meal)

- Additional vitamin D supplement (as directed by test results; if you are vitamin D deficient, you may need up to 6000 mgs per day)

Add the following if symptoms persist:

- Full-spectrum digestive enzyme (if desired)

- Coenzyme Q10, a powerful antioxidant (100 mgs per day with food)

- Chromium (additional 100-mg tablet before meals, especially if you are insulin-resistant)

- Acetyl-L-Carnitine (500 mgs per day) to improve mitochondrial function and breakdown of fatty acids

- Additional fatty acid supplements to soothe inflammation, including gamma linoleic acid (GLA) from evening primrose (400 mgs), alpha linoleic acid (ALA) from flax or hemp (400 mgs)

Additional (for use under medical guidance; see Appendices for more information):

- Betaine HCl for low gastric acidity taken midmeal

- Medical food for support in healing inflammation and inflammation-related symptoms, such as joint pain. Discontinue use of other supplements, except EFA and probiotic, if using a medical food.

Vitamin D

This essential nutrient is called a vitamin, but vitamin D is actually a precursor hormone—the building block of a powerful steroid hormone in your body called calcitriol. Vitamin D works in concert with other nutrients and hormones in your body to support healthy bone renewal—the ongoing process of mineralization and demineralization that, when it goes awry, shows up as rickets in children and osteomalacia ("soft bones") in adults. Links have also been discovered between vitamin D deficiency and obesity, insulin resistance, heart disease, certain cancers, and depression. I test all of my patients and have been surprised to find that 85 percent come up with a vitamin D deficiency.

Researchers are discovering that vitamin D promotes normal cell growth and differentiation throughout the body, a key factor in stabilizing insulin, maintaining a healthy immune system, and losing weight. It might just be the secret diet ingredient in dairy products. Importantly for inflammatory issues, vitamin D is actually a potent anti-inflammatory with the ability to turn off a prolonged inflammatory response.[7]

Your body can't create vitamin D on its own. Instead, it's designed to make it through sun exposure—in theory, as little as a couple of hours per week in the sun. You can also ingest D through food, especially eggs and certain fish. But many people, especially those like me who live in northern climates, aren't getting enough. And those who live in southern latitudes are dutifully using their sunscreen, so they too may be deficient. I recommend upping your daily intake of vitamin D to 1000 mgs during the winter months, but always have your vitamin D levels tested—especially before you increase any supplement dosage. The best way to get vitamin D is as nature intended: during the summer, or if you live in a sunny area, you can bare your unscreened extremities to the sun for 15 minutes—enough to feel warm but not get burnt. Do this in the mornings and late afternoon, never at midday when the sun is highest.

A Day in the Life of the
Inflammatory Issues Custom Plan

Time	Activity
6:30 A.M.	Wake up gently. Lie in bed and take several deep belly breaths—at least ten. Set a positive intention for the day.
7:00	Make breakfast. Take multivitamin, probiotic, glutamine, EFA tablets, and additional supplements. If you are using medical food, follow your practitioner's guidelines instead.
7:15	Breakfast. Eat slowly and chew your food well. Take your time. If you are taking a digestive enzyme supplement, remember to take it mid-meal. Floss.
8:00	Walk to work or gentle stroll outdoors. If it is sunny, try to expose your extremities to the sun for 15 minutes to initiate the creation of vitamin D.
9:00	Drink two big glasses of water or a cleansing herbal tea (see page 65).
10:00	Snack.
12:00 P.M.	Lunch, take appropriate supplements. Give yourself time to digest. Practice deep breathing. Floss or use a toothpick.
2:00	Tea break.
3:00	Snack.
5:00	Exercise or walk. If you can, try to meditate or breathe deeply.
6:00	Dinner.
6:30	Self-care ritual.
7:00	Drink two more glasses of water or soothing herbal tea. Take calcium and magnesium supplements now to help you sleep. Relax. Floss.
9:00	Bedtime. Breathe deeply into the belly at least ten times, then let go of your day. It's done. Sleep.

The Core Balance Menu Plan for Inflammatory Imbalance

Snack Ideas:

- Rice cakes with cashew or almond butter
- Celery, red pepper, or cucumber sticks with hummus
- Boiled egg
- A handful of nuts
- A small piece of fruit
- Half a serving of previous day's entrée

* Recipes start on page 259.

Inflammatory Imbalance Menu

DAY ONE

BREAKFAST

2 eggs, any style
2 Homemade Turkey Patties*
½ cup sliced strawberries

MORNING SNACK

½ pear spread with
1 tablespoon cashew butter

LUNCH

baked or broiled chicken
breast, salt and pepper to taste
Spinach with Lemon
and Garlic*
½ millet roll

AFTERNOON SNACK

2 unsweetened rice cakes or 8
rice crackers spread with
1 tablespoon cashew butter

DINNER

Dilled Salmon*
Stir Fry Broccoli with Ginger*
¼ cup wild rice

Inflammatory Imbalance Menu

DAY TWO

BREAKFAST

Confetti Scramble*
½ cup raspberries

MORNING SNACK

1 small baked apple sprinkled
with cinnamon and
2 tablespoons crushed pecans

LUNCH

Easy Chicken Florentine*
2 cups mixed salad greens
with 1 teaspoon olive oil
and juice of ½ lemon

AFTERNOON SNACK

Avocado and Pear Dip*
with ½ cup sliced cucumber
or zucchini

DINNER

roast turkey breast
½ sweet potato with ½
tablespoon butter, sprinkled
with cinnamon if desired
Brussels Sprouts with
Mushrooms*

Inflammatory Imbalance Menu
DAY THREE

BREAKFAST

2 Salmon Cakes*
½ cup sliced strawberries

MORNING SNACK

Lemony Hummus* with ½ cup
sliced vegetables

LUNCH

Turkey Hash*
2 cups mixed salad greens
with 1 teaspoon olive oil
and juice of ½ lemon
½ gluten-free roll

AFTERNOON SNACK

1 hardboiled egg
¼ cup blueberries

DINNER

Chicken and Asparagus Sauté*
2 cups mixed salad greens
with 1 teaspoon olive oil
and juice of ½ lemon
Minty Cantaloupe Balls*

Inflammatory Imbalance Menu
DAY FOUR

BREAKFAST

2 eggs, any style
Zucchini Cakes*
½ cup sliced strawberries

MORNING SNACK

Lemony Hummus* with ½ cup
sliced vegetables

LUNCH

Sweet Arugula Salad
with Chicken*
½ millet roll

AFTERNOON SNACK

2 unsweetened rice cakes or
8 rice crackers spread with
1 tablespoon cashew butter

DINNER

Rosemary Lamb*
Zucchini Ribbons*
½ sweet potato with
½ tablespoon butter, sprinkled
with cinnamon if desired

Inflammatory Imbalance Menu
DAY FIVE

BREAKFAST

Cheeseless Artichoke Omelet*
½ cup cantaloupe

MORNING SNACK

Guacamole* with ½ cup
sliced vegetables

LUNCH

Chicken and Asparagus Sauté*
1 cup mixed salad greens with
1 teaspoon olive oil
and balsamic vinegar
½ millet roll

AFTERNOON SNACK

1 small apple, sliced and
spread with 1 tablespoon
cashew butter

DINNER

Turkey Frittata*
1 cup mixed salad greens
with 1 teaspoon olive oil
and balsamic vinegar
½ cup steamed broccoli

Inflammatory Imbalance Menu
DAY SIX

BREAKFAST
Spinach Scramble*
½ cup raspberries

MORNING SNACK
½ pear spread with
1 tablespoon cashew butter
1 tablespoon almonds

LUNCH
leftover Turkey Frittata*
2 cups mixed salad greens
with 1 teaspoon olive oil
and juice of ½ lemon

AFTERNOON SNACK
Olive Tapenade* with ½ cup
sliced vegetables

DINNER
Sherry Chicken*
½ cup steamed green beans
¼ cup wild rice

Inflammatory Imbalance Menu
DAY SEVEN

BREAKFAST
Turkey Hash*
½ cup sliced strawberries

MORNING SNACK
2 unsweetened rice cakes or
8 rice crackers spread with
1 tablespoon cashew butter

LUNCH
baked or broiled chicken
breast, salt and pepper to taste
Crunchy Snow Peas*
½ gluten-free roll

AFTERNOON SNACK
Avocado and Pear Dip*
with ½ cup sliced cucumber
or zucchini

DINNER
Cheeseless Artichoke Omelet*
1 cup mixed salad greens
with 1 teaspoon olive oil
and juice of ½ lemon
½ cup sliced strawberries

Inflammatory Imbalance Menu
DAY EIGHT

BREAKFAST
2 Salmon Cakes*
¼ cup blueberries

MORNING SNACK
1 hardboiled egg
½ cup cantaloupe

LUNCH
leftover Sherry Chicken*
Gazpacho*

AFTERNOON SNACK
1 unsweetened rice cake or
4 rice crackers spread with
1 tablespoon almond butter

DINNER
Ginger Salmon*
Asparagus with a Zing*
⅓ cup wild rice

Inflammatory Imbalance Menu
DAY NINE

BREAKFAST

2 eggs, any style
Zucchini Cakes*
½ cup sliced strawberries

MORNING SNACK

Olive Tapenade* with ½ cup
sliced vegetables

LUNCH

Mushroom Scramble*
2 cups mixed salad greens
with 1 teaspoon olive oil
and juice of ½ lemon
¼ cup blueberries

AFTERNOON SNACK

1 small baked apple sprinkled
with cinnamon and
2 tablespoons crushed pecans

DINNER

Sweet Chicken Marsala*
⅓ cup wild rice
½ cup steamed broccoli

Inflammatory Imbalance Menu
DAY TEN

BREAKFAST

Confetti Scramble*
¼ cup raspberries

MORNING SNACK

½ baked pear sprinkled with
cinnamon or nutmeg and
1 tablespoon crushed pecans

LUNCH

leftover Sweet Chicken
Marsala* on 2 cups
mixed salad greens
½ cup sliced strawberries

AFTERNOON SNACK

2 stalks celery, each stuffed
with 1 tablespoon Lemony
Hummus*

DINNER

Fillet of Fish Amandine*
⅓ cup wild rice
½ cup steamed broccoli with
½ tablespoon butter

Inflammatory Imbalance Menu
DAY ELEVEN

BREAKFAST

Onion Tomato Scramble*
½ cup sliced strawberries

MORNING SNACK

2 unsweetened rice cakes or 8
rice crackers spread with
1 tablespoon cashew butter

LUNCH

Turkey Hash*
½ cup steamed green beans
½ cup cantaloupe

AFTERNOON SNACK

Lemony Hummus* with
½ cup sliced vegetables
1 tablespoon almonds

DINNER

Summertime Grilled Chicken*
¼ cup wild rice
½ cup sliced strawberries

Inflammatory Imbalance Menu
DAY TWELVE

BREAKFAST

Spinach Scramble*
½ cup raspberries

MORNING SNACK

1 small baked apple sprinkled
with cinnamon and
2 tablespoons crushed pecans

LUNCH

Spinach Salad*
½ millet roll

AFTERNOON SNACK

Avocado and Pear Dip*
with ½ cup sliced cucumber
or zucchini

DINNER

baked or broiled turkey
breast, salt and pepper
to taste
½ cup steamed green beans
with juice of ½ lemon
1 cup mixed salad greens
with 1 teaspoon olive oil
and juice of ½ lemon

Inflammatory Imbalance Menu
DAY THIRTEEN

BREAKFAST

2 Salmon Cakes*
½ cup sliced strawberries

MORNING SNACK

2 unsweetened rice cakes or 8
rice crackers spread with
1 tablespoon cashew butter

LUNCH

Sweet Chicken Salad*
½ gluten-free roll

AFTERNOON SNACK

1 hardboiled egg
2 tablespoons almonds

DINNER

Red and Green Turkey
Stir Fry*
¼ cup brown rice
½ cup sliced strawberries

Inflammatory Imbalance Menu
DAY FOURTEEN

BREAKFAST

Cheeseless Artichoke Omelet*
½ cup blueberries

MORNING SNACK

Avocado and Pear Dip*
with ½ cup sliced cucumber
or zucchini

LUNCH

Garlic Poached Haddock*
½ cup steamed broccoli
½ millet roll

AFTERNOON SNACK

Guacamole* with ½ cup
sliced vegetables

DINNER

Tarragon Chicken*
Rosemary Green Beans*
¼ cup wild rice

Inflammatory Issues FAQ

I don't have insulin resistance. Can I still be inflamed?

Yes. You can still be on the way to insulin resistance—as many of us in the industrialized nations are—without a full-blown diagnosis. You can also be inflamed to a lesser or greater degree, depending on your story. And trust me, if you are inflamed, you are on your way to insulin resistance—the two conditions are interlinked. Follow the plan for the next two weeks and see how you feel. The good news is that early intervention will normalize your insulin sensitivity and restore metabolic balance, which helps cool inflammation.

I'm finding it really hard to give up
the foods I love. Can I modify this plan?

I sympathize, believe me. However, if you can follow the plan for the next two weeks as it's written, you will begin to feel differently about your favorite foods (which are the most likely inflammatory culprits, in fact). I know it's hard to break old habits and tastes, but if you give yourself 14 days, you won't miss those foods anymore. Plus, know that you will have ample opportunity to reintroduce them—you just might not want to. I know you can do this for two weeks, so try your hardest, and instead of a favorite snack, treat yourself to an activity you enjoy.

I'm not feeling any different and
I'm not losing weight. What's going on?

If you've been following the Inflammatory Imbalance Custom Plan menu for a week or more and don't feel any improvement, it's probable that another core imbalance is to blame. Go back and look at your answers to the quiz. Are there other areas that had a high score or a tie? Many imbalances overlap with an inflammatory imbalance, including digestive issues, adrenal imbalance, detoxification issues, and hormonal imbalance. Try following the menu for another high-scoring imbalance and see if you feel any better. Or stick with this for another week. Your body may just need the extra time to heal. Also, you may want to try a medical food if you aren't already doing so. I've found medical foods intended to support the healing of inflammatory issues to be extremely helpful for my patients.

chapter thirteen

THE DETOXIFICATION IMBALANCE CUSTOM PLAN

Those of you who scored highest on the Detoxification Imbalance section of my quiz are probably dealing with detoxification systems that are functioning poorly or gummed up with too many toxins. Any hiccups in your detox balance lead to inflammation, a condition shared with your sisters in Chapter 12. In fact, poor detox function and inflammation often go hand in hand. How does the detoxification balance tip? Some women may be having difficulty detoxifying properly because of genetic or lifestyle influences, while others may be suffering from high levels of environmental toxins that are simply overwhelming their detoxification organs.

Barbara came to me desperate to lose weight. At 59 years old, she was 25 pounds overweight and nothing she did made any difference. All conventional tests were normal. On her first visit, we also discussed other symptoms, and Barbara reported fibromyalgia, anxiety, atrial fibrillation, panic attacks, and fatigue. She told me, "I feel like I have the flu all the time. I wake up and it feels as if I never slept." Barbara also said she was under huge, unremitting stress that had not let up for 15 years. She was worried that she might have a stroke if things didn't change—and her weight felt like the first place to start. I ran a battery of tests: Barbara's adrenals were on overdrive, she was positive for bacteria and yeast, but the most telling thing was that Barbara's liver was enlarged and her liver enzymes were elevated (a hepatitis screen was negative). This led me to the conclusion that Barbara's detoxification system was crying out for some help—but first we had to clear her digestive tract. I put her on the Core Balance Detox Imbalance Custom Plan with extra support provided by a medical food for digestion and inflammation. She also took a probiotic and betaine HCl to boost her stomach acids.

Once Barbara became more stable, I treated her parasites with Candex and uva ursi and added some adrenal support. She continued on the Detox Imbalance Custom Plan and began to lose weight. Then it was time to deal with her liver health. She switched to a medical food that supports the liver's metabolic process. She's been following the Detox Imbalance Custom Plan since then. When I saw Barbara a few months ago, her symptoms were completely gone. Her liver and enzymes were back to normal. No more anxiety. No more atrial fib. No more pain. And no more extra weight. "I feel so good!" she said. "My thinking is clear and I have more energy than ever. I didn't think it could happen. Thank you!" I reminded her that it was her body doing the work—only now she knew how to give it the right tools.

How a woman detoxifies is as important to her overall health and her weight as almost any biological system I can think of. New research shows that detox enzymes occur in most parts of the body, including brain cells—which means that efficient detoxification may play a larger role in Alzheimer's, Parkinson's, and mood disorders than previously thought. Difficulty detoxifying is often the underlying core imbalance that creates imbalances everywhere else and seriously undermines your health. Nature knows this; that's why we have a formidable waste-management system in place, backed up by our digestive tract and immune system. Until about 150 years ago, this was enough. But the modern age, with its synthetic chemicals, empty calories, and labor-saving devices, has changed the game (and you can see it in our thickening waistlines).

Each day we bathe in a toxic soup of air pollutants, heavy metals, PCBs, and other frightening environmental toxins.[1] We ingest vast amounts of man-made chemicals, including over-the-counter and prescription drugs, pesticides, stimulants, refined sugar and carbohydrates, and processed fats. Even naturally occurring chemicals in foods can be toxic if we have undiagnosed food sensitivities, bacterial or yeast infections, or parasites that interfere with the digestive process and/or immune response. And on top of all this, to cope with chronic stress, we engage in even more taxing behavior by smoking, taking recreational drugs, and drinking alcohol and caffeine in excessive amounts (all the while failing to exercise, stool, and sleep regularly—three potent detox boosters).

What this adds up to is a highly evolved cleaning system that is perpetually overtaxed and getting more so. If you don't help it clean house by detoxifying deliberately, clearing out dietary, environmental, and emotional clutter on a regular basis, your body just gets overwhelmed by the mess. You know by now that your core physiology relies on a conversation that takes place between your organs, your biochemicals, your DNA, and your cells. And in the absence of good detox, you can imagine the clutter and junk that's getting in the way of your conversation! When your inner conversation gets muddled, you feel sick and tired. Often, you gain weight that your body doesn't want to let go.

Generally speaking, our bodies do a heroic job of stemming the toxic tide, but every woman has a tipping point. If you are reading these lines, you can be fairly confident that your body has reached yours and taken out an insurance policy in the form of extra weight.[2] The good news is that much of the damage can be undone, just by boosting your body's natural detox capabilities with a clean diet, periodic rest, and internal cleansing. Now, I can almost hear the groans—and I've often heard them in my office. But I am not talking about aggressive colon cleanses or fasting on lemon juice. The best detox plans work with whole, easily digested foods (you don't starve!), tons of filtered water, lots of sleep, gentle exercise, taking away offending foods and substances, and adding restorative supplements.

An Inside Look at the Detox Process

Your metabolism exists to break down substances into usable forms (energy) and nonusable forms (waste). Detoxification is how your body handles the waste. Your detoxification system, which includes your liver, kidneys, digestive tract, circulation and lymph systems, lungs, and skin, has to process toxins in the environment, from your diet, and your emotions. This means that you are detoxifying all the time—you'd die if you weren't. Every time you exhale, sweat, or go to the bathroom you are naturally detoxifying. In fact, almost every system in your body has some detox component.

The lymph system, which rivals your circulatory system in its expanse and complexity, acts as your body's sewer system. When blood circulates, it brings nutrients to cells and removes waste, but this is not a direct exchange. Rather, a buffer of fluid surrounding the cells, called interstitial fluid, acts as a medium for the exchange. Lymph fluid is essentially extra interstitial fluid, a clear fluid that contains much of the metabolic debris created by cells as they go about their business. Like tributaries trickling into a stream that feeds a slow-

Symptoms of Toxicity

- Acne, chronic breakouts, and skin rashes

- Bad breath

- Bloating, gas, GI distress

- Canker sores

- Cognitive difficulty (fuzzy thinking, inability to concentrate)

- Constipation or diarrhea

- Dark circles under eyes

- Excessive thirst

- Fluid retention

- Food cravings and sensitivities

- Headaches

- Insomnia

- Muscle and joint pain

- Noticeably reduced tolerance to alcohol and caffeine

- Postnasal drip

- Scratchy throat

- Significant reactions to odors, cleansing agents, perfumes, etc.

- Sinus congestion

- Stubborn weight gain

- Worsening symptoms of PMS and menopause

201

moving river, the lymph system transports lymph fluid through ever-widening vessels, moving it through 500 filtration and "dumping" points—your lymph nodes. At each successive node the lymph fluid is filtered and bacteria is removed. If lymph fluid is blocked in one lymph node it will usually take a detour, but when blockage is extreme it can cause the lymph fluid to back up and cause swelling in the surrounding tissue, a condition known as lymphedema.

Lymph vessels merge at certain points to form lymphatic trunks. You have six major lymph trunks in your body, each responsible for draining filtered fluid from one region of the body. Purified lymph travels up your torso and finally returns to the bloodstream through the thoracic duct located just below your collarbone. The lymph system has no pump; instead, lymph moves through breathing, exercise, and massage.

Because lymph cleanses nearly every cell in your body, symptoms of chronic lymph blockage are diverse, but they can include worsened allergies and food sensitivities, frequent colds and flu, joint pain, headaches and migraines, menstrual cramps, arthritis, fibrocystic breasts, breast tenderness, sinusitis, loss of appetite and other GI issues, muscle cramping, tissue swelling, fatigue, mental fuzziness, cellulite, and depression. In the absence of particular symptoms, you may feel generally tired and toxic, with a heaviness in your abdomen.

The Heroic Liver

Some toxins you take in are mobilized, neutralized, and excreted right away; others are stored in your fat cells. When you lose fat, you release the toxins back into your system, which can cause symptoms and inadvertently encourage you to keep weight on. Your liver is responsible for neutralizing, converting, and excreting up to 99 percent of bacteria and body toxins when it is working properly—and it's also the organ that metabolizes fat! When your liver is damaged, stressed, or fatty, its efficiency declines rapidly. A healthy liver filters almost two quarts of blood per minute. The liver removes bacteria, chemicals, heavy metals, bacterial endotoxins, antigen-antibody complexes, and excess sugar and fats and excretes this waste through bile into the small intestine, where it binds with digestive chyme to create stool. It does so with the assistance of antioxidants and phytonutrients that in turn power a two-phase enzymatic process whose well-being is crucial to your long-term health.

During phase one, most unwanted chemical compounds, like drugs, pesticides, and gut toxins, are converted into highly unstable intermediate substances along the pathway—along with excess hormones and histamines (a byproduct of inflammation). This first phase calls on some 50 to 100 different nutrient-fueled enzymes alone! You can measure how well your phase one detoxification is working by how well you tolerate caffeine, perfumes, and other airborne fumes. The intermediate substances formed in phase one are further processed and neutralized during phase two in a process called convergence. Phase two convergence calls upon many helpers, primarily an important enzyme called glutathione and certain amino acids. Again, these substances depend on access to the right nutrients for their existence and optimal function. Much more is involved, and difficulties can occur at a number of points—but for now, this is enough to show you why a full roster of nutrients is vital to liver health, and why, for detoxification, supporting the liver is crucial.

Severe Environmental Sensitivities

One growing subset of people who must pay especially strict attention to detox and their liver health are those people with severe environmental sensitivities, or "pathological detoxifiers." These women have difficulty moving toxins from phase one to phase two; often they are missing essential nutrients or lack a certain genetic variation, also called a "snip" or SNP (which stands for Single Nucleotide Polymorphism), that bridges the two. This leaves them extremely vulnerable to the host of half-converted and highly toxic phase one compounds. These women always need to be mindful to keep their livers healthy.

For the most part, individuals without this problem are able to keep their heads above water thanks to the heroic efforts of their livers—but this can change quickly if they are exposed to toxins in large quantities or over a prolonged period, and this includes persistent stress. For some women, the hormonal shifts of menopause tip them over the edge; for others it may be an emotional crisis, such as a divorce; for most of us, however, the change creeps up slowly, the residue of a lifetime of poor nutrition and unhealthy lifestyle.

As I've said, effective detoxification is so important to our survival that we would die within hours if we couldn't detoxify. This is good news for those of you with detoxification imbalance, because it means that your body will be working hard to back up your detox efforts over the next two weeks. You already have such an elegant detoxification system in place; now's your chance to help it do its job! Once you've restored balance to this system, you'll be amazed at how much clearer, cleaner, and lighter you feel.

The Detoxification Imbalance Eating and Action Plan

In many ways, this plan is the easiest and the hardest of all. It is easiest because you already have a ferocious detoxification system in place that is poised to kick into high gear once you clear away some of the extraneous debris. This means you will see and feel results very quickly if you are diligent. It's the hardest because it requires the most significant changes in your lifestyle—as well as your diet. The plan focuses on removing the most obnoxious, offensive allergens and toxins—or what I call stressors. Stress is different for everyone—what really bothers me might not bother another woman, and vice versa. So think of it as anything that doesn't work well for you. And don't forget electromagnetic pollution from electronics, cell phones, clock radios, digital personal devices, and power lines. Removing or severely limiting things that don't work for you lifts your "body burden," but in order to heal, you have to add the right kind of support.

The challenge for you will be to identify which stressors are impacting your detox capabilities. You have to look at all aspects of your life: your diet, your water supply, your work, your home, your relationships—even your dentist! People with mercury amalgam fillings may want to consider getting their fillings replaced. Mercury is a highly toxic heavy metal and can be extremely inflammatory, especially if it becomes unstable or degrades. Think about how long you've had your fillings and how often you chew on them—it's the vapors that are released, not the fillings themselves, that cause problems. I had a patient tell me recently that ever since she got the mercury out of her mouth, she feels better every day. (You can find out more about mercury-free dentistry in the Referrals and Resources section.)

Please note that if you have any dietary sensitivities, you will want to deal with those first (by either eliminating the offensive food or following the Digestive Sensitivities menu). This plan focuses on liver detoxification and support; if you don't heal your gut first, it won't be up to the task of neutralizing the additional toxins that get dumped from your healing liver. Also, when we begin to lose weight, fat releases fat-soluble toxins into the bloodstream and can make symptoms temporarily worse. That's why it's crucial that you also focus on flushing out toxins by drinking a lot of water.

I've designed a hypoallergenic, detoxifying menu for you, but you must take responsibility for identifying and clearing away the chemicals and pollution in other areas of your life. And this includes your emotions. Emotions can be highly irritating, especially the kind that are stuck and/or hidden. For help in dealing with toxic emotions, please read Stage IV as you cleanse over the next two weeks. And be kind and patient with yourself. I recommend trying to find an alternative therapy that you like, such as acupuncture, massage, or a mindful exercise that helps rid the body of toxins. This will help you significantly in your process and keep you feeling well. Finally, detoxification follows your circadian rhythm, so plan to sleep—a lot.

Marcelle's Prescription for
DETOXIFICATION IMBALANCE

1. Follow the menu starting on page 211 and purchase supplements.

2. Schedule appointment for diagnostic tests. Talk to your health-care practitioner about your plan to detox. Discuss any concerns, especially if you are currently on any medication.

3. Add gluten-free psyllium husks or other fiber supplement if you aren't having one to two easy bowel movements a day.

4. Buy certified organic produce as often as possible and be sure to wash all produce thoroughly with a veggie wash.

5. Examine your surroundings and make them as "green" and clean as possible. Go through your house, your kitchen, your refrigerator, your bathroom cabinets and shelves, your garage, and your work-space and remove any product that has ingredients you cannot pro-nounce or that has a noxious odor. For more ideas, see page 209.

6. Take a hot bath with Epsom salts, a sauna, or a steam bath for 15 minutes, two to three times a week, to help sweat out toxins. You can also use a dry brush on your skin before you shower to loosen dead skin and remove buildup. For the same reason, work up a good sweat when you exercise.

7. Use glass whenever you can for storage and heating, especially in the microwave. Limit use of plastic wrap—the softer the plastic, the more likely it is to leach harmful chemicals like PCBs into food and other items.

8. Don't drink water out of plastic bottles left in the sun or washed in the dishwasher. High temperatures create a volatile situation in which dangerous phthalates and the endocrine disrupter bisphenol A can leak into your food and beverages. Try a stainless steel ther-mos or water bottle (see the Resources section for information).

9. Up your intake of pure, filtered water to 10 eight-ounce glasses a day. Remember that your skin is your largest detox organ, so don't forget the water that you bathe in. Consider investing in a reverse-osmosis filter for your house to insure that you are bath-ing in clean water as well as drinking it.

10. Give yourself a 10 p.m. bedtime and stick to it. Efficient detoxifi-cation requires seven to nine hours of sleep per night.

11. Start walking or engage in moderate, mindful exercise 30 to 60 minutes each day, either all at once or split in two sessions.

12. Organize your social life ahead of time so that during your detox you are engaged in only positive, joyful encounters. Schedule less than you normally do and plan to leave plenty of time to rest, nap, and journal while you detox.

13. Read Stage IV and consider enlisting help in dealing with toxic relationships.

Diagnostic Testing for Detoxification Imbalance

- ALCAT for food sensitivities and allergens
- Complete Blood Count (CBC with differential) to test for anemia, infection, or other blood disorders
- Comprehensive Digestive Stool Analysis (CDSA) to test digestion and absorption and bacterial balance
- Standard Comprehensive metabolic Profile (CMP) to test electrolytes, blood sugar, blood protein, pH level, and liver and kidney function
- Comprehensive Metabolic Profile (CMP) to test for amino acid deficiency
- Comprehensive Parasitology 2 (CP x 2) to test for parasites
- Urine heavy metal test to test for heavy metal toxicity
- Blood Lipid Panel to test HDL, LDL, and triglycerides
- Genova liver detoxification profile to test for phase one and phase two liver detoxification capabilities and estrogen metabolism

Foods to Include for Detoxification Imbalance

- Aloe vera
- Alfalfa sprouts
- Algae and other green chlorophyll powders (very cleansing)—start slowly
- Brown rice
- Chile peppers
- Dark green vegetables
- Fruit
- Garlic
- Leafy greens—especially liver-loving dandelion
- Lemon
- Mung beans
- Millet
- Oats (gluten-free)
- Root vegetables
- Seeds
- Wheat grass juice

Foods to Avoid for Detoxification Imbalance

- Alcohol

- Artificial chemicals, sweeteners, preservatives, additives, colorings

- Caffeine

- Dairy

- Processed food

- Grilled or charbroiled meats

- Refined grains

- Gluten and grains—wheat, barley, spelt, kamut, rye, triticale

- Sugar, syrups, honey

- Eggs may be a problem for some women, but they are included in these menus because they are an excellent source of protein for breakfast. If you feel symptomatic after eating eggs, try a gluten-free whole grain cereal with a whey or rice protein fruit smoothie for breakfast instead.

Supplements for Detoxification Imbalance

Basic:

- High-potency multivitamin with calcium and magnesium

- Antioxidant combination (Co-enzyme Q10, 100 mgs, and alpha linoleic acid from flax or hemp, 500 mgs)

- Probiotic (take 5 to 15 minutes before meal with water)

- Glutamine (1000 mgs three times daily)

- Taurine (500 mgs)

- A green drink, such as wheat grass or chlorophyll-based; start with ½ a serving (about 4 ounces) and see how you feel. If it agrees with you, drink the full amount.

Additional (as desired):

- Fiber supplement, such as gluten-free psyllium husks, or shake (see page 74 for recipe)
- Activated charcoal tablets—take as needed to neutralize ingested toxins
- Deglycerized licorice
- Liver-loving herbs, such as milk thistle, kudzu, turmeric, and dandelion

If medical tests warrant (use only under medical guidance):

- Medical foods to support active detoxification
- Chelation supplements to remove heavy metals, as directed by a practitioner

Green Your Scene

Here are some easy ways to reduce chemicals and pollutants in your food and environments. For a list of my favorite products, see the Referrals and Resources section.

- Invest in some houseplants for every room.

- Buy a central water and air filter for your home. Nikken air filters are great.

- Change humidifier filters and vacuum bags often.

- Replace bed linens with organic cotton variety—and if you can afford it, consider investing in a "green" mattress set. Or cover your mattress, pillows, and duvet with hypoallergenic covers.

- Recycle all your old plastic storage containers and buy glass.

- Replace your plastic water containers with glass or stainless steel.

- Replace cleaning solvents with natural brands or use baking soda and vinegar.

- Start composting to make fertilizer for your garden. Contact your local recycling center for instructions.

- Don't forget your beauty products! Organic shampoos, conditioners, and moisturizers are available at most natural food stores. Mineral makeup is a chemical-free alternative to toxic cosmetics.

- Do not dump unused medications down the toilet or sink. They run off into the water supply and expose us all! Return unused medications to pharmacies or medical practitioners.

- Replace all Teflon-coated pans.

- Test the air in your office. If you work in a sick building, you have the right to object.

- Subscribe to Clean Eating magazine at www.cleaneatingmag.com.

- Be careful when disposing of light bulbs, mercury thermometers, and anything else that contains toxic metals or ingredients. Call your local recycling center for more information.

A Day in the Life of the
Detoxification Imbalance Custom Plan

Time	Activity
6:30–7:00 A.M.	Wake up slowly and breathe deeply into the belly ten times. Exhale fully, pumping the diaphragm to get the lymph moving. Drink two full glasses of filtered water or warm water with lemon and a dash of cayenne pepper to stimulate the liver to create bile.
7:00	Self-care ritual.
7:30	Make breakfast, take supplements and fiber.
8:00	Jump on trampoline, do breathing exercises, or walk to get your breath, circulation, and lymph moving. Aerobic exercise and weight training are great because you sweat!
9:00	Work, household duties, chores, errands, and so on. Keep a thermos of water with you. For plastic-free alternatives, see the Resources section.
10:00	Snack/tea or broth break.
12:00 P.M.	Lunch. Breathe deeply and walk for 20 minutes.
2:00	Cleansing herbal tea or broth break.
3:00	Snack.
4:00	Cleansing tea or broth break—or drink more water.
5:00	Walk or exercise vigorously enough to break a sweat. When you get home, dry brush skin or take a hot bath. Alternatively, take a steam bath or sauna at the gym. Or try hot yoga.
6:30	Dinner.
7:30	Connect with loved ones, engage in a favorite activity. Resist the impulse to use electronics.
8:30	Time to wind down. Drink a sleep-inducing cup of herbal tea. Dim lights. Stretch lightly before bed. Don't forget to floss and clean out bacteria from your gums.
9:00	Bedtime.

The Core Balance Menu Plan for Detoxification Imbalance

Snack Ideas:

- Rice cakes/apple slices with almond or cashew butter
- Celery/carrot/pepper slices with hummus
- One piece of fresh fruit
- Handful of nuts or seeds
- Half a serving of previous evening's entrée

* Recipes start on page 259.

Detoxification Imbalance Menu
DAY ONE

BREAKFAST

Cheeseless Artichoke Omelet*
½ cup raspberries

MORNING SNACK

2 hardboiled eggs
½ cup cantaloupe

LUNCH

Sweet Arugula Salad
with Chicken*
½ cup sliced strawberries

AFTERNOON SNACK

½ baked pear sprinkled with
cinnamon or nutmeg and
1 tablespoon crushed pecans

DINNER

Dilled Salmon*
Sautéed Swiss Chard*
¼ cup wild rice

Detoxification Imbalance Menu
DAY TWO

BREAKFAST

2 eggs, any style
2 slices nitrate-free bacon
⅓ cup blueberries

MORNING SNACK

Avocado and Pear Dip*
with ½ cup sliced cucumber
or zucchini

LUNCH

2 Homemade Turkey Patties*
2 cups mixed salad greens
with 1 teaspoon olive oil
and juice of ½ lemon
½ cup sliced strawberries

AFTERNOON SNACK

Olive Tapenade* with ½ cup
sliced vegetables

DINNER

Sherry Chicken*
Rosemary Green Beans*
¼ cup wild rice

Detoxification Imbalance Menu
DAY THREE

BREAKFAST

Turkey Frittata*
½ cup cantaloupe

MORNING SNACK

1 small baked apple sprinkled
with cinnamon and
2 tablespoons crushed pecans

LUNCH

Not Your Mom's Chicken Salad*
on 1 cup mixed salad greens
½ cup sliced strawberries

AFTERNOON SNACK

Guacamole* with ½ cup
sliced vegetables

DINNER

Rosemary Lamb*
½ sweet potato with
½ tablespoon butter, sprinkled
with cinnamon if desired
½ cup steamed kale

Detoxification Imbalance Menu
DAY FOUR

BREAKFAST

Spinach Scramble*
½ cup sliced strawberries

MORNING SNACK

2 unsweetened rice cakes or
8 rice crackers spread with
1 tablespoon cashew butter

LUNCH

leftover Rosemary Lamb*
2 cups mixed salad greens
with 1 teaspoon olive oil
and juice of ½ lemon

AFTERNOON SNACK

2 stalks celery, each stuffed
with 1 tablespoon Lemony
Hummus*

DINNER

Cashew Chicken*
½ cup steamed broccoli
¼ cup brown rice

Detoxification Imbalance Menu
DAY FIVE

BREAKFAST

Turkey Hash*
⅓ cup blueberries

MORNING SNACK

Guacamole* with ½ cup
sliced vegetables

LUNCH

Confetti Scramble*
½ gluten-free roll

AFTERNOON SNACK

Avocado and Pear Dip*
with ½ cup sliced cucumber
or zucchini

DINNER

Garlic Poached Haddock*
Asparagus with a Zing*
½ cup wild rice

Detoxification Imbalance Menu
DAY SIX

BREAKFAST

Onion Tomato Scramble*
½ cup sliced strawberries

MORNING SNACK

Olive Tapenade* with ½ cup
sliced vegetables

LUNCH

Steamed Fish*
Zucchini Ribbons*
¼ cup wild rice

AFTERNOON SNACK

1 small baked apple sprinkled
with cinnamon and
2 tablespoons crushed pecans

DINNER

Red and Green Turkey Stir Fry*
½ cup brown rice
⅓ cup raspberries

Detoxification Imbalance Menu
DAY SEVEN

BREAKFAST

2 eggs, any style
Zucchini Cakes*
½ cup raspberries

MORNING SNACK

Avocado and Pear Dip*
with ½ cup sliced cucumber
or zucchini

LUNCH

leftover Red and Green
Turkey Stir Fry*
¼ cup brown rice
½ cup sliced strawberries

AFTERNOON SNACK

1 small apple, sliced and
spread with 1 tablespoon
cashew butter

DINNER

Tarragon Chicken*
Crunchy Green Beans*
½ sweet potato with
½ tablespoon butter, sprinkled
with cinnamon if desired

Detoxification Imbalance Menu
DAY EIGHT

BREAKFAST

Turkey Hash*
½ cup blueberries

MORNING SNACK

2 hardboiled eggs
½ cup cantaloupe

LUNCH

Mushroom Scramble*
½ cup cantaloupe
2 cups mixed salad greens
with 1 teaspoon olive oil
and juice of ½ lemon

AFTERNOON SNACK

2 unsweetened rice cakes
or 8 rice crackers spread with
1 tablespoon cashew butter

DINNER

baked or broiled chicken
breast, salt and
pepper to taste
Brussels Sprouts
with Mushrooms*
¼ cup wild rice

Detoxification Imbalance Menu
DAY NINE

BREAKFAST

Spinach Scramble*
⅓ cup blueberries

MORNING SNACK

1 small baked apple sprinkled
with cinnamon and
2 tablespoons crushed pecans

LUNCH

Spinach Salad*
½ millet roll

AFTERNOON SNACK

Lemony Hummus* with ½ cup
sliced vegetables

DINNER

Chicken and Asparagus Sauté*
¼ cup brown rice
⅓ cup raspberries

Detoxification Imbalance Menu
DAY TEN

BREAKFAST

Spicy Fiesta Eggs*
½ cup blueberries

MORNING SNACK

Olive Tapenade* with ½ cup
sliced vegetables

LUNCH

Simple Sautéed Fish*
Zucchini Ribbons*
¼ cup wild rice

AFTERNOON SNACK

Avocado and Pear Dip*
with ½ cup sliced cucumber
or zucchini

DINNER

Ginger Salmon*
Squash Medley*
½ gluten-free roll

Detoxification Imbalance Menu
DAY ELEVEN

BREAKFAST

2 eggs, any style
2 turkey sausages
¼ cup blueberries

MORNING SNACK

Guacamole* with ½ cup
sliced vegetables

LUNCH

Sweet Chicken Salad*
½ millet roll

AFTERNOON SNACK

2 tablespoons almonds
½ cup raspberries

DINNER

Baked Salmon with
Hazelnut Butter*
Stir Fry Broccoli with Ginger*
¼ cup wild rice

Detoxification Imbalance Menu
DAY TWELVE

BREAKFAST
Onion Tomato Scramble*
⅓ cup blueberries

MORNING SNACK
2 unsweetened rice cakes or
8 rice crackers spread with
1 tablespoon cashew butter

LUNCH
Turkey Frittata*
2 cups mixed salad greens
with 1 teaspoon olive oil
and juice of ½ lemon

AFTERNOON SNACK
Lemony Hummus* with
½ cup sliced vegetables

DINNER
Quick and Easy Chicken*
Spinach with Lemon
and Garlic*
¼ cup wild rice

Detoxification Imbalance Menu
DAY THIRTEEN

BREAKFAST
Cheeseless Artichoke Omelet*
½ cup blueberries

MORNING SNACK
Avocado and Pear Dip*
with ½ cup sliced cucumber
or zucchini

LUNCH
Sweet Arugula Salad
with Chicken*
½ millet roll

AFTERNOON SNACK
1 small apple, sliced and
spread with 1 tablespoon
cashew butter

DINNER
Spicy Crunchy Chicken*
Rosemary Green Beans*
½ cup brown rice

Detoxification Imbalance Menu
DAY FOURTEEN

BREAKFAST
2 eggs, any style
2 Homemade Turkey Patties*
½ cup raspberries

MORNING SNACK
1 small baked apple sprinkled
with cinnamon and
2 tablespoons crushed pecans

LUNCH
leftover Spicy
Crunchy Chicken*
½ cup steamed green beans
¼ cup wild rice

AFTERNOON SNACK
Olive Tapenade* with ½ cup
sliced vegetables

DINNER
Cinnamon Lamb Chops*
Crunchy Snow Peas*
¼ cup brown rice

Detoxification Imbalance FAQ

I feel worse! What's going on?

As I said before, when you detoxify and begin to lose weight, toxins stored in your fat and liver circulate in the bloodstream and may aggravate symptoms. The first step is to up your fluid intake significantly and flush your kidneys. Consider buying a mini-trampoline to help get your lymph moving or try a lymph massage and drainage therapy. And be sure to rule out any GI issues or dietary sensitivities. You need to heal these first (see Chapter 8). Try to keep to the plan and rest often, including taking a nap. You should feel better within two to three days. If you don't, investigate a medical food supplement with your health-care practitioner.

This is too much change! Do I have to do it all?

Of course not. But you do need to follow the menu and take your supplements if you want to lose weight and feel better. The changes to your environment can come slowly, if you so choose. But know that the cleaner your diet and environment are, the faster you will see results. So do what you can and relax! Read Stage IV and consider whether some of your frustration has to do with stuck patterns of thinking.

I'm not losing weight and/or I don't feel different. What's going on?

Continue the plan for the full two weeks and then some—restoring balance can take some time. If you haven't tried a medical food to support active detox, consider doing so. If you don't feel any positive shift after this, go back to the Core Balance Quiz and look at your scores. You could be dealing with overlapping issues, such as digestive issues, adrenal imbalance, or hormonal imbalance. My best advice is to work with a practitioner who can advise you on doing a full-scale detox including heavy metals, which may include getting the mercury taken out of your mouth. If your urine heavy metal test shows that you do have high levels of heavy metal toxicity, consider enlisting the help of a specialist who works with nutrients and chelation. Chelation therapy is a somewhat controversial alternative practice that rids the body of heavy metals; talk to a functional medical practitioner about whether or not it might work for you.

Now What?

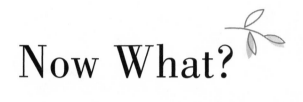

First off, give yourself a big hug for following the Core Balance Program this past month to the best of your abilities. If you are reading these lines, it shows you have a motivated heart and the willingness to try new things. Good for you. In my opinion, willingness to make changes and seek different solutions is more than half the ball game and a terrific predictor of success. Willingness leads to experimentation, which leads to permanent change. So take a big breath in and fill your whole body with a sense of satisfaction that you've gotten this far.

But now what? We are at a crossroads here at the end of 28 days. If you are anything like my patients, your present results are going to guide your future path—and there are several to choose from. I will lay out a few options and ask you to trust your symptoms and your intuition to tell you where you need to go.

Most of you should be feeling the benefits of the physical body returning to Core Balance: increased body wisdom; boundless reserves of energy and vitality; and steady and safe weight loss. However, there will always be some patients who don't respond predictably to the month-long program. There are many reasons for this, and most of them come down to entrenched imbalances that are highly individual and may need further testing and guidance to identify.

Choose Your Next Step

1. You are seeing and feeling the results you want but still wish to lose more weight . . .

If you're at this point, I encourage you to continue with your Core Imbalance Custom Plan for another two to four weeks, or until you achieve your healthiest self. If you are feeling physically stronger, now is the time to begin paying more attention to the other corners of your puzzle: your instinctual, emotional, and thinking selves. Read Stage IV as you continue with your eating and action plan and consider adding some of the alternative healing therapies I recommend there. You may also want to consider adding more physical activity to your routine.

2. If you are making good progress but feel frustrated and hemmed in by the food restrictions on your Custom Plan . . .

If you feel this way, you may begin to slowly reintroduce some of your favorite foods by adding them one at a time, in a significant quantity, and seeing how you feel. I recommend adding one food on day one, then repeating that food two days later. It helps to keep a food journal as you reintroduce potentially allergic and addictive foods and chronicle how you feel after you eat them. If you sense a negative reaction, you've just gotten a valuable piece of information about yourself. From here, only you can make the choice whether or not it is worth it to you to continue eating those reactive foods that could be undermining the integrity of your health. I find in my practice that many women learn to judge whether or not they want a "food hangover"; more often than not, awareness leads to healthier choices. Alternatively, you can choose to revert to the Core Balance Essential Plan, which will expand your food choices somewhat, and continue rotating meals for the next two to four weeks, or until you achieve your optimal weight and fitness level. Read Stage IV and consider implementing some alternative therapies to help support this next stage of your discovery.

3. If you have not made any progress (in other words, you aren't losing any weight or feeling any better) or if you are losing weight but feel worse . . .

For this condition, further medical inquiry may be required. Continue on your Core Imbalance Custom Plan, if you can, or revert to the Essential Plan if it is easier and does not trigger increased symptoms. If you have not already scheduled the appropriate diagnostic tests for your Core Imbalance, please do so. I recommend the following tests in addition, which are also explained fully in the Appendices, if they aren't already on your list:

- ALCAT test for allergies and food sensitivities

- Adrenal Stress Index (ASI) to test cortisol levels throughout the day

- Breath test for small intestine bacterial and fungal overgrowth

- Complete Blood Count (CBC with differential) to test for anemia, infection, or other blood disorders

- Comprehensive Digestive Stool Analysis (CDSA) to test digestion, absorption, and bacterial balance

- Standard Comprehensive Metabolic Profile (CMP) to evaluate electrolytes, blood sugar, blood protein, pH level, and liver and kidney function

- Comprehensive Metabolic Profile to test for amino acid deficiency

- Comprehensive Parasitology 2 (CP x 2) to test for parasites

- Urine heavy metal test to test for heavy metal toxicity

- Blood lipid panel to measure HDL, LDL and triglycerides

- Genova liver detoxification profile to test for phase one and phase two liver detoxification capabilities and estrogen metabolism

- Hormone Panel and estrogen metabolism tests, appropriate for age

- 24 hour Urine Iodine test

- Thyroid testing: TSH, Free T4 and free T3, thyroid antibodies

- Neurotransmitter test

- Celiac test for gluten sensitivity/allergy

I strongly advise seeking the counsel of a functional medical practitioner to help you get to the individual root of your imbalance. This book covers the most common obstacles to weight loss in most women, but there are many unique genetic variations and individual tendencies that will become obvious when you work one-on-one with a trusted practitioner. I've listed referrals in the Resources section to help you find a practitioner in your area. I also encourage you to call the Women to Women Clinic at 800-798-7902 or visit us on the Web. We are happy to provide in-depth phone consultations or schedule an appointment for you.

Don't forget that our feelings and our physical health are intertwined, so you may be dealing with subterranean emotional issues that are complicating your imbalances. Please read Stage IV and consider trying some of the alternative therapies therein.

4. You are feeling better, and perhaps even great, but you haven't lost weight . . .

Oh, the frustration! And you've been so diligent. I'm sorry you haven't seen the results you hoped for, but I also want you to focus on how much better you are feeling in your skin. This is a great accomplishment on its own. However, I know you bought this book because you really want to lose weight, so here are a few options that actually cover all of the above and then some.

Continue on your Core Imbalance Custom Plan for the next two to four weeks—and get strict with yourself if you haven't been. It will only help you in this next stage. You can enlist the help of a functional medical practitioner in your area and schedule the above tests if you haven't already had them (and in addition to whatever diagnostics I prescribed in your Custom Plan). You may also be dealing with more than one core imbalance, a fact that further diagnostic testing and individualized attention will reveal.

It may be helpful to go back and retake the Core Imbalance Quiz; your answers may have changed in a surprising way. Sometimes the symptoms of one imbalance will mask other symptoms that reveal themselves only when the imbalance starts to right itself—think of it as peeling layers from an onion. You've just gotten through the first layer. It's not uncommon for some of my patients to follow one eating and action plan for a month and then switch to another for the next month—or combine them.

It's also possible that your body is still on defense because of deep emotional issues that need attention. Read Stage IV and remember: this is a process! It's taken you a lifetime to get where you are; it may just take a little more time to get you where you want to be. But if you are open and willing, I promise you your hard work will pay off in spades (and lost pounds).

5. If you began the Core Balance Program more than 25 pounds overweight, have been on the Core Balance Program for two months, and have tried all of the above recommendations . . .

If all of your tests are optimal and if the weight still will not budge (not if you are losing weight slowly), you may be interested in pursuing a somewhat controversial hormone therapy. It uses tiny doses of HCG (human chorionic gonadotropin), a peptide hormone synthesized by the body during pregnancy, by injection or nasal spray. Larger doses of HCG are widely used as a fertility drug in women without any serious side effect. Still, the therapy is controversial.[1]

HCG therapy appears to be most effective for weight loss when used in combination with a severely restricted calorie diet (500–800 calories per day) under medical guidance. I have witnessed amazing results in patients who have been unable to lose weight any other way—particularly those past menopause. They have shed tens of pounds—quickly and efficiently—without feeling hungry, depressed, or fatigued or experiencing loss of muscle or a lot of sagging skin.

You should be advised that the medical community considers use of HCG for weight loss "off-label" use and is extremely skeptical of its benefits in this area—so don't expect a lot of support from your mainstream practitioner. There is also some evidence that misuse may up the risk of autoimmune disorders. For this reason, I don't recommend it lightly, nor do I advise that anyone try it unless she has more than 25 stubborn pounds to lose. However, it's a fact that many women are happily using it for weight loss and it is working—so I would feel remiss if I didn't mention it as a last resort. If you can honestly say you've followed the Core Balance Diet religiously for two months, including my recommendations for achieving some emotional freedom, without any weight loss, this may be an encouraging option for you. Do your research and discuss what you find with a caring practitioner. Know that there are risks that may be associated with HCG use.

Whatever else you do now, I hope you will read the following section, Stage IV: Core Balance for Life, if you have not done so already. We have focused largely on the physical up to this point, but now we are heading deeper into the core, piecing together the center of your puzzle to reveal the vibrant picture that is at the root of your Core Balance. This is critical for every woman's ability to maintain her Core Balance through life—no matter how many plates she finds herself juggling at any one time.

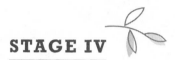

Core Balance for Life: Transformation Inside and Out

chapter fourteen

YOUR ISSUES ARE
IN YOUR TISSUES

We are about to enter into a part of our journey where many Western practitioners fear to tread: the spiritual and emotional terrain that forms the backbone of true wellness. You simply cannot heal the body if you don't heal the mind, and you cannot heal the mind if you don't heal the spirit. But this isn't easy. It requires a leap of faith.

Remember my patient Sally from the Hormonal Imbalance Custom Plan, who came to me with symptoms including hot flashes and night sweats? In Sally's case, healing her core hormonal imbalance was the first step on an arduous journey that began long before she was born. Sally's grandmother died when her mother was very young. Deprived of any maternal affection, Sally's mother was herself an absent parent. As a girl, Sally never received the physical affection or unguarded love that she needed. As so often happens in this scenario, Sally began to look elsewhere for love and validation during her teenage years and found herself pregnant at 16 years old. She took the pregnancy to term and put her infant son up for adoption.

Fast-forward 30 years. Sally is in perimenopause and experiencing hormonal symptoms, severe anxiety, and, it turns out, symptoms of extreme adrenal burnout. Sally attributed her exhaustion to day-to-day stress and her worry for her daughter, a compulsive eater. Somewhere along the line, Sally had begun to realize that she was trapped in a cycle of abandonment that was undermining her—and her daughter's—happiness. Sally is a life coach, so she is perhaps more keenly attuned to these kinds of things.

Even so, what brought Sally to me were her physical symptoms. And just as we have done in this book thus far, Sally and I worked to rebalance her physical core for the better part of a year. Each time something stabilized, we would add another piece. At first Sally said, "No way, I can't do this." But little by little, she began to make the positive changes that restored her physical balance. During that time, Sally admitted that she had tried to find the son she put up for adoption for about eight to ten years, but had run into one roadblock or another. Once she was feeling better, Sally began to seriously delve into her emotional and instinctual issues—all those unfelt, scary places that had grown inside her since she was a girl. Up until that point, every therapist she'd been to had focused only on her intellect. They asked her why she couldn't stop thinking about her son—but nobody helped her unlock her hidden feelings about being abandoned as a child and then abandoning her own children (literally and metaphorically).

Sally enrolled in a powerful program for inner change—the Quadrinity Process at the Hoffman Institute, which I'll tell you more about shortly—and there she got in touch with all of the secrecy, shame, and anger that had been tapping her adrenals and causing her anxiety. Ultimately, Sally found the right avenue to find her now-adult son and the right help for her daughter, which included looking at her own mothering through a different lens. It included forgiving herself and her mother—and her grandmother. After fifty years on the planet, Sally finally began to undo all the damage she had inherited from her childhood, and her physical body reacted to the release by letting go of its defensive posture. She was no longer plagued by anxiety or hormonal symptoms and her fatigue and fuzzy thinking never came back. Today Sally is healthy, lean, and actively engaged in her own—and her children's—healing. "I never knew there could be any other way," she says. "I now realize that my pervasive anxiety came from being cut off from my own essence. No one ever honored what I thought was important—touch, unconditional love, mothering—and it took a lot of psychic energy to stuff all that need away. It was physically exhausting. It took years, and a lot of work, to finally come out. But it all started when I began to heal my physical symptoms. All of a sudden I felt in my core that there were other possibilities."

Peeling Back the Layers

Like Sally, you have many pieces that fit into your individual health puzzle—some of them are physical, others are intellectual, emotional, and spiritual. Figuring out the shape and texture of these pieces is sort of like peeling an onion. Up until now, the pages in this book have been dealing with the first layer—your core imbalances. This is far and away the most crucial first step of any long-lasting wellness plan because quite often emotional and psychological issues are compounded or triggered by physical imbalances and vice versa. For instance, if you have a dietary sensitivity to gluten and you begin each day with a bagel or a bowl of cereal, you are going to trigger a biochemical chain reaction that keeps you craving carbs all day. You'll simply kill for carbs! And, like so many of my patients, this inability to stop eating carbs leads to a downward emotional spiral that only makes the bingeing—and the self-blame—worse.

If you think about it, it's not surprising that food is such a powerful link in the connection between our physical and spiritual selves. In his book *It Must've Been Something I Ate,* food critic Jeffrey Steingarten aptly measures the emotional weight that our meals are made to carry. "In all of Nature's kingdom, only mammals, female mammals, nourish their young by giving up a part of their own bodies," he writes. "For us, food is not just dinner. Our attitudes toward food mirror our feelings about mothers and nurturing, about giving and sharing, about tradition and community—and whether the natural world seems inherently benign or hostile."[1]

Listen to my patient Kathy as she describes this typical no-win situation:

"I wake up feeling slightly queasy and want something solid for breakfast, so I eat a toasted bagel. By the time I get to work, I'm still feeling hungry. When a couple of colleagues go out for coffee, I join them and buy a danish. As I eat the danish, I start feeling guilty because I know it's fattening, but it just tastes so good. I vow not to eat lunch to make up for it. By 3ε β,Ι'm exhausted and starving, but I force myself to wait until I get home. When I get home, I basically clean out the cabinets and the fridge: chips, cookies, leftover pasta, yogurt. Whatever I can get my hands on. I can't stop myself. I eat until I'm stuffed and then I spend the rest of the night hating myself for doing it. I feel depressed, bloated and, strangely, sort of wired. I think constantly of making myself throw up, but I don't. Instead, I pinch the rolls of my stomach, disgusted. I promise myself that 'tomorrow I'll be good.' I vow to eat only salad for the next five days. But then the next morning, I wake up and the same thing happens. I have no self-control!"

Kathy had no idea that she was suffering an adrenal imbalance and gluten sensitivity, made worse by a neurotransmitter roller-coaster ride triggered by her binge eating—a cycle of soaring cortisol followed by a serotonin crash. Once we got her on the right eating and action plan, she began to eat protein for breakfast and lunch, watched her gluten and simple carb intake, and took the right supplements. Within weeks, Kathy was no longer hitting the fridge at the end of the day like a ravenous wolf. She began to understand that her "weakness" was not the fault of lackluster willpower: She suffered from a sensitivity to gluten that contributed to her need to eat certain foods. Did this solve her compulsive eating challenges completely? No, of course not, because Kathy is a complex and unique woman with a complicated health puzzle—like all of us. But it was a start, and it gave her the energy to peel back the next layers, exploring her emotional, intellectual, and spiritual selves. She continues that journey to this day.

I recommend reading this section during the first two weeks of The Core Balance Program, while you follow the Essential Eating and Action Plan. As you begin your customized eating and action plan during the last two weeks, you can decide to experiment with certain concepts or therapies then or wait until you've completed the full four weeks. Or you can take these steps whenever you feel fit and well enough to go to the next level. And go there you should, because as hard as you are working to heal your physiological imbalances that cause stubborn weight to stick, you won't keep weight off or stay in balance very long if you don't address the deeper emotional challenges that undermine your balance.

The Endless Conversation

Perhaps the easiest way to grapple with this idea is to remember the idea of a conversation: think of everything you eat, absorb, breathe, think, believe in, experience, do, or don't do as voices that participate in the conversation happening all the time inside you. Your physical body and all it entails participates, but—in this scenario—so do your thoughts and emotions. They are simply other forms of input among many that the body must process, similar to the way it metabolizes food. The question you must answer when it comes to your emotional health is: How does your body process your emotions and thoughts? Do you efficiently "metabolize" them, using the good and eliminating the bad? Or do you hold on to this input, storing it away, as the body holds on to fat to insulate itself from threat? Do you know where this conversation began? Is the voice in your head your own, or that of your parent or other caregiver? Remember that your conversation is uniquely yours: We all know that certain events are stressful for everyone, like death, divorce, financial worries, and illness, but we all react to them differently. And of course certain stressors are different for every woman. One woman might go into full stress mode at the mere thought of getting up and speaking in front of an audience, while another looks forward to it.

Remember: stress is medically defined as any trigger that precipitates a fight-or-flight response, or in my words, any informational input that adds a new burden to your internal conversation. And some of these triggers may be buried so deep you barely know they're there. If we look at Core Balance, which includes maintaining your optimal weight for the rest of your life, as the product of your internal conversation, then sustaining Core Balance for life comes down to the ease and speed by which all information relevant to you is exchanged. If the conversation is muddled, one-sided, or disrupted, as it is when you have a physical core imbalance, your health and weight will suffer. But your conversation will also get disrupted, and your health will also suffer, if the psychological information being exchanged is intrinsically, chronically stressful. In other words, if the conversation is loaded with painful personal events, memories, or negative thoughts and feelings, you'll be constantly triggering the brain to initiate the stress response and interrupt the informational flow.

In the book *Healing Mind, Healthy Woman,* Dr. Alice Domar estimates that the average woman experiences about fifty brief fight-or-flight episodes a day due to stress![2] And this problem is compounded by the tendency for women to react to life stress by internalizing it. Internalized stress leads to fatigue, depression, insomnia, IBS, and chronic pain, and, of course, stubborn, toxic weight. In other words, all that stress, all those emotional issues, get stuck in your tissues. Or as the title of one of my favorite books sums up: *Feelings Buried Alive Never Die.* How people cope with stress—both internal and external—has proven to be a significant factor in their longevity. As I tell my patients, the one common characteristic of people who live to be 100 or more is the tendency to be able to move on from stress. This doesn't mean living a stress-free life. It means facing adversity, grieving, and letting it go, moving the stress out of your tissues, so you can be the joyful, balanced person you were born to be.

For this reason, I've come to believe firmly that if you don't clean your emotional house, eventually you will get drawn back into old, sticky, negative patterns, lose your Core Balance, and put back on all the defensive weight you lose. Backsliding into these unhealthy emotional patterns that trigger physiological imbalances is the real reason why so many successful dieters regain lost weight. It's not that they are bad or undisciplined (after all, they had the discipline to lose the weight in the first place); it's the pull of entrenched (and often inherited) biochemical wiring and emotional ruts. Like the chicken or the egg—no one's sure which comes first. The secret, of course, is to heal them both!

Often, emotional healing requires more professional intervention because most of us aren't aware of how deep and how entrenched our negative patterns are or what to do once we become aware. In fact, we may not even realize there are any dysfunctional patterns. We may just think, *This is who I am. This is what I do.* (To get you started thinking about the patterns that may be affecting you, I've listed some common dysfunctions on page 232.) The big "Aha!" moment comes when you realize that everything is connected. Your emotions and your thoughts are just as influential, and just as connected to your core balance, as, say, cholesterol levels or overwork or the bag of chocolate chip cookies in the back of the cabinet. In fact, your feelings about the chocolate chip cookies are as important to your core balance as whether or not you actually eat them.

Self-Destructive Behavior Patterns

- **Codependency:** being psychologically addicted to or dependent on another person in an unhealthy way; making excuses and changing one's own behavior to enable poor or addictive behavior in someone else; changing one's behavior out of fear of losing another's affection, love, or presence

- **Transference:** process through which emotions and desires originally associated with one person (like a parent or sibling) are unconsciously shifted to another person

- **Avoidance:** changing behavior to avoid difficult or confrontational emotions, situations, or relationships

- **Control:** exercising authoritative or dominating influence over others

- **Perfectionism:** being displeased with anything that is not perceived to be perfect or that does not meet extremely high standards

---

And that's the big monkey wrench! Often your current feelings about a seemingly neutral object like a chocolate chip cookie are loaded with meaning from forgotten childhood experiences, for better or for worse. If you associate chocolate chip cookies with warm kitchens and baking with a loving mother, you will have a different attachment to those cookies as an adult than a woman who was spanked each time she stole a cookie from the cookie jar or a woman who was never allowed cookies at all. You may not be conscious of why you feel the way you do (memory is a slippery thing, after all); all you may know is that you feel either cozy and safe or vaguely guilty or insatiable when confronted with a chocolate chip cookie. And this will influence whether you eat chocolate chip cookies at all, when you eat them, and how many you have to eat. Your emotional response is conditioned from your childhood experience—just as Pavlov's dogs were conditioned to salivate whenever the doorbell rang. We learn as children how to behave by watching our parents and caregivers. We adopt and adapt our own behavior to earn love from them. As adults, we may unconsciously continue this behavior, even when it no longer serves us. As Sally's story demonstrates, if we grow up feeling abandoned, we unconsciously reenact the abandonment or overcompensate with codependent behavior. We echo behavior that was normal and acceptable for us in childhood—even if that behavior puts us into direct conflict with who we are as adults. In other words, some of us are unwittingly living a life that is either a tribute or a reaction to our parents. It's not really who we are at all. It's a masquerade—and with time it takes its toll on every layer of our health. Andrew Harvey, the religious scholar and writer, describes it like this:

"Very few, if any, of us develop entirely healthy egos; mostly our ego development is conditioned by parental, social, and religious restrictions. Many of us also will be marked at an early age by various forms of trauma—whether abuse or abandonment or other forms of psychological difficulty. In some cases this experience of trauma will be so severe that any further unfolding of the personality will be aborted; in most cases, wounds will be afflicted on the psyche around which defenses will be built like hardened scars. These in turn will come to seem essential parts of our innate character—and not 'accidental traits' that a great deal of inner work can dissolve and undo."[3]

So where do we begin? It's pretty simple, actually. In order to lift the burdens of emotional baggage that disrupt your internal conversation, we need to begin improving the kind of information that gets exchanged and the speed of the conversational flow. The easiest place for most women to begin is with the body. And the good news is you've already started! By following the Core Balance Eating and Action Plans you are already changing your internal biochemical conversation for the better. Now it's time to go further.

Healing the Conversation

Dr. Candace Pert, in the *Molecules of Emotion,* describes a disrupted conversation between thoughts and physical response as a "feedback loop that's gone out of control."[4] One way to promote healing and restore lifelong balance is to figure out a way to break any dysfunctional feedback loops and encourage a healthier conversation. This is where many alternative and talk therapies come in. Biofeedback is a medically proven therapy that trains patients to use thoughts to influence their nervous system responses. Essentially, biofeedback helps us recondition our patterns of reaction to stress by teaching us how to rewire our autonomic responses through repetitive exercises. Hypnotherapy works on this concept as well, and, importantly, so do meditation and many forms of mindful exercise, like yoga and tai chi. Then there's the range of practices known as energy healing: if you simply exchange the word "information" for "energy," you will begin to understand how these therapies work. Acupuncture, Reiki, massage, craniosacral therapy, Rolfing, emotional freedom techniques (EFT), and other modes of healing energetic work strive to open up channels of communication in the body and influence the flow of information—or energy—that's being communicated. These therapies will also help you understand how your biography becomes your biology by getting you back in touch with your essence. What matters most is that you find therapies that work for you and your individual needs.

In addition to following the Core Balance Diet, I encourage you to investigate the holistic therapies listed in the Appendices that work with touch, emotional freedom, and energy. These techniques cultivate the positive in the mind-body connection and help the body process and release the negative—toxic emotions and blocked energy—from your tissues. There is a lot of research out there, and most of it concludes that the power of touch is real. Touch therapy is known to lower heart rate and blood pressure and improve recovery rates; one study from Duke University in North Carolina showed that touch can cut levels of stress hormones, increase levels of melatonin, and boost serotonin.[5] Hugging increases the levels of oxytocin in the blood (the "love" hormone synthesized by the hypothalamus). Hugging is a good example of how the power of touch can help guide the biochemical conversation back on to a healthier track, and other massage, touch, and energy therapies work along the same lines. Any practice is worth pursuing if it connects you to the most important emotional "foods": love of others, connection with nature, connection with animals, and connection with spirit.

As physical creatures, we like to linger in the realm of the body—we prefer to see results in tangible form. When you have physical symptoms, it's easy to know when they are getting better. Emotional healing is a bit harder to measure. Sometimes we feel a lot worse before we feel better; other times we make great strides but then fall back into old habits when we are under acute stress. This is normal. It happens to everyone—I imagine it even happens to the Dalai Lama. Eventually, however, emotional healing leads to a deep and lasting transformation of your spirit that will nourish and sustain your core balance, regardless of life events. Your spiritual self may not be as familiar to you as your body and your mind (that is, your thoughts and emotions), but she does exist, whether you know her or not.

Many women are strangers to their spiritual selves. One of my patients reacted to this idea by saying, "Are you kidding? I don't have a spirit!" As I told her, every person resides in a house with all of these rooms—body, spirit, intellect, and emotions—but some of the doors are shut. Emotional healing is meant to throw all the doors of all the rooms in your house wide open so a fresh breeze can blow through. That breeze is the energy that connects you to all living things and gives you a sense of being part of something larger than yourself. You can call this energy God, or love, or chi, or *prana*—even "the Force." The important thing is that you learn to trust in it. It is the voice of your own authentic self—the you that is free from your painful legacies and inherited trauma.

When it comes to addressing toxic emotions that threaten your Core Balance, you may be entering into deep, fearful water. And this is where that great deal of inner work—and honesty—is required. Each woman has a different life story, different family histories, and different relationships that shape her inner landscape. The trials and tribulations we carry with us from childhood are the mysterious pieces in our health puzzles. Until we learn how our past experiences have shaped us and how to fit these experiences into our puzzles, the picture will never be complete. When we are dealing with weight gain—particularly a lot of weight gain—these past experiences are always involved, whether you are aware of them or not. Many women gain weight to physically insulate themselves from their emotional pain; other women gain power and solidity by getting big, even when they feel small and powerless inside. The point is, weight loss is more than a physical process. Weight loss is the byproduct of healing your core, and that means healing all the parts of yourself and working constantly to keep them whole. If you don't open your heart and mind to this truth, your issues will remain in your tissues—no matter how much weight you lose and relose—sabotaging your core balance and keeping you from real happiness.

The Quadrinity Process

At my practice, I refer many of my patients who are ready to the Quadrinity Process at the Hoffman Institute. I have been through it myself and it was the most profound emotional healing experience I've ever encountered. The Quadrinity Process addresses all four corners of health, all the rooms in your house, at once—that's the "quad." It helps the body register emotional change at a cellular level and changes the mind-body conversation for good. It stays with you, permanently altering how you are with yourself and with everyone around you. It reconnects you with your authentic self.

The Hoffman Quadrinity Process is an eight-day residential course designed to inspire powerful personal change. Participants work in small ratios with a band of trained staff members in a retreatlike atmosphere. Before entering the program, you must fill out an extensive, comprehensive questionnaire that goes over every aspect of your physical, mental, and spiritual health. Teachers read these questionnaires carefully before you begin, so upon entering the process they already have an in-depth understanding of your issues. No electronics, newspapers, cell phones, or extraneous reading material is allowed—no distractions from getting in touch with your primary creative force. Through certain physical and psychological exercises, soothing rituals, and plenty of time to reflect and journal—I myself wrote pages and pages—the Quadrinity Process opens all your inner closets and clears out the clutter of beliefs, distortions, and emotional needs adopted from early life experiences; misperceptions that block our ability to be fully present and open to life's creative energy. Many of these beliefs come from something Hoffman founder Bob Hoffman calls "negative love syndrome," or the tendency all children have to try and win parental affection by imitating their parents' moods, behaviors, and attitudes, including their negativities. Upon graduation from the Process, you gain the community and tools you need to heal the self-sabotaging effect of negative love and to finally let go of what is not working for you. You emerge fully integrated—your physical, emotional, intellectual, and spiritual aspects in balance—and finally, truly, free.

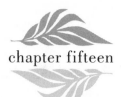

chapter fifteen

REVISING YOUR
NEGATIVITY SCRIPT

I saw a patient at the clinic the other day—attractive, successful, professional—someone who, if you judged her by appearance only, looked as if she had the world on a string. But once the door to my office closed and we began talking, another side emerged. As this patient answered my questions, it became clear that she was suffering. First we discussed her physical symptoms, which had to do with GI issues, joint pain, and fatigue. She admitted to frequently stealing a catnap on the floor behind her desk because she was so tired after lunch. She had come to see me because lately the fatigue was worse and her weight was creeping up: her workouts made her feel more tired, instead of refreshed, and she had barely any energy to get through the evenings with her family. Her mother had recently been diagnosed with Hashimoto's disease (a thyroid disorder) and she was concerned that something might be wrong with her thyroid, too.

As I dug a little deeper, this patient, whom I'll call Anna, also revealed that even though she was a highly accomplished woman, she had very little joy in the day-to-day. She expected a great deal from herself and everyone around her—and though she didn't come right out and say it, I could sense she was a serious perfectionist, like so many women these days. "If I don't exercise every day, I feel disgusting," she told me, offhandedly. When I said that "disgusting" was a pretty strong word, she shrugged. When I asked her if she had any hobbies or activities that were purely pleasurable, she replied, "Not really." I then began to explain the principles behind Core Balance and the possible imbalances she might be dealing with. I ordered all the appropriate diagnostic tests and suggested some supplements and specific diet and lifestyle changes, which she seemed very eager to try.

Up to this point, Anna was willing to try everything I had suggested and comfortable with the parts many patients find challenging, like diet changes—this particular woman had no difficulty with self-discipline. But as the appointment drew to a close, I gently added that she might want to investigate her emotional and spiritual patterning and how that might be impacting her symptoms. She visibly bristled and became very defensive. I explained to her everything I've told you so far, and added that certain stuck emotions and thoughts might possibly be contributing to her exhaustion and her perfectionism; it might be useful to know what they were, where they came from, and, eventually, how to move past them. Anna was dubious; in her mind, there was nothing to explore. Her family life had been "average—nothing special." But she listened as I explained. I ended by asking, "What kind of conversation do you have with yourself when no one else is listening?" She couldn't really say. So I sent her home with homework. I asked her to try and catch the voice in her head talking to her—the voice of her thinking mind—and write down what it said.

When Anna came in six weeks later, she sheepishly told me, "I had no idea I was such a bully. I never let up." We then had a conversation, which became an ongoing conversation at each visit, about how she could investigate this further. As Anna began to get into her emotional self, she remembered how high her father's expectations of her were. She told me about one instance of bringing home her sixth grade yearbook. Her father glanced at it and said, casually, "I see you didn't join any clubs." By the time Anna graduated from high school, she ran the yearbook, sang in the choir, played on several teams, and was an active participant in a variety of clubs. She was also the valedictorian of her class—yet she had never made the connection between her need for accomplishments and that one comment until she went through the healing process. She also began to realize the impact of only seeing her father only on weekends (her parents had divorced when she was very young). He was not a naturally affectionate or loving man, and so Anna unconsciously behaved in a way that would elicit the most praise from him as quickly as possible. It took a lot of unraveling for Anna to begin to understand that the voice that had been driving her actions all those years had never been her own—it was her father's. No wonder she felt exhausted: For years she'd been marching to someone else's tune.

What Does Your Script Say?

Most of the women I meet, including myself, have an endless loop of negative thoughts that plays in our heads, a negativity script scrolling on our inner teleprompter that was written so long ago, and plays so continuously, that most of us are hardly aware it's there. Personally, before I did the Quadrinity Process, my negativity script played loudest in the wee hours of the morning when I couldn't sleep. The negativity script eats up an incredible amount of energy, goodwill, and self-esteem. Feeding this well of negativity often leaves us with an insatiable emotional hunger, which we frequently misinterpret as physical hunger (especially if our biochemical conversation is off). This script is the sound of your inner conflict, and the louder it plays, the more stressful it is on your body.

You may be tempted to think you don't have a negativity script, like Anna, but let's try this exercise. Below, I've listed just a few of the most universal statements that I hear from my patients. Read them and circle any that sound familiar—any that you've ever said about yourself.

- If I could lose weight, I'd be happy.

- I hate the way I look. How did I let this happen?

- I hate my hair/skin/legs/breasts/thighs [fill in your own body part].

- I have to do it all myself. Nobody gets it.

- Nothing looks good on me.

- My life is such a mess.

- If it's not perfect, why bother?

- Bad things always happen to me.

- Nobody loves me.

- I'm a wreck.

- It figures.

- I feel so unappreciated.

- I don't have any time for me.

- I can't do anything right.

- I can't trust anyone.

- I'm lazy.

- No one will ever love me/want me because I'm so fat.

- I feel so unattractive.

- My life is over.

- Everything feels out of control.

- I'm old.

- I'm ugly.

- I'm a slob.

- I have nothing to give anyone.

- I wanted to do so much more with my life.

- I'm just so tired/angry/anxious/sad.

- I'm a _____ [pig, idiot, loser, liar, faker, worrywart, shrew, bad mother, bad wife, bad friend—fill in your own self-criticism].

How many of these statements sound like something you've said to yourself? How often do you find your inner voice (the sound of your intellect) giving you a good drubbing? Now take another minute to circle any of the following statements that you feel are sincerely true about you:

- I am an amazing woman.
- I take terrific care of myself.
- I am getting the love/appreciation I deserve.
- I set clear and firm boundaries.
- I am sexy.
- I am beautiful.
- I am a great daughter/wife/mother/friend.
- I appreciate the here and now.
- I am a good friend to others.
- I take time to play every day.
- My actions reflect my values.
- I'm capable of providing for myself.
- I'm honest with myself and others.
- I am my own best friend.
- I know how to say no.
- I'm good enough.
- I've accomplished a lot.
- I know how to relax.
- I am worthy of love/money/commitment/pleasure/_____.
- I know who I am.

- I can trust myself.
- I try my best most of the time.
- I have nothing to feel guilty about.
- Things are good.
- I am content.
- I am happy.

How do the two lists compare? If you circled many more positive statements than negative statements, congratulations! You are one of the very lucky few and you've probably done a lot of work to get here. The vast majority of women are far more familiar with negativity—and though it may surprise you to hear me say it, that's not necessarily a bad thing in itself. In fact, it's one of the ways that females bond—by sharing our mutual disappointments in ourselves, our appearance, and our lives. It lends us humility and has other useful aspects for society. As subversive as it sounds, my suspicion is that negative thinking lends us compassion and the ability to plan—characteristics that make us uniquely human. At one point in our collective history, this tendency may have even been a survival tool. Strong negative feelings about one's self and one's abilities keep a member of a society weak and dependent on the group, a useful thing when leaving the group could lead to starvation and death, or when a family's or society's survival depends on a strong matriarchal web and keeping the population of the group high. Today, seeing our faults clearly promotes change and growth and can propel us into taking beneficial action to help ourselves.

But there's one important link missing here: whether or not what you perceive about yourself is true. In some cases it may be—perhaps at heart you really are untrustworthy or greedy or lazy. Or perhaps—and this is the case far more often than not— it's just your thinking brain repeating words and phrases that have no basis in reality but have come to have meaning for you. Do you, like Anna, have a negativity script written by someone else that you are living out, whether you like it or not? If you don't, you are one of the rare exceptions. A more likely scenario is that living with your negativity script feels so normal, you can't imagine any other way to be.

Sometimes the negativity script is written from wounds inflicted in childhood. Other times it contains echoes of things other people have said about you that you think are true. And most sinister of all, some of its self-abasements are the result of a kind of mass cultural brainwash by advertisers and marketers who profit from women's dissatisfaction with themselves. There is a multibillion-dollar industry out there selling women false and unattainable images of who they should be and keeping them from celebrating who they really are. (More on this in the next chapter.) In other words, the negativity script comes from everywhere: your past, your subconscious, your relationships, your culture. And once you have internalized these thoughts, they become influential participants in the mind-body conversation, changing your biochemistry and your tissues.

The negativity script wouldn't be a big deal if we didn't secretly believe all those terrible things we say about ourselves. But we do. Without a meaningful, powerful counter to these negative thoughts, is it any wonder that they become what you believe about yourself deep down inside? We unwittingly set a place at the table for these core negative beliefs and they keep us stuck, frustrated—and often fat. And who can blame our loyal bodies from trying to insulate us from this negativity in the only way they know how? Think about it! It's like trying to juggle all your plates in the air while a heckler stands on the sidelines telling you how badly you're doing it. What a crazy thing to sign up for! And we all do it! That is, until we come to a point in our journey where we just don't want to do it anymore. For many women, this juncture coincides with menopause—it's one of the many gifts that transition has to offer. But it can happen whenever you are ready to do the inner work that real transformation requires. My sincere hope is that that moment is now.

Your negativity script can change. Just as you can "talk" to your cellular DNA with food, you can "talk" to your conditioned psychological responses through different kinds of therapies and change them. But you have to take the time to unearth the root cause. It takes a lot of work, but if you do it, you'll find that the internal heckler finally shuts up. You just don't have to listen to her anymore. You will come to see that you have a choice in how much meaning you attach to those self-defeating thoughts; how much power you give those childhood experiences; and whether or not you find strength and validation from within or continue to allow others to tell you who you are and what you are capable of.

This concept can be put into cold, hard scientific terms, such as "cognitive restructuring." Retraining the mind to let go of negative thoughts has its roots in cognitive therapy, which was first developed by Aaron T. Beck, Ph.D. At its best, learning how to think differently puts us on the right track to changing how we feel, which changes our biochemical state, which in turn changes our physiology. This is the mind-body connection at work—but be careful when it comes to dealing with the thinking mind. Often we engage the intellect without moving on to integrating the spirit, the emotions, and the body. Cognitive restructuring is a proven scientific therapy for revising your negativity script—it's a great place to start this process—but I encourage you not to bypass other forms of alternative healing, as we discussed in the former chapter.

The Power of Positive Thinking

I bet you expect that I'm going to tell you to stop thinking negative thoughts because they attract negativity to you (à la the secret behind the blockbuster book *The Secret*) and replace them with positive affirmations. Affirmation is the practice of repeating supportive sayings to yourself, such as "I am talented and beautiful and I will succeed." Like a mantra, these sayings sink into your subconscious, countering your negativity script and drowning it out. Do good things necessarily follow? I'm sure. It stands to reason that if you turn the volume down on your negativity script, it requires less energy and maintenance, which certainly helps you cope. For some, though, this just isn't enough.

I think daily affirmations really can work wonders for your emotional state, especially when used in combination with other mind-body therapies, like EFT, but only if you come to truly believe them—and that can be a big step for some women. Some practitioners will tell you it doesn't matter whether you believe them or not, as long as you continue to say them; like hypnosis, the repetition will seep into your consciousness and eventually you will believe. But I think that your emotional self knows when it's being sold a bill of goods. Affirmations may help you feel better temporarily (not a bad thing), but you also have to debunk the untruths in your negativity script. In other words, the power to believe good things about ourselves is directly related to how firmly we hold the beliefs about what is bad. We have to do both: affirm the positive and unravel the negative to get at where and how and why our negativity script was written.

Let's look at a typical negativity script cycle. At every step, I will point out what's going on in this woman's thinking by referring to certain common "cognitive distortions." These distortions, over time, transform temporary negative thinking into disruptive, dysfunctional thinking.

Janet has had a busy week. She's been on the road for her job for the past two days and has gotten home just in time to drive her son to soccer. She sits in the car before the game as he warms up, not wanting to hover like her mother did. This brief respite gives her a moment to focus on her car, which has been her mobile office during her trip. Used cups and food wrappers are on the floor. Her son's lunch box is open in the backseat, and it smells stale. Crumpled paper, hair elastics, and other debris cover the floor. Janet thinks, *I'm such a slob! A big, fat, slob* (labeling and mislabeling). She remembers that she hasn't done laundry in over four days. Her mother did laundry every night—and ironed. Janet remembers how wonderful it was to get a pile of freshly pressed clothes at the foot of her bed each evening. Her own kids never have that. They're lucky if she folds the laundry; she just doesn't have the time. Usually they have to sift through the jumbled pile of washed clothes themselves. She's such a terrible mother (magnification). True, she has been away for two days and landed a huge client—but if only she could be more organized at home things would be under control (disqualifying the positive). What's her problem? Other people seem to manage just fine, but she can't keep it all together (overgeneralization). If her son loses the soccer game this afternoon, it will probably be because his mother is such a wreck (personalization). Things just have to change, she thinks. She has to try harder, find more time (all-or-nothing thinking).

Janet puts her head against the steering wheel, craving a glass of wine. She reaches into the backseat to fish out the uneaten sandwich from her son's lunch box.

Cognitive Distortions

- **All-or-nothing thinking:** You see things in black and white; there is no gray. If your performance falls short of perfect, you see yourself as a total failure.

- **Overgeneralization:** You see a single negative event as a never-ending pattern of defeat.

- **Mental filter:** You pick out a single negative detail and dwell on it to the exclusion of all else.

- **Disqualifying the positive:** You reject positive experiences by insisting they "don't count" for some reason or other.

- **Jumping to conclusions:** You make a negative interpretation even though there are no definite facts that convincingly support your conclusion.

- **Mind reading:** You arbitrarily conclude that someone is reacting negatively to you and don't bother to check it out.

- **False predictions:** You anticipate that things will turn out badly and feel convinced that your prediction is an already established fact.

- **Magnification or minimization:** You exaggerate the importance of things or you shrink things until they appear tiny, whichever makes you feel bad about yourself.

- **Emotional reasoning:** You assume that your negative emotions reflect the way things really are.

- **Should statements:** You motivate yourself with shoulds and shouldn'ts, with the emotional consequence of guilt. Or you direct should statements toward others and feel anger, frustration, and resentment.

- **Labeling and mislabeling:** You attach a negative, emotionally loaded label to yourself or someone else.

- **Personalization:** You see yourself as the cause of some negative external event for which, in fact, you were not primarily responsible.

(Adapted from Dr. David Burns, *The Feeling Good Handbook*. New York: William Morrow and Company, Inc. 1989)

Now your negativity cycle may look like Janet's, or it may be completely different. The interesting thing here is to note how much negativity was triggered by a very minor event (the dirty car). At each turning point, Janet's thinking mind led her deeper into a negative place, one that shows unfinished business between Janet and her mother. Never once did Janet counter with a positive thought. She did not "count" in her motherhood tally the fact that she'd raced back from her business trip to take her child to his game or that she was contributing to her family's income as well as taking care of the children (unlike her mother). More profoundly, Janet was falling into a self-serving kind of negativity that discounted others: for instance, her partner as someone she could lean on, her son's ability to win at soccer regardless of her, or her family's self-reliance and resilience in her absence (her son had a lunch box filled with lunch by someone!). She also failed to observe that her family might be learning a valuable lesson by folding their own laundry. The unfortunate outcome for Janet was an emotional need spawned by negative thinking that translated into a physical craving for wine and a hit of food.

Luckily, there are many fantastic people out there who have done a lot of research into how to retrain the mind to let go of the negative and revise scripts like Janet's. My friend and colleague Byron Katie, author of *Loving What Is*, comes immediately to mind. She has done so much to educate people on the power of turning negative thinking around through a process of inquiry she calls The Work. Doing "the work" requires paying attention to negative feelings you have about yourself and others and then asking questions that turn these thoughts around. Famed author Julia Cameron, who wrote *The Artist's Way* in the 1990s, also offers a method of freeing our creative selves from the shackles of negativity by, among various wonderful exercises, drafting a positivity script. What these wonderful women teach is the ability to retrain your mind by cultivating awareness of your negative mind chatter—and then rescripting it into something truer. The first step, as you work through the Core Balance program, is to begin to listen to what your thinking mind is saying to (or yelling at) you.

Listening to the Mind

The first place to begin listening to your mind is to find a quiet spot and do nothing. Just hold an imaginary glass up to the wall of your mind and listen in. Meditation is very useful for this, as the mind never gets busier than when you ask it to be quiet! It helps to have a journal or some paper on hand to write down what you hear. In *The Artist's Way*, Julia Cameron recommends getting up a half hour earlier than normal and journaling at least three stream-of-consciousness pages. She calls these the morning pages. You can also use journaling as your ritual practice in your eating and action plan. As you write, I'm sure you will begin to see some patterns emerge. Are there certain negative statements that always appear? In my pages, I often wrote: "I have no time to do this."

As you begin to hear what your thinking mind is saying to you when you are quiet, try to catch it in action at other times during the day. What does it say when you are running late, or forgot something, or strayed from your eating plan? What does it say when the bills are due at the end of the month or after a parent-teacher conference? What does it say after sex? Psychotherapy is very useful in exploring the source of your negativity script—it's the fastest way to begin to revise it. So I encourage anyone struggling with toxic weight to investigate counseling, and specifically the Quadrinity Process at the Hoffman Foundation. If that's not possible for you right now, I suggest you read further on this topic (see sidebar) and begin to practice your own ways to turn the volume down.

Every woman is unique, and a practice that works for one may not work for another. However, one tried-and-true method you can begin working on now is to simply ask yourself if the negative thing you are thinking is really true or a distortion of the truth. Take Janet's thought that she's a slob. Is she really? Yes, her car is dirty after a long road trip, but whose wouldn't be? She also admits to not doing laundry for four days—hardly an eternity. Moreover, it seems she was raised in a very neat household and appreciated her mother's efforts, which might incline her naturally toward tidiness. When I asked Janet this very question, she thought about it and agreed that, no, she wasn't really a slob. She just happened to have a messy car that day! Once Janet was relieved of the need to call herself a slob, the label fell off her negativity script. She believed *more* that she was a neat person who occasionally had to deal with mess than that she was a slob. Without that label messiness had less of a hold on her; it wouldn't trigger her negativity script or her impulse to use food and alcohol for comfort. Now that's the real power of positive thinking at work!

Suggested Reading List

- *The Hoffman Process: The World-Famous Technique That Empowers You to Forgive Your Past, Heal Your Present, and Transform Your Future*– Tim Laurence

- *You Can Heal Your Life*– Louise Hay

- *No One Is to Blame*– Bob Hoffman

- *Loving What Is*– Byron Katie

- *The Artist's Way*– Julia Cameron

- *Healthy Woman, Healing Mind*–Alice Domar, MD

- *Fat is a Family Affair*– Judy Hollis

- *Change 101: A Practical Guide*–Bill O'Hanlon

- *Codependent No More*– Melody Beattie

- *Truth Heals: What You Hide Can Hurt You*– Deborah King

- *Transitions*– William Bridges

Think of your negativity script as a tape in a tape player. When it begins to play, visualize the tape player and mentally press the pause button. You can do this anytime, anywhere. It only takes a second or two. With time, I hope, you can press stop, and even eject, and never have to listen to that tape again.

Let's take a lesson out of Byron Katie's process. At home, try writing down a list of negative core beliefs that you hold about yourself (or use the ones you circled above). Julia Cameron calls these your "blurts." Now ask yourself if each statement is really true. What are the circumstances that lead you to say it? Is there a counterpoint to the statement that is more true? Katie tells her clients to ask themselves the following four questions: 1) Is it true? 2) Can you absolutely know that it's true? 3) How do you react, what happens, when you believe that thought? and 4) Who would you be without the thought? These are immensely powerful questions!

For example, say you often tell yourself how much you hate your legs. Ask yourself: Is that really, absolutely true? How does it feel to hate your legs? What happens to your mood, your body, when you have that feeling? Who would you be if you weren't the person who hated her legs? Now ask yourself if there is something more true than that thought. Wouldn't you hate to not have the use of your legs, regardless of their shape? Isn't it closer to the real truth to say that you don't like the way your legs look to you, but you appreciate what they do for you, their power and stamina and their ability to hold you up? Write down five great, true things about your legs to say to yourself when you begin to obsess over their shape. (For instance, *I walk my children to school on these legs*). As you let go of the burden of being the person who hates her legs, you may find that once your mind is free, it considers your legs quite useful and wonderful, and that your body appreciates being carried in style to the gym, to work, and toward the rest of your life.

A Walk on the Spiritual Side

The spirit is the hidden source of the most healing energy we have. It is this energy that binds the body and mind as one and all living things to one another. If your spirit is sick, no amount of physical or mental doctoring will truly heal you. When we are cut off from our spirit, our emotions are largely reactive. We feel as if they control us, not the other way around. When we have a sense of the spirit, our emotions emanate from a deeper place. We may feel very passionately, but we stop trying to use emotion as a shield or distraction. We no longer try to manipulate other people with our emotions. And, importantly, we are able to judge emotions for what they are—passing biochemical surges—and stop letting them rule our lives.

These days, many people consider spirituality and religion the same thing. But I don't. When I talk about your spiritual self, I'm talking about a sense of loving space and stillness that resides in all of us, that is collective and broad and nondenominational. Depending on who you are, you may access this space at different times: in nature, playing a sport, praying, holding a baby, meditating, or simply sitting in the sun. During these times, you are connecting to your spirit, a connection that often comes with a sense that there exists a benevolent, harmonious universal force connecting you to all living things. How you define this unifying energy is your personal decision, but drawing upon it is one of the most powerful balancing tools you have at your disposal.

One of the key ways to access the spirit is through personal ritual. All spiritual endeavors incorporate ritual—lighting candles, chanting, praying, repeating sacred texts, music, laying on of hands, honoring nature and the change of seasons, fasting, feasting, and purifying are only a few examples. I will not even try to suggest a ritual that might resonate for you; I'll only suggest that you actively seek one out. Be fearless in this and commit to as if your life happiness depended on it—because it very well might. Ritual is the practice of welcoming the spirit, and the more you repeat it, the more profound it becomes. Talk to your friends, your health-care practitioners, and people at your place of worship and find out what they are doing. Try a meditation class or go on a spiritual retreat. Be open to the universe and kind to yourself and see what miracles ensue.

Practicing Loving-Kindness

Some of us don't have a lot of tools to deal with troubled emotional states, yet all of us have the capacity to "sweeten" our minds. *Metta*, or loving-kindness, meditation was a practice taught by the Buddha to develop the mental habit of selfless love. Like all Buddhist meditations, loving-kindness can transform habituated negative patterns of mind.

The practice begins by developing a loving acceptance of yourself. Sit quietly and visualize yourself smiling, or repeat an affirmation or positive mantra or prayer, as you steadily breathe in and out. If feelings of self-loathing or unworthiness arise, know that your thinking mind and its negativity script are at work. Keep at it, continuing to bring your thoughts back to a positive image or sound. Then, when you are ready, send your prayer of loving-kindness out toward others in this order:

1. A respected, beloved person, such as a spiritual teacher

2. A dearly beloved, who could be a close family member or friend

3. A neutral person—somebody you know, but have no special feelings toward

4. A hostile person—someone you are currently having difficulty with

Take your newfound sense of loving acceptance into your life, your work, your community, and your relationships. You may be surprised to find how quickly it comes back to you.

The Core Balance Diet begins with physical changes that help to heal your physiological imbalances, but by no means does it end there as so many other diets do. In fact, I see all of the physical, emotional, and intellectual changes you've been making this month as a gateway to deep, integral changes ahead. These lasting changes are at the heart of true wellness in you—as well as in those around you and the planet we all share, because, in the end, we are all connected.

If there is light in the soul,
There will be beauty in the person.
If there is beauty in the person,
There will be harmony in the house.
If there is harmony in the house,
There will be order in the nation.
If there is order in the nation,
There will be peace in the world.

— Chinese proverb

chapter sixteen

WRAPPING IT UP

In my own life and in my 25 years of practice, I've experienced core balance as the best gift that a woman can give to herself. It is a gift that keeps on giving through thick and thin, during good times and bad, wellness and illness, prosperity and misfortune, joy and grief. The music of life is always changing: core balance gives you the resilience and energy to keep dancing, whatever the beat. Does this mean you will never miss a step or fall down? Of course not. You're human. Life happens. Everyone has days, months, and even years when the dance is a struggle. We go on vacation and overeat; we slack off exercise for a while; we face economic hardship; we leave a relationship or it leaves us; we age. As the years pass, we may fall ill, lose loved ones, or have to make infinitely difficult decisions that leave us weeping and winded, wondering if anything will ever be the same. No wellness program in the world can alleviate the often harsh reality of being human. But it can give you the tools you need to heal and stay healthy. The Core Balance Diet is designed to reveal the root strength that lies within every woman, a profound power that will get you back up again and again to dance to whatever tune is playing—and not put on weight.

Marcelle's Prescription for
ONGOING CORE BALANCE

1. Do a total body check several times a day. Scan your body, your intellect, your emotions, and your spirit. Take time to register what's going on.

2. Do not skimp on your self-care—even in times of extreme stress. It's even more important then.

3. Continue taking a daily multivitamin, EFA supplement, and probiotic.

4. If your weight begins to creep up or your clothes feel tight, go back to the Core Balance Essential Plan for a couple of weeks.

5. Work with a functional medical practitioner or health-care professional versed in integrative medicine.

6. Consider consulting an image consultant (you'll learn more about this presently) to help you look your best all the time, regardless of where your weight is at.

7. Reach out and make connections with others. Take a class or join a support group.

8. Spend some time each day doing something that is purely pleasurable.

9. Exhale. Deeply. Often.

10. Be kind to yourself. You are a luminous being walking a human path. It's not easy.

Up until now, we've talked a great deal about the changes you can expect as you begin to restore core balance to your body, mind, and soul. For most of us, the anticipation of who we will be and what we will look like at the end of the Core Balance Diet is intoxicating. It's tempting to think that if we just lose the weight, everything in our lives will suddenly be better. We'll finally get the love, money, respect we secretly know we deserve. You know how this goes! Do you have a pair of jeans or a skirt in your closet that you're saving for the day when you finally reach your goal weight? I certainly did. Or perhaps there's a trip or a class you want to take or a piece of clothing you want to buy, but you won't allow yourself to do so until you've whipped yourself into shape first. At my practice, I like to call this the waiting room effect. Many of my patients, as well as many of the other women I meet, seem to be waiting in the wings of their lives—putting off celebrating who they are at this very moment for the dream of who they will be someday.

We all see the pictures in the magazines and catalogs, the starlets on the red carpet, and wish that we had a face or a body or a marriage or a career like theirs. It is the bane of our culture that our sex seems doomed to chase an unattainable (and ever-changing) ideal of perfect beauty; to count our flaws before our virtues; and to always compare ourselves to (often retouched) photos of an impossible ideal. No matter what we look like, how deep our pockets are, how loved we are, or how much we've accomplished, we seem to never think we're enough—and this is true for all women, even those seemingly perfect females on the cover of *Vogue*. If you've ever seen a before-and-after picture of a celebrity, you know that a movie star looks very much like everyone else when she wakes up in the morning. It's just that she gets her picture taken under good lighting after sitting for four hours in Hair and Makeup. No one is perfect or has a perfect life. But media is in the business of selling advertising. Period. Marketers and advertisers will do whatever it takes to keep you yearning for the impossible. Longing motivates purchasing—after all, if you could achieve satisfaction, why would you ever need to buy another thing?

If you've read this far, you know by now that many of us use food to feed hungers that have nothing to do with physical need. A hunger for a more perfect outer appearance, or a picture-perfect life, can become insatiable. And, of course, this need for perfection works like a finger pressing the Play button on your negativity script, which, ironically, sabotages the ability to truly get well and lose weight. I think back now to all those years when my skinny skirt hung in my closet, and I realize that every morning when I opened the closet door that skirt berated and humiliated me. It made me focus on everything I wasn't at that time, instead of what I already had going for me. It was depressing and defeating to open the closet each morning—not motivating! As I said in the last chapter, dissatisfaction—with one's appearance, marriage, career—is not all bad; it can be a source of great motivation and inspiration for beneficial, even life-saving, change. But it's equally important, when talking about change and the future, not to dismiss the present.

I won't lie to you. It feels fantastic to lose those toxic pounds; it's worth every ounce of energy, time, money, and emotional commitment you put toward it. But it's not the secret to happiness. If you are in a bad marriage and you are overweight, you won't instantly have a better relationship when you're skinny. If you haven't figured out the childhood roots of your emotional burdens, you will still carry that weight regardless of what the scale says. The key to happiness is appreciating and making the most of who you are right now. Not the ideal you, but the real you. I'm sure you know women in your life who exemplify what I'm talking about. They may not be the youngest, the most beautiful, or the most shapely, but they have a special allure, a style and presence that draws people toward them. Every stage of life has its unique beauty; one of the gifts of age is the ability to embrace who you really are and what your body needs to thrive as it matures. Whether you lose five pounds or fifty on the Core Balance Diet, your inner beauty will always be there to draw on. Now, whether or not you make this beauty visible to the outside world depends largely upon the choices you make each day.

I bring this up now because, honestly, what the world sees does matter. Women have always known this: impressions count. We have been working hard on the inside to restore harmony to your physiology, balance to your thoughts and emotions, and strength to your spirit, but now I want to move to the surface and talk about the outside: the you the world sees; the wrapping on the gift you give yourself every day. Tending to your image is not vanity; it is a necessary—and enjoyable—part of self-care. Remember, everything is connected. Taking care of your outer self helps your inner self and vice versa. When we look better, we feel happier. And when we feel happier, we change our emotional state, which changes our physiology. Taking care of the outside also doesn't hurt in the compliment department, a bonus that can encourage you to stay centered and committed to the more challenging aspects of the Core Balance program (as long as you don't become too reliant on external validation!). If everyone keeps telling you how great you look, you'll stay motivated and energized to follow your Eating and Action plan.

As a functional medical practitioner, I've been trained to cultivate health in the body and mind at all times, even in the presence of grave illness. I want to take that concept to a more practical level in this chapter and teach you how to make the best of who you are, right now—regardless of whether or not you ever fit into your skinny clothes. It's time, in the words of my colleague and image consultant Julie Cunningham, to make your image work for you and not the other way around. It's time to step out of the wings of your life and take the stage, even if you haven't lost a pound.

Ready for Your Close-up

Whether you've been on the Core Balance Diet for a week or a month, you may be feeling some internal shifting—and with this shift you may be seeing an improvement in your appearance. This is a kind of magic bonus to the Core Balance program. Often the first signs that your body is responding to proper care are clearer skin, stronger, healthier nails, and restored luster and vitality to your hair. If you've noticed these changes, it is a great sign that you have accurately diagnosed your imbalance, that you are filling in any nutritional gaps, and that weight loss is soon to follow.

Your skin is the largest organ in your body and the most visible. It is linked to all the body's major functions, including the immune, respiratory, circulatory, lymph, and neurotransmitter systems. It is the body's primary defense against the elements, our greatest sensor and a unique communicator between the emotions and the body. Whatever is going on inside will quickly show up on the outside: we blush when we're ashamed, get goose bumps when we're cold, and blanch with fear. A woman's complexion is intimately connected with her feelings of self-confidence and power: it's the "face" she shows to the world. As your body returns to its natural Core Balance, you may find that certain skin conditions—like acne and dermatitis—resolve on their own; others, like wrinkles, skin discoloration, and rosacea, may take a little more pampering. To this end, I recommend starting a holistic skincare regime using organic products. This is crucial for any woman with dietary, inflammatory, or detoxification imbalances and helpful for everyone else. Artificial preservatives and additives in nonorganic products are absorbed through the skin as easily as they are from food, and they become part of the toxic load your body has to deal with, which exacerbates toxic weight gain and the aging process.

Let's do a quick skin check: walk over to a mirror and look at your face, neck, and hands. Now roll up your sleeve and look at the underside of your elbow or forearm. Any difference you see between the two is the result of aging, sun exposure, and your internal environment. Now, when it comes to wrinkles, you may think that there's not much you can do about them. You can't help getting older every year. But there is something you can do about it. Aging can be measured chronologically, but when it comes to your skin, cellular—or biological—aging is far more relevant. Cellular aging means that the DNA inside a healthy cell has become fragmented or shortened, which affects, and ultimately kills, the mitochondria inside the cell. (Remember, mitochondria are those mighty energy-making powerhouses I described in Stage I.) How well we age is based in part on how healthy our mitochondria are. And what causes mitochondria to self-destruct? No one knows for sure, but there is convincing evidence that points toward the aging effects of free radicals and inflammation, which are exacerbated by our Western diet and the chemical soup

Acute skin conditions and allergic responses, such as eczema, hives, rashes and/or unusual thickening, mottling/bruising, or mole growth are very individual. Some may indicate a more serious underlying condition. If you notice any sudden or extreme change in your skin or moles, you should make an appointment with your health-care professional.

we are exposed to in our environment. Moreover, many of the chemicals in cosmetics and creams may themselves actively damage mitochondria when you slather them on, making their claims of enhancing youth less truthful. For more information on natural alternatives and healthy skin care, please see Referrals and Resources.

Marcelle's Prescription for
CORE BALANCED SKIN

1. Cleanse your skin morning and night with a gentle, soap-free cleanser. Do not scrub! Scrubbing actually breaks capillaries and damages cell tissue, which encourages invasive bacteria. Use a wad of cotton or your fingertips. Rinse thoroughly with clean, tepid water and dry gently. Use a natural toner and moisturize when your skin is still wet.

2. Try to keep your hands off your skin unless they are clean; your fingers can transmit oil and bacteria. Don't pick blemishes—it damages tissue and permanently widens pores.

3. Use an all-natural exfoliant two to three times a week to remove excess dead skin cells.

4. Moisturize and protect with an all-natural moisturizer/sunscreen. Find a product that contains valuable topical antioxidants like CoQ10, ALA, DMAE, and Vitamin C serum. See Referrals and Resources for suggestions.

5. Use sunscreen with an SPF of 30 when out in the sun for more than fifteen minutes.

6. Discuss the usefulness of a regular facial peel with a responsible aesthetician. Glycolic or hydroxy (alpha or beta) peels can help the texture and appearance of surface skin while stimulating new cell growth underneath.

7. Consider switching to mineral-based makeup. You should be able to replace your favorite lipsticks, mascara, and foundation with chemical-free alternatives that work just as well.

8. Remember that beauty starts deep within! Follow your Core Balance eating and action plan and drink lots of fresh, purified water.

9. Additional measures: If you have made all the positive diet and lifestyle changes to support your glowing health (and skin) but still feel your outside doesn't reflect your inside, there are other steps you can take.

10. Investigate dermabrasion to resolve deep scarring and imperfections.

11. Talk to a professional aesthetician about pulsed laser technology for unwanted hair, sun damage, spider veins, rosacea, melasma, and other discoloration.

12. If your acne is not improving, talk to your medical professional about what will work best for you, and support your body by following your Eating and Action Plan the whole time.

Dressing the Part

No matter what size you are, if you aren't wearing the right clothes it will detract from your appearance. The dilemma is, what is "right"? Too many of us get our fashion advice from magazines and TV shows, without really understanding what clothes look best on our figure or harmonize with our personalities. Many years ago, I began working with Julie Cunningham, who was training specialists for an image consultant company called Color Me Beautiful. It was there that I first learned how to choose a wardrobe that worked with my blessings, even during the time when I was seriously overweight. Once I figured out which colors were right for me and which silhouettes fit my personality best, the number on the scale really didn't matter. I swear. I could rely on my clothing to work for me, even during stressful times, even when I didn't feel my best, which freed me up to stop fretting about my image and focus on more important changes. Since then, I've recommended Julie's work, now called Julie Cunningham Colors, to many, many patients—all of whom experienced a similar transformation. It is difficult to believe it until you experience it yourself, so I encourage you to try a visit with a color specialist or image consultant in your area (I've included some contact information in Referrals and Resources). With the help of an image consultant, you will learn which colors to use in makeup and clothing and which styles suit you the best. The goal is to use your clothing to your best advantage, the way the right setting brings out the luster of a diamond. Don't wait to do this! Even if you've just begun The Core Balance Diet, honor who you are today. Don't hide your light under a bushel (or the wrong clothes).

Which reminds me. Unless you really have nothing to wear, I want you to go to your closet right now and take out your "skinny" article of clothing. Now go give it to Goodwill or another needy cause—regardless of what the scale says.

And while you're at it, do a closet detox! Get rid of any other clothes that make you feel bad about yourself, as well as anything that you haven't worn in over a year. Pitch the frumpy bridesmaid's dress. Toss the T-shirt that makes you feel beefy. Lose the trendy belt that always makes you feel fat. Unburden your image in the same way you are clearing clutter from your diet, your habits, and your emotional life. From now on, you are only going to buy well-made clothing that fits, clothing that embraces who you are right now, not who you once were or who you may be someday. If you don't like the way the size sounds, cut the tag out. If your bra is too small, buy a bigger one. Allow yourself to feel and look good now and to trust in the unique, complicated conversation that is you—always changing, always growing, and learning not to be afraid to be present, just the way she is.

Now, take a bow.

The Recipes

Please note: I have written these recipes with family cooking and leftovers in mind. Quantities can easily be halved or doubled; please adjust as desired. I encourage you to freeze leftovers to have on hand for those nights you haven't gone shopping or just don't feel like cooking. If a recipe appears in your menu plan, it's okay to substitute it for a similiar meal (i.e., a dinner entrée for a dinner entrée)—and preferable to eating something not on your menu plan. It's also useful to keep leftovers on hand as an emergency snack measure for when cravings strike. If you are ravenous and about to binge, you'll be far better off reaching for leftovers of one—or any—of these healthy choices than you would chips, crackers, or sweets. And who knows? If you cook these recipes for your entire family, you may just help your loved ones get healthier and leaner over the next month, too.

Throughout the book, I've told you that you will not have to count calories or be held to any exact portion sizes. My goal is to get you to eat consiously and intuitively. On some of the following recipes, I've included serving sizes. The aim of these serving sizes is not to give you a strict regulation on what you can and cannot eat but to provide some general guidance on which to base your helping size when dividing the recipe may not be straight forward. These serving sizes are all approximate. Please use them loosely.

SNACKS

AVOCADO AND PEAR DIP

Serving Size

2 tablespoons

2 fresh average avocados, peeled and mashed

1 medium fresh pear, peeled and finely chopped

2 fresh green onions, white and green parts finely chopped

Mix all ingredients until well combined. Serve.

8 servings

CHEESE BALLS WITH PARSLEY

1½ cups cream cheese, softened

¼ cup grated cheddar cheese

¼ cup scallions, finely chopped

1 tablespoon Worcestershire sauce

½ cup parsley

Mix all ingredients together except for parsley. Form into 15 balls and roll in parsley. Refrigerate for up to three days.

15 servings

GUACAMOLE

Serving Size
2 tablespoons

½ jalapeño pepper, finely chopped

½ medium tomato, chopped

2 green onions, finely chopped

1 ripe avocado

1½ teaspoons fresh lime juice

1 tablespoon chopped fresh cilantro

Place pulp of ripened avocado, onions, pepper, tomato in medium bowl. Add lime and cilantro. Salt and pepper to taste. Mix well. Refrigerate extra for up to three days.

8-10 servings

LEMONY HUMMUS

Serving Size
2 tablespoons

1 15-ounce can chick peas

¼ cup tahini

1 clove of garlic, finely chopped

⅓ cup lemon juice (or to taste)

2 tablespoons water

1 tablespoon olive oil

Salt and pepper, to taste

Purée all ingredients.

12 servings

MINTY CANTALOUPE BALLS

1 cantaloupe
1 cup fresh mint, finely chopped
1 tablespoon lime juice

To prepare melon balls, cut cantaloupe in half, remove seeds. Using a ½ inch melon baller, scoop melon from rind. Toss with mint leaves. Add lime juice and toss well. Refrigerate 4-6 hours. Refrigerate extra.

Approximately 6 servings

OLIVE TAPENADE

Serving Size

2 tablespoons

½ cup roasted garlic*
½ cup pitted green olives
½ cup pitted Kalamata olives
3 teaspoons fresh lemon juice
1 tablespoon olive oil

* To roast garlic, place 3 whole unpeeled garlic heads in a shallow pan and bake at 350 degrees for 40 minutes or until soft. Let cool, then peel and mash.

Puree garlic, lemon juice, and olive oil. Add minced olives and mix well. Refrigerate.

12 servings

TROPICAL PROSCIUTTO ROLLS

   6 very thin slices of prosciutto
   ½ large mango cut into 6 pieces

Wrap each slice of mango with a strip of prosciutto.

2 servings

SOUPS AND SALADS

ASPARAGUS SOUP

Serving Size

Approx. 1½ cups

1½ pounds chopped asparagus
1 14.5-ounce can organic chicken broth
1 medium onion, chopped
1 cup water
1 tablespoon butter
⅓ cup heavy whipping cream
Salt and pepper to taste

In large saucepan, sauté onion in melted butter until golden. Add asparagus and stir frequently for 5 additional minutes. Add cup of water, broth, heavy whipping cream, salt and pepper. Bring to a boil. Lower heat to simmer and cover. Cook 10 minutes until asparagus is softened. Puree in small batches in blender until smooth.

4 servings

BEST EVER EGG DROP SOUP

1 14.5-ounce can organic chicken broth
2 eggs
2 green onions, finely chopped
2 thin slices ginger

In a small pan bring broth and ginger to a simmer. Drip egg mixture slowly, in a steady stream, into simmering broth. Add green onions, Remove ginger and serve immediately.

1 serving

GAZPACHO

3 cups tomatoes, very ripe, seeded and diced

2 cups red bell pepper, diced

1½ cups red onions, diced

½ cup celery, diced

¾ cup cucumber, diced

1 teaspoon garlic, minced

¼ cup red wine vinegar

1¾ cups organic vegetable juice

Pinch cayenne

1 teaspoon cumin

Mix diced tomato, peppers, red onions, celery, and cucumber together in a medium bowl. Divide the mixture in half and separate into two bowls. Add garlic and vinegar to one of the batches and puree in blender until smooth. Add vegetable juice, cayenne, and cumin to the blender. Gently blend all ingredients. Pour puree over remaining batch of diced vegetables and mix well with a wooden spoon. Refrigerate overnight. Freeze leftovers.

8 servings

MUSHROOM SOUP

Serving Size

Approx. 1 cup

3 cups fresh mushrooms, chopped

3 tablespoons butter

¾ cup chopped onion

2 cloves minced garlic

2 teaspoons wild mushroom powder

1 teaspoon dry mustard

4 cups organic chicken broth

2 tablespoons Madeira wine

¼ cup heavy cream (at room temperature)

Melt butter in dutch oven. Stir in mushrooms, onion, and garlic and cook for 15 min until mushrooms soften and mixture begins to thicken. Add mushroom powder and dry mustard. Mix well and cook for 10 minutes on low heat. Add wine and broth. Bring mixture to a slow simmer. Remove from heat and allow to cool for 10 minutes. Slowly whisk in heavy cream. Reheat gently, stirring constantly.

6 servings

POTASSIUM BROTH

3 quarts water

4 large potatoes with skin, washed well, chopped or sliced

2 cups carrots, chopped

2 cups celery

1 cup onion, chopped

Additional leftover vegetables, such as kale, chard, leeks, beets and beet tops, turnips,
  green or yellow beans

Fresh herbs. such as parsley, sage, rosemary, thyme, and garlic

2 tablespoons lemon juice, or to taste

Salt and pepper to taste

Optional: 2 teaspoons miso paste or a vegetable bouillon cube

Place all of the vegetables and herbs in a large pot and cover with water. Season with lemon juice, salt, and pepper. Cover and cook slowly for 45 minutes or until all vegetables are very soft. Remove from heat and strain through a colander, catching the liquid in a large bowl or pan. Refrigerate liquid. Warm before serving, adding miso paste or bouillion, if desired.

CREAMY PARMESAN DRESSING

Serving Size

2 tablespoons

3 tablespoons grated Parmesan

3 tablespoons mayonnaise

2 tablespoons fresh lemon juice

1 teaspoon Dijon mustard

1 teaspoon Worcestershire sauce

¼ teaspoon Tabasco sauce

Whisk all ingredients together. Refrigerate extra and use as a tasty dip for vegetable slices.

4 servings

SWEET ARUGULA SALAD WITH CHICKEN

1 cup cooked diced chicken
1 cup arugula torn into pieces
½ pear, peeled and cut into small pieces
1 tablespoon olive oil
Juice of 1 lemon
Salt and pepper to taste

Combine chicken, arugula, and pear in bowl. Toss well. Add olive oil and lemon juice. Toss again, coating well.

2 servings

EGGS

CHEESELESS ARTICHOKE OMELET

5 artichoke hearts, chopped
½ tablespoon olive oil
¼ tablespoon salt
5 eggs
6 egg whites
1 tablespoon unsalted butter
1½ tablespoons fresh, finely chopped thyme

In large skillet, heat oil over high heat. Add artichokes and sprinkle with salt. Sauté artichokes, stirring occasionally for ten minutes. Mix eggs and egg whites in bowl and combine artichokes and thyme. In large skillet, heat 1 tablespoon olive oil. Pour in egg mixture. Cook for 5 minutes. Carefully lift edges and flip frittata. Cook for one more minute. Slice into four wedges.

4 servings

CONFETTI SCRAMBLE

½ tablespoon olive oil
¼ cup red pepper, diced
¼ cup spinach, washed, trimmed, and chopped
1 tablespoon onion, diced
4 eggs
Salt and pepper to taste

Beat eggs in small bowl and set aside. In small skillet, sauté onion, pepper, and spinach until desired doneness. Pour eggs over mixture and scramble until set. Add salt and pepper to taste.

2 servings

CRAB AND SWISS PIE

1 cup Swiss cheese, shredded
8 ounces crabmeat (fresh is best)
¾ cup heavy cream
4 eggs, well beaten
½ teaspoon salt
¼ teaspoon nutmeg
1 tablespoon olive oil

Preheat oven to 325 degrees. Lightly coat deep-dish pie pan with olive oil. Place cheese in even layer over bottom of pan. Follow with an even layer of crab. Mix remaining ingredients and pour over top. Bake 40-50 minutes until knife inserted in center comes out clean. Remove from heat, slice into four wedges, and serve.

4 servings

CREAMY CHEESY SCRAMBLE

10 large eggs
¾ cup scallions, minced
4 ounces cream cheese
2 tablespoons butter
1½ tablespoons chopped shallots
Pinch salt
Pinch pepper

In medium skillet, melt butter until a light foam forms. Add scallions and shallots and sauté until tender, approximately 2 minutes. In separate bowl, whisk remaining ingredients. Pour egg mixture into skillet; cook, stirring continuously. Once eggs are cooked through, spread in pan to uniform thickness and divide into 6 even portions.

6 servings

CREAMY SALMON OMELET

2 tablespoons butter

4 eggs, beaten

½ cup cream cheese

⅛ cup sweet onion, chopped

½ cup smoked salmon, chopped

Heat butter in large skillet. Sauté onion until soft. Remove onion from pan and set aside. Pour beaten eggs into pan. As eggs set, gently lift cooked edges with spatula, allowing uncooked eggs to move to bottom of pan. Cook 3 minutes. Once egg mixture has set, add cream cheese, salmon, and cooked onion. Fold omelet in half. Remove pan from heat; allow omelet to stand for 3 minutes before slicing in half and serving.

2 servings

DELICIOUS CRUSTLESS SEAFOOD QUICHE

1 tablespoon and 1 teaspoon butter

10 eggs, beaten

1 cup light cream

8 ounces shredded cheese of your choice

¼ teaspoon black pepper

6 ounces fresh or canned crabmeat

6 ounces chopped fresh shrimp

6 scallions, thinly sliced

¼ teaspoon Tabasco sauce

¼ teaspoon salt

Grease 8" glass pie dish with ½ teaspoon butter. Mix all ingredients together and pour in dish. Bake at 350 degrees for 35-45 minutes, or until center is set. Let stand 5 minutes and slice into six even wedges. Leftovers can be refrigerated or frozen.

6 servings

EGGS FLORENTINE

4 eggs
2 cups fresh spinach, chopped
¼ cup heavy cream
⅓ cup grated Parmesan cheese
1 clove garlic, sliced

In small saucepan heat cream, Parmesan, and garlic 3-4 minutes until warm. Add spinach, stirring well. Pour mixture into large skillet. Create four evenly spaced wells in mixture. Break 1 egg into each well. Cook over medium heat until eggs reach desired doneness. Cut in half and serve.

2 servings

MUSHROOM SCRAMBLE

1 tablespoon olive oil
1 tablespoon onion, finely chopped
1 red pepper, minced
½ cup sliced mushrooms
6 eggs

Heat olive oil in large skillet over low heat. Sauté onions, mushrooms, and pepper until vegetables reach desired doneness. In separate bowl, beat eggs until frothy. Add egg mixture to pan and scramble until set. Divide in half and serve.

2 servings

NOT YOUR EVERYDAY EGG SALAD

4 hardboiled eggs, chopped

2 ounces tofu, drained and chopped

¼ cup diced celery

¼ cup diced onion

4 tablespoons mayonnaise

1 tablespoon fresh chopped dill

1 teaspoon Worcestershire sauce

Salt and pepper to taste

½ cup green peas

In large bowl, combine all ingredients and mix well. Cover and chill well. Divide in ½ and serve.

2 servings

ONION TOMATO SCRAMBLE

3 cherry tomatoes, chopped

½ medium sweet onion, chopped

2 eggs, beaten

1 tablespoon fresh basil, chopped

1 tablespoon olive oil

In small skillet, sauté onion until translucent. Add tomatoes and cook for 3-4 minutes or until tomatoes soften. Add eggs and basil. Cook, gently turning the mixture constantly, until eggs set.

1 serving

PEPPER AND ONION BREAKFAST OMELET

½ teaspoon olive oil
¼ cup chopped red or green pepper
¼ cup chopped onion
2 eggs, beaten
1 oz cream cheese, cut into small pieces

Heat olive oil in small skillet over medium heat. Sauté onions and peppers until desired doneness and remove from skillet. Add egg mixture to skillet. Top with cream cheese pieces and cooked onions and peppers. Lift corners of egg mixture, allowing uncooked portion to flow onto hot pan and cook. When eggs are fully cooked and cheese is melted, fold omelet in half. Remove from pan and serve.

1 serving

RICOTTA AND LEEK FRITTATA

2 eggs, well beaten
1 tablespoon whole-milk ricotta
1 tablespoon butter
½ leek, white part only, chopped
Salt and pepper to taste

In a small skillet, sauté chopped leek in ½ tablespoon butter for 2 minutes until softened. Remove pan from heat and allow mixture to cool. Mix all other ingredients together. Melt remainder of butter in pan. Stir in egg mixture and cook over medium heat until egg mixture sets. Wrap handle of skillet in an oven proof mitt or foil and turn oven to broil. Place skillet under broiler heat for 2 minutes or until frittata turns golden brown. Remove from heat and serve.

1 serving

SPICY FIESTA EGGS

    4 eggs
    1 yellow pepper, diced
    1 jalapeño pepper, seeded and chopped
    2 medium-size ripened tomatoes, seeded and chopped
    2 tablespoons olive oil
    1 teaspoon chili powder, or to taste
    ½ teaspoon ground cumin
    ¼ teaspoon salt

In large skillet, heat oil over medium heat. Add peppers. Cook for 2 minutes. Add tomatoes, chili powder, cumin, and salt. Cover and simmer over heat for about 7 minutes. Whisk eggs in separate bowl; add slowly into pan. Cover and cook over low heat until eggs are set. Divide in half and serve.

2 servings

SPINACH QUICHE

    6 scrambled eggs
    10 ounces washed spinach
    6 tablespoons light cream
    2 tablespoons olive oil
    ¾ cup parmesan cheese
    1½ tablespoons lemon juice
    ½ teaspoon minced garlic
    ¼ cup diced onion
    ½ teaspoon nutmeg

Mix all ingredients except onion in large bowl. In large skillet, sauté onion in olive oil until soft. Pour mixed ingredients into pan, reduce heat to low and cover. Cook until eggs have set. Gently lift cooked edges with spatula, remove pan from heat, and let sit, covered, for five minutes before slicing into thirds and serving.

3 servings

SPINACH SCRAMBLE

½ cup spinach
2 tablespoons water
1 tablespoon onion, chopped
1 tablespoon red pepper, chopped
2 eggs, beaten
½ teaspoon olive oil
Salt and pepper to taste

In medium skillet over medium heat add water and spinach. Cook, stirring until spinach wilts. Drain any remaining water from pan. Push spinach to the outer edges of pan. Add ½ teaspoon olive oil. Sauté onions and peppers until tender, slowly mixing cooked spinach in with the cooking vegetables. Add eggs and continue stirring until eggs set.

1 serving

TOMATO AND ASPARAGUS FRITTATA

½ pound fresh asparagus (thin spears work best), cut into 2-inch pieces
2 fresh sliced plum tomatoes
⅔ cup Swiss cheese
4 eggs, beaten
¼ teaspoon salt

Spray large skillet with non-stick spray. Mix all ingredients together. Cover and cook over low heat for 25 minutes or until mixture is set. Divide in half and serve.

2 servings

VEGETABLES AND SIDE DISHES

ASPARAGUS WITH A ZING

½ cup fresh asparagus spears, with tough ends removed
½ cup white medium onion, chopped
¼ cup celery, finely chopped
½ tablespoon balsamic vinegar
Pinch cayenne pepper
Salt to taste

Steam asparagus until almost completely cooked, moving to skillet when done. Add remaining ingredients and mix well. Cover and cook on medium heat until asparagus reach desired doneness. Divide in half and serve.

2 servings

BRUSSELS SPROUTS WITH MUSHROOMS

Serving Size

Approx. ¾ cup

4 cups brussels sprouts, trimmed and halved
½ pound whole mushrooms
5 tablespoons butter
½ cup chopped fresh parsley
Salt and pepper to taste
Fresh lemon juice

Cook brussels sprouts in a pot of lightly salted boiling water for 15 minutes, or until tender when pierced with a fork. Drain. Melt butter in a large skillet over medium high heat. Cook mushrooms until lightly browned and set aside. Gently add drained brussels sprouts to mushrooms, and sprinkle with parsley and lemon juice, stirring constantly. Add lemon juice to taste. Serve immediately.

6 servings

CHEESY CAULIFLOWER BAKE

2 cups chopped cauliflower

4 slices cooked bacon, crumbled

2 eggs, beaten

½ medium onion, finely chopped

2 tablespoons olive oil

1 cup grated parmesan cheese

2 cloves garlic, minced

Preheat oven to 350 degrees. Heat olive oil in large skillet. Add onions and garlic and cook until lightly browned. Remove from pan and mix with remaining ingredients in large bowl. Spray 9 x 13 baking dish with non-stick cooking spray. Pour in mixture. Bake 50-60 minutes or until golden brown. Cut into six equal squares. Refrigerate leftovers for up to three days.

6 servings

CRUNCHY GREEN BEANS

Serving Size

Approx. ½ cup

1½ cups cut fresh green beans

2 tablespoons chopped pecans

1 teaspoon olive oil

¼ teaspoon salt

⅛ teaspoon pepper

Steam green beans until desired crispiness. In skillet, sauté the pecans in oil until golden, 2-3 minutes. Drain the green beans and add to skillet. Toss well. Add salt and pepper to taste.

6 servings

CRUNCHY SNOW PEAS

Serving Size

Approx. ½ cup

1½ cups snow peas, strings removed

1½ teaspoons soy sauce (use Bragg Liquid Aminos for gluten free)

¼ teaspoon sesame oil

1 teaspoon toasted sesame seeds

Mix all ingredients well and steam to desired crispiness.

6 servings

EDAMAME MIX

½ red pepper, chopped

1 cup shelled edamame beans (if you have whole edamame, steam for about 3 minutes
   and shell beans from pod)

1 cup yellow beans, cut into thirds

Juice from 1 lime

2 teaspoons dried oregano

⅛ teaspoon sea salt

¼ teaspoon cayenne pepper

Mix all ingredients and serve. Leftovers can be refrigerated for up to three days.

4 servings

FESTIVE BLACK BEAN SALSA

Serving Size

Approx. ½ cup

1 cup black beans
1 peeled lime, segmented and cut into small pieces
1 medium tomato, seeded and diced
½ medium onion, diced
1 tablespoon balsamic vinegar
2 cloves garlic, minced
1 cup fresh cilantro, chopped
1 tablespoon flaxseed oil
¼ teaspoon salt

Mix all ingredients together. Refrigerate 4-6 hours. Serve over fish, beef, or chicken. Leftovers may be frozen.

8 servings

GREEN BEANS WITH WALNUTS AND GARLIC

1 pound fresh green beans, trimmed
2 garlic cloves, mashed
¾ cup walnuts, chopped
2 tablespoons olive oil
Tamari or Bragg Liquid Aminos, to taste

Blanch the beans for 3 minutes. Cut into small pieces. In medium skillet, heat the oil and add the garlic, beans, walnuts, and a few drops of tamari. Sauté quickly until heated through.

4 servings

ROSEMARY GREEN BEANS

1 pound green beans
2 tablespoons olive oil
3 shallots, chopped
1½ teaspoons fresh rosemary, chopped

Steam green beans until desired doneness. Set aside and allow beans to cool. In large skillet, heat olive oil. Add shallots and rosemary to skillet and sauté until shallots are tender, approximately 5 minutes. Add green beans to pan and toss thoroughly. Add salt and pepper to taste. Leftovers can be refrigerated up to three days.

4 servings

SAUTÉED GREEN BEANS

2 cups green beans, trimmed
⅓ cup water
1 chicken bouillon cube
½ cup thinly sliced onion
1½ tablespoons oil

Place onion and bouillon cube in saucepan. Add the green beans, water, and oil and bring to a boil over high heat. Reduce heat and cook uncovered until liquid is reduced to 1 tablespoon, stirring constantly. Remove from heat and let stand 5 minutes before serving.

4 servings

SAUTÉED SWISS CHARD

2 tablespoons olive oil

2 cloves garlic, sliced very thin

1 pound red Swiss chard, trimmed and sliced

1 pound green Swiss chard, trimmed and sliced

Salt and pepper to taste

In large skillet, heat oil. Cook garlic until light golden brown, approximately 2 minutes. Add Swiss chard and cook until soft. Salt and pepper to taste.

4 servings

SPINACH SALAD

1 cup spinach leaves, washed and dried

½ cup strawberries, sliced

2 hard-boiled egg whites, chopped

4 ounces chicken, cooked

⅓ teaspoon olive oil

Balsamic vinegar to taste

Toss spinach, strawberries, and egg whites. Mix olive oil and balsamic vinegar and drizzle over salad. Add chicken and serve.

1 serving

SPINACH WITH LEMON AND GARLIC

2 10-ounce bags spinach, washed and trimmed
3 cloves garlic, minced
1 to 1½ tablespoons fresh lemon juice, or to taste
1 tablespoon olive oil

In large skillet, heat oil. Add garlic and stir until garlic is lightly browned. Add spinach in small bunches. Cook 2-3 minutes or until spinach wilts. Remove from heat. Add lemon juice and salt to taste.

4 servings

SQUASH MEDLEY

1 pound broccoli florets
1 medium yellow summer squash cut lengthwise and then sliced
Juice from ½ lemon
2 tablespoons olive oil
1 garlic clove, minced
½ teaspoon dried oregano

Steam for broccoli and squash 5-8 minutes or until vegetables reach desired crispness. Combine oil, garlic, and oregano. Remove vegetables from steamer; toss with oil mixture, coating well. Drizzle lemon juice over vegetable mixture.

4 servings

STIR FRY BROCCOLI WITH GINGER

1 pound broccoli cut into bite-size pieces; discard tough stem ends

3 cloves garlic, crushed

1½ tablespoons fresh ginger, grated

1 tablespoon Bragg Liquid Amino Acids or soy sauce

Heat olive oil in heavy skillet over high heat. Add garlic and broccoli, stirring constantly until broccoli is desired tenderness. Add ginger and soy sauce, stirring gently. Continue stirring until all ingredients are heated through, approximately 1 minute.

4 servings

STUFFED RED PEPPERS

¾ pound whole-milk ricotta cheese

2 large sweet red peppers

⅓ cup kalamata olives pitted and chopped

⅓ cup chopped raw walnuts

⅓ cup grated Parmesan cheese

¼ cup minced fresh parsley

2 teaspoons lemon zest

Preheat oven to 350 degrees. Halve peppers and remove seeds. Boil peppers until crisp, tender, approximately 10 minutes. Combine all ingredients except Parmesan cheese. Mix well. Fill pepper halves. Sprinkle with Parmesan. Place peppers in baking pan. Fill pan with ¼ inch water. Bake 20-25 minutes or until heated through. Place under broiler for 2 minutes to brown top, if desired.

4 servings

TASTY TOMATOES

2 large tomatoes
1 tablespoon butter, melted
1 tablespoon Parmesan cheese, grated
¾ teaspoon garlic salt
⅛ teaspoon black pepper

Preheat oven to 350 degrees. Cut tomatoes in half. Brush with butter. Mix remaining ingredients. Spoon evenly over tomatoes. Bake for 40 minutes.

2 servings

VEGETABLE CONFETTI

2 large sweet red peppers, diced
½ cup onion, minced
2 garlic cloves, minced
¼ cup olive oil
1½ pounds fresh cut green beans, trimmed
1 tablespoon fresh basil, finely chopped
½ teaspoon salt, or to taste
½ cup shredded Parmesan cheese

In skillet, sauté the peppers, onions, and garlic in oil until vegetables are tender. Add the beans, basil, and salt; toss to coat. Cover and cook over medium-low heat for 7-8 minutes or until beans reach desired tenderness. Stir in cheese. Spread mixture evenly in pan, divide into 6 equal portions, and serve immediately.

6 servings

ZUCCHINI CAKES

1 cup grated zucchini

1 tablespoon oil

2 eggs, slightly beaten

½ clove garlic, minced

1 tablespoon onion, grated

Mix all ingredients in large bowl and divide into four equal portions. Heat oil over medium-high heat in large skillet. Drop mixture by serving portions into hot oil. Press lightly with spatula to form cake shape and cook on each side until browned and heated through.

2 servings

ZUCCHINI RIBBONS

2 medium zucchini

3 cloves garlic, crushed

2 tablespoons fresh parsley, chopped

½ tablespoon salt

1 tablespoon oil

Juice of ½ lemon

Pull zucchini into ribbons with vegetable peeler. Heat oil in large skillet and cook garlic until lightly browned. Add zucchini and salt. Stir constantly until zucchini cooks (about 2 minutes). Remove from heat and add parsley and lemon juice.

4 servings

CHICKEN AND TURKEY

CASHEW CHICKEN

6 boneless, skinless chicken breast halves
Salt and freshly ground black pepper
1 tablespoon olive oil
½ cup sliced raw cashews
⅔ cup dry white wine
¾ cup water
2 garlic cloves, finely minced
¼ cup butter
2 tablespoons fresh lemon juice

Season chicken breasts with salt and pepper to taste.

In a large skillet heat oil over medium-high heat. Brown chicken breasts on each side. Reduce the heat to medium-low, cover, and cook chicken for about 10-12 minutes or until cooked through. Remove from pan.

Heat drippings left in skillet over medium heat and add cashews, stirring, for 1 minute. With a slotted spoon, transfer cashews to a paper towel to drain. Keep any remaining liquid in pan and add wine, water, and garlic; boil until liquid is reduced by half. Remove skillet from heat, stir in butter, lemon juice, and cashews. Spoon cashew sauce over chicken and serve. Refrigerate leftovers.

6 servings

CASHEW CILANTRO CHICKEN

1 pound boneless, skinless chicken breasts, cubed

4 cups Chinese cabbage, finely shredded

1½ cups fresh cilantro leaves, chopped

¼ cup raw cashews, chopped

4 teaspoons reduced sodium soy sauce or Bragg Liquid Aminos

2 teaspoons rice vinegar

⅛ teaspoon crushed red pepper

2 tablespoons toasted sesame oil

In large skillet, heat 1 tablespoon sesame oil, add chicken, and stir occasionally for 3-4 minutes or until chicken is cooked through.

Add soy sauce, rice vinegar, remaining oil, and red pepper to skillet. Cook, stirring continuously, for two or more minutes. Remove from heat and stir in cilantro. Divide mixture into 4 equal portions and serve over cabbage. Sprinkle with cashews. Refrigerate or freeze leftovers.

4 servings

CHICKEN AND ASPARAGUS SAUTÉ

6 boneless, skinless chicken breast halves
¼ cup chicken broth
1½ pounds asparagus, cut into pieces, tough ends removed
1 clove garlic, chopped
2 tablespoons olive oil
2 tablespoons lemon juice
Salt and pepper to taste

Rub chicken breast with 1 tablespoon lemon juice and salt and pepper to taste. Cut into pieces.

In large skillet, bring chicken broth to a boil. Add chicken, stirring frequently until chicken browns, about 4 minutes. Add asparagus. Cover and cook for 5 minutes, stirring occasionally until chicken is done and asparagus reaches desired tenderness. Remove from skillet and toss with garlic and tablespoon of lemon juice. Refrigerate or freeze leftovers.

6 servings

CHICKEN CACCIATORE

1 tablespoon olive oil

3 cloves garlic, minced

1 28-ounce can crushed tomatoes

¾ cup fresh mushrooms, sliced

1 bay leaf

1 tablespoon dried oregano

2 tablespoons red wine

2 pounds boneless, skinless chicken thighs, sliced into strips

1 medium onion, thinly sliced

2 green peppers, thinly sliced

½ cup grated Parmesan cheese

Sauté garlic and chicken in oil. Cook over medium heat until chicken is evenly browned on both sides. Add onion and peppers. Stir. Add tomatoes, mushrooms, spices, and wine. Cover and simmer for 45 minutes. Sprinkle with Parmesan cheese. Refrigerate or freeze leftovers.

8 Servings

CREAMY CILANTRO CHICKEN

4 boneless, skinless chicken breast halves
1 tablespoon olive oil
4 ounces cream cheese, cubed
¾ cup heavy cream
¾ cup fresh cilantro
Juice from 1 lime
Salt and pepper

Season chicken with salt and pepper. In large skillet, brown chicken in olive oil, 3-4 minutes on each side. Remove chicken from pan and set aside. Add cubed cream cheese, heavy cream, lime juice, and ½ cup fresh cilantro to pan. Reserve ¼ cup cilantro for garnish. Stir all ingredients over medium heat until mixture is melted and smooth. Add chicken back into pan. Cover and cook on low heat for an additional 10-15 minutes or until chicken is cooked through. Sprinkle with additional cilantro. Remove from heat and serve. Leftovers may be refrigerated for up to three days.

4 servings

CHICKEN LYONNAISE

4 boneless, skinless chicken breast halves
2 tablespoons olive oil
2 cloves garlic, minced
3 tablespoons dry white wine
3 tablespoons soy sauce or Bragg Liquid Amino Acids
2 tablespoons Dijon mustard

Heat oil in large skillet over medium heat. Sauté garlic until lightly golden brown. Add chicken breasts, browning each side. While chicken cooks, combine wine, soy or Bragg, and mustard in small bowl and mix well.

Pour mixture over chicken and cover. Continue cooking, covered, for 12–15 minutes or until chicken is done. Refrigerate or freeze leftovers.

4 servings

CURRIED CHICKEN SALAD

Serving Size

Approx. 1 cup

1 pound cooked boneless, skinless chicken breasts, diced
¾ cup sour cream
½ cup apple, chopped
¼ cup celery, chopped
½ teaspoon curry powder
Salt and pepper to taste

Combine all ingredients in large bowl. Mix well. Chill before serving. Leftovers may be refrigerated for up to three days.

6 servings

EASY CHICKEN FLORENTINE

3 boneless, skinless chicken breast halves

2 tablespoons olive oil

10 ounces fresh spinach

2 cloves garlic, minced

⅓ cup heavy cream

¼ cup Parmesan cheese, grated

Heat 1 tablespoon olive oil in large skillet. Add chicken and cook until lightly browned. Cover and cook 9-12 minutes or until chicken is cooked through. Remove chicken from skillet and set aside. Add remainder of olive oil, spinach, and garlic. Cook until spinach wilts (approximately 3 minutes). Gently stir in cream and cheese. Turn heat to low, add chicken, and cook until chicken is cooked through. Refrigerate leftovers.

3 servings

GREEK STUFFED CHICKEN BREASTS

4 boneless, skinless chicken breast halves

⅓ cup feta cheese, crumbled

1½ tablespoons dried tomatoes, chopped

2 tablespoons cream cheese, softened

1 teaspoon dried basil

½ tablespoon olive oil

Place tomatoes in small bowl. Cover with boiling water. Let stand for 15 minutes. Remove from water and place between layers of paper towels to dry. Slice a pocket along the meatiest side of each chicken breast, taking care to not cut through the entire breast. Combine tomatoes, crumbled feta, cream cheese, and basil. Divide mixture into 4 portions. Place one portion of mixture into pocket of each chicken breast. In large skillet, heat olive oil over medium heat. Add chicken breasts and cook for 7-9 minutes, or until heated through. Refrigerate or freeze leftovers.

4 servings

HOMEMADE TURKEY PATTIES

1 pound turkey, ground
4 egg whites
¼ cup green onion, minced
⅔ cup dried parsley
⅜ teaspoon dried marjoram
½ tablespoon olive oil
Salt and pepper to taste

In a mixing bowl, crumble turkey. Mix in egg white, green onions, parsley, and marjoram. Add salt and pepper to taste. Shape turkey mixture into 12 small patties. In a large skillet, heat olive oil and add patties. Cook for 5-6 minutes on each side or until cooked through. Refrigerate or freeze leftovers.

12 servings

LEMON CHICKEN

3 tablespoons olive oil
4 boneless, skinless chicken breast halves
⅓ cup white wine
1 tablespoon freshly squeezed lemon juice
½ teaspoon dried dill
Pinch salt

Heat oil in large skillet. Cook chicken on both sides until a light golden brown. In medium bowl, mix wine, lemon juice, dill, and salt. Pour mixture over chicken. Cover and simmer chicken until cooked through (approximately 10-12 minutes). Remove chicken from skillet and plate. Add wine mixture to skillet and heat to boiling. Continue to boil until liquid is reduced by half. Pour sauce over chicken and serve. Refrigerate or freeze leftovers.

4 servings

NOT YOUR MOM'S CHICKEN SALAD

Serving Size

Approx. ¾ cup

1½ cups cooked chicken breast, chopped

½ cup apple, diced

¼ cup walnuts, chopped

1 cup celery, diced

1 cup green onions, chopped

1½ tablespoons balsamic vinegar

2 tablespoons olive oil

Place first five ingredients in large bowl. Using whisk, blend oil and vinegar. Pour over chicken mixture and mix well. Chill. Mix before serving. Leftovers may be refrigerated for up to three days.

4 servings

ORANGE CHICKEN STIR FRY

4 boneless, skinless chicken breast halves, cut into bite-sized pieces

1½ pound asparagus, trimmed and cut into ½-inch pieces

2 navel oranges

1 clove garlic, minced

4 tablespoons water

1 tablespoon olive oil

From one orange, grate 1 teaspoon zest and squeeze ⅓ cup fresh juice. Peel remaining orange and separate segments and cut into small pieces.

In large skillet, heat olive oil over medium-high heat. Add chicken. Stir continuously until chicken is cooked. With a slotted spoon, remove chicken pieces from skillet and set aside. Add asparagus, orange peel, and garlic to remaining juices in skillet. Cover, stirring occasionally, until asparagus reaches desired tenderness. Add chicken, orange pieces, and orange juice to skillet. Stir to incorporate all ingredients. Once mixed, spread evenly in pan, divide into 4 equal portions, and serve. Refrigerate or freeze leftovers.

4 servings

QUICK AND EASY CHICKEN

2 tablespoons olive oil

4 boneless, skinless chicken breast halves

1 14.5-ounce can Italian style stewed tomatoes

⅔ cup sliced black olives

1½ teaspoons grated lemon zest

Heat oil in large skillet. Cook chicken several minutes on both sides until lightly golden brown. Add remaining ingredients and bring to a boil. Cover, reduce heat, and simmer 18-20 minutes or until chicken is cooked through. Refrigerate or freeze leftovers.

4 servings

RED AND GREEN TURKEY STIR FRY

1½ tablespoons olive oil

1 boneless turkey breast, cut into strips and seasoned with salt and pepper to taste

1 red pepper, cut into strips

1 yellow bell pepper, cut into strips

¼ sweet onion, diced

1 pound Swiss chard leaves, stalks removed and chopped

2 tablespoons apple cider vinegar

Heat ½ tablespoon oil in large skillet over medium high heat. Sauté turkey strips for 3-5 minutes until no longer pink. Remove turkey from pan. Add remaining ½ tablespoon olive oil to pan and sauté peppers and onion until tender. Gently stir in Swiss chard to pan and toss lightly. Reduce heat to low and add vinegar. Gently stir until vegetables reach desired tenderness. Return turkey to pan and continue to stir gently until all ingredients are heated through. Divide mixture into four equal portions and serve. Refrigerate or freeze leftovers.

4 servings

SHERRY CHICKEN

4 skinless chicken breast halves, bone-in
10 green olives, pitted and chopped
2 tablespoons onion, finely chopped
1 clove garlic, minced
Heaping ½ teaspoon grated lemon peel
1 tablespoon olive oil
1 cup chicken broth
3 tablespoons dry sherry
¼ teaspoon salt
¼ teaspoon pepper

Combine olives, onion, garlic, lemon peel, olive oil, salt, and pepper in large bowl. Mix well.

Heat oven to 375 degrees. Place chicken breasts in roasting pan, meaty side up. Spread olive mixture over each breast. Roast for 30-40 minutes until chicken is no longer pink and juices run clear.

Remove chicken from pan. Place pan drippings in saucepan. Add broth and sherry, heat to boiling over medium heat. Serve over chicken breasts. Refrigerate or freeze leftovers.

4 servings

SNAPPY ONE SKILLET TURKEY DINNER

Serving Size

Approx. 1 cup

2 tablespoons olive oil
1 pound turkey slices, approximately ¼-inch thick
2 tablespoons Dijon mustard
4 tablespoons honey
¾ cup carrots, thinly sliced
1½ cups snap peas, strings removed

Pierce turkey slices several times with fork. Marinate turkey slices in honey and Dijon mustard for 20 minutes. Heat oil in large skillet. Remove turkey slices from marinade. Cook turkey slices in oil 3-4 minutes on each side until light golden brown. Add carrots, cover, and simmer for 5 minutes. Add snap peas and cook for 3 more minutes or until turkey is cooked through. Refrigerate or freeze leftovers..

6 servings

SPICY CRUNCHY CHICKEN

1½ cups cooked chicken breast, chopped

1 cup boiling water

¾ cup unpeeled apple, chopped

½ cup onion, chopped

1 teaspoon granulated chicken bouillon

2 tablespoons curry powder

1 cup raw sliced almonds, chopped

¾ tablespoon olive oil

½ cup plain, full fat or 2% yogurt

In skillet, heat olive oil, add almonds, and cook, stirring continuously until nuts are lightly browned. Sprinkle with 1 tablespoon curry powder, covering nuts completely. Remove almonds and drain on paper towels. In same skillet, sauté apple and onion until softened. Add 1 tablespoon curry powder and continue cooking over low heat for 3 minutes. Dissolve bouillon in hot water. Add bouillon, lemon juice, and yogurt to skillet. Stir continuously over low heat until mixture thickens slightly (approximately 5 minutes). Add chicken and cook until heated through. Once fully cooked, spread mixture evenly in pan, divide into 4 equal portions. Refrigerate or freeze leftovers.

4 servings

SUMMERTIME GRILLED CHICKEN

4 boneless, skinless chicken thighs, approximately 1 pound
4 yellow summer squash, quartered
⅓ cup fresh chives, chopped
1 lemon
1½ tablespoons olive oil
Salt and pepper to taste

Grate 1 tablespoon lemon zest and squeeze the juice from the lemon. Mix oil, lemon juice, and zest together. Pierce chicken thighs several times with fork. Add chicken to 2 tablespoons of above marinade, cover and refrigerate for one hour. Remove chicken from marinade. Grill or broil chicken and squash. Cook until chicken is cooked throughout and squash reaches desired doneness. Remove chicken and squash from grill. Cut each squash slice in half, then cut chicken into strips. Toss with remaining marinade. Sprinkle with chives. Refrigerate or freeze leftovers.

4 servings

SUMPTUOUS CHICKEN STEW

Serving Size

Approx. 1½ cups

1½ tablespoons olive oil
4 boneless, skinless chicken breast halves, cubed
1 medium onion, thinly sliced
4 cloves of garlic, thinly sliced
1 28-ounce can crushed tomatoes
2 medium heads escarole, chopped
2 cups cooked brown rice

In large pan or Dutch oven, brown the chicken pieces, seasoning with salt and pepper to taste. Set aside.

Sauté onion, garlic, and oregano until onion is slightly brown. Add tomatoes. Simmer for 10 minutes. Add chicken and cook for another 5 minutes or until chicken is cooked through. Add escarole, stirring until tender (approximately 5 minutes). Serve over brown rice. Refrigerate or freeze leftovers.

6 servings

SWEET CHICKEN MARSALA

1 tablespoon olive oil
1 pound boneless, skinless chicken breasts
2 Anjou pears, peeled and cut into bite-size pieces
⅔ cup Marsala wine
1 cup organic chicken broth
1 tablespoon cornstarch
2 teaspoons sage leaves, finely chopped
Salt and pepper to taste

Sprinkle chicken with salt and pepper to taste. In large skillet, heat oil over medium-high heat. Cook chicken until no longer pink (approximately 10-12 minutes depending on thickness of chicken).

Remove chicken from pan. Add pears and cook over medium heat until browned on all sides.

Whisk together broth, cornstarch, wine, and sage. Slowly add wine mixture to skillet. Heat until boiling, boil for 1 minute, then turn heat down. Add chicken to skillet. Heat until all ingredients are warmed through. Once cooked, spread mixture evenly in pan, divide into 4 equal portions, and serve. Refrigerate or freeze leftovers.

4 servings

SWEET CHICKEN SALAD

Serving Size

Approx. ¾ cup

2½ cups cooked chicken breasts cut into small pieces

¾ cup celery, chopped

1 cup seedless red grapes, chopped

¾ cup mayonnaise

1 tablespoon lemon juice

½ cup slivered almonds

Mix all ingredients together in large bowl. Chill well and serve. Leftovers may be refrigerated up to three days.

6 servings

TARRAGON CHICKEN

4 skinless chicken breast halves, bone-in

2 tablespoons olive oil

Salt and pepper to taste

3 tablespoons dried tarragon leaves, crumbled

⅔ cup dry white wine

Heat oil in large skillet over medium high heat. Add chicken, season with salt and pepper, and brown evenly on all sides.

Add garlic and wine, then sprinkle with dried tarragon. Simmer for 30 minutes, covered, until chicken is cooked through. Refrigerate or freeze leftovers.

4 servings

TARRAGON TURKEY SALAD

½ cup mushrooms, sliced
½ cup zucchini, thinly sliced
½ cup black olives, sliced
1 red bell pepper, chopped
¼ onion, chopped
2 teaspoons dried tarragon
⅔ cup olive oil
⅓ cup balsamic vinegar
1 cup turkey, cooked and chopped
4 cups mixed greens

In large bowl, gently toss together sliced mushrooms, sliced zucchini, sliced black olives, sliced red bell pepper, and chopped onion and tarragon. Add oil and vinegar, tossing to coat evenly. Cover and refrigerate 4 hours.

Mix turkey, mixed greens, and marinated vegetables together. Divide into 4 equal portions; serve cold. Leftovers may be refrigerated for up to three days.

4 servings

TURKEY FRITTATA

½ pound ground turkey

2 tablespoons chicken broth

5 eggs

3 cups kale, finely chopped

1 tablespoon olive oil

⅓ cup onion, finely chopped

1-2 cloves garlic, minced

Heat olive oil on medium heat in large skillet. Sauté onion until lightly golden brown. Add garlic, crumbled turkey, kale, and broth, Stir well to mix ingredients. Cover and continue to cook for approximately 4-5 minutes or until turkey is cooked through. Turn heat to low.

In separate bowl, beat eggs and season with salt and pepper to taste. Pour egg mixture evenly into skillet. Do not mix. Cook for 2 minutes.

Turn oven to broil. Wrap handle of skillet with ovenproof mitt or tinfoil. Place skillet under hot broiler on middle rack of oven. Cook until eggs are set but not browned (approximately 2 minutes). Remove from heat and divide into four equal wedges.

4 servings

TURKEY HASH

1 cup cooked turkey, diced
1½ tablespoons onion, diced
½ cup red pepper, diced
½ tablespoon fresh dill, chopped
½ tablespoon olive oil
2 eggs

Mix turkey, onion, pepper, and dill together. Heat oil in large skillet. Spread turkey mixture evenly in pan. Cook until golden brown on each side. Top with two eggs prepared any style. Remove from heat and divide in half. Serve.

2 servings

FISH AND SHELLFISH

BAKED SALMON WITH HAZELNUT BUTTER

1 pound salmon, cut into 4 fillets
3 tablespoons toasted hazelnuts, finely chopped*
4 tablespoons butter
1½ tablespoons freshly squeezed lemon juice
Salt and pepper to taste

* To toast hazelnuts: Place hazelnuts in single layer in shallow pan. Place in preheated 350-degree oven and bake for 9–11 minutes, gently shaking pan midway through cooking time.

Mix toasted hazelnuts and butter in small bowl.

Season salmon fillets to taste. Lightly coat shallow baking dish with olive oil and place fillets in pan. Bake fillets in 350-degree oven until cooked to preferred doneness. Top with lemon juice and hazelnut butter.

4 servings

CREOLE FISH

1 tablespoon olive oil

1 medium onion, chopped

½ cup celery, chopped

¼ cup red pepper, seeded and chopped

2 teaspoons dried parsley

1-2 teaspoons hot sauce or to taste

1 bay leaf

1 28-ounce can tomatoes with liquid, chopped

1 pound fish (haddock, halibut, or tilapia) cut into small pieces

Sauté onion, celery, and pepper in oil until soft. Add tomatoes, parsley, and bay leaf. Simmer, covered, for 25 minutes. Add fish and simmer until cooked thoroughly, approximately 6-9 minutes. Remove bay leaf. Divide into 4 equal portions and serve.

4 servings

DILLED SALMON

4 tablespoons softened butter

Juice of 1 lemon, or more to taste

1½ tablespoons fresh dill, chopped

4 salmon steaks, approximately 1 pound

2 tablespoons olive oil

Mix butter, lemon juice, and dill together until creamy. Chill well for 2-4 hours.

Generously rub both sides of each steak with olive oil. Broil or grill salmon on high heat for 5-6 minutes or desired doneness. Top each steak with butter and serve.

4 servings

FILLET OF FISH AMANDINE

1 pound white fish fillets (haddock, halibut, or swordfish)
¼ cup butter
¼ cup sliced raw almonds
2 teaspoons freshly squeezed lemon juice
Salt and pepper to taste

Preheat oven to 350 degrees.

Place butter, almonds, and lemon juice in pan and sauté until nuts are lightly browned. Remove almonds and set aside. Place fish fillets in 9 x 9-inch pan. Pour butter mixture over fillets. Bake for 10-14 minutes until fish flakes easily. Sprinkle almonds on fish.

4 servings

GARLIC POACHED HADDOCK

1 pound haddock
2 cups dry white wine
2 cloves garlic, crushed
2 green onions, chopped
½ teaspoon whole black peppercorns

In a large skillet, combine wine, garlic, green onions, and peppercorns. Add haddock. Bring to a boil, then lower heat and simmer for approximately 12-15 minutes or until fish flakes easily.

4 Servings

GINGER SALMON

1 pound salmon, cut into 4 fillets
Juice from 1 lemon
3 tablespoons sliced ginger
3 tablespoons olive oil
Salt and pepper to taste

Place salmon in steamer basket. Rub with ½ of lemon juice and salt and pepper to taste. Lay slices of ginger across fillets.

Cover and steam for approximately 7 minutes or until salmon reaches desired doneness. Salmon is done when it flakes easily with a fork.

Mix olive oil and lemon juice. Drizzle over fillets.

4 servings

JAZZY CAJUN JAMBALAYA

Serving Size

Approx. 1½ cups

1 tablespoon olive oil

1 pound shrimp, cleaned and deveined

3 sweet Italian sausages, chopped

1 19-ounce can whole tomatoes, chopped, with juice

1 red pepper, seeded and chopped

½ cup uncooked long grain rice

1 garlic clove, minced

1 teaspoon chili powder (or to taste)

½ teaspoon dry mustard

¼ teaspoon hot sauce (or to taste)

2¼ cups water

In Dutch oven, cook sausage over medium-high heat for 3 minutes until no longer pink. Drain off fat. Add tomatoes and juice. Add 2¼ cups water, rice, chili powder, dry mustard, and cayenne pepper. Cover mixture and bring to a boil. Simmer, covered, for 15 minutes. Stir in pepper and shrimp. Simmer, covered, for 5 more minutes. Serve. Refrigerate or freeze leftovers.

6 servings

MEDITERRANEAN SCALLOPS

1½ pounds sea scallops

1 pound plum tomatoes, chopped

¾ cup Kalamata olives, pitted and chopped

1 tablespoon red wine vinegar

2 tablespoons olive oil

1 small onion, chopped

2 cloves garlic, minced (or more to taste)

¼ cup water

Heat 1 tablespoon olive oil in large skillet. Add onion and cook until translucent. Add garlic to skillet, cooking approximately 1-2 minutes until garlic is slightly golden brown. Add chopped tomato, red wine vinegar, and water. Cook on medium-high heat, stirring occasionally, until mixture thickens. Stir in olives and remove mixture from skillet. Season olives with salt and pepper on both sides. Add 1 tablespoon olive oil to skillet and cook scallops until opaque. Spoon olive and tomato mixture over cooked scallops. Divide into 6 equal portions, counting scallops if necessary, and serve.

6 servings

SALMON CAKES

2 cups fresh salmon, flaked
1 tablespoon mayonnaise
1½ tablespoons grated Parmesan cheese
1½ tablespoons onion, finely chopped
1 tablespoon fresh dill, chopped
1 egg
Salt and pepper to taste

Remove all bones from salmon. Combine salmon, mayo, Parmesan, dill, onion, and egg and mix well. Form into 6 patties and chill for at least 2 hours.

Heat olive oil in large skillet over medium heat. Cook patties in single layer, about 6-8 minutes, turning once, until golden brown. Season with salt and pepper and serve with lemon wedges or sour cream.

6 servings

SALMON WITH DILLED BUTTER

1½ pounds salmon, cut into 6 fillets
3 tablespoons melted butter
3 tablespoons fresh dill, chopped
Salt and pepper to taste

Combine butter and dill in bowl. Season each fillet with salt and pepper. Brush top of each fillet with butter mixture.

Preheat oven to 500 degrees. Lightly coat shallow baking dish with olive oil. Place fillets in baking dish and bake for 12-20 minutes or until salmon achieves desired doneness at the thickest part. Refrigerate or freeze leftovers.

6 servings

SALMON WITH FRESH THYME

1 pound salmon, cut into 4 fillets
4 tablespoons fresh thyme, chopped
Salt and pepper to taste
Olive oil

Preheat oven to 200 degrees. Mix thyme, ½ teaspoon salt, and ½ teaspoon pepper. Lightly coat a shallow baking dish with olive oil. Place salmon skin-side down and rub with a light layer of oil and dash of salt and pepper. Bake for approximately 40 minutes or until salmon flakes easily.

4 servings

SIMPLE SAUTÉED FISH

3 tablespoons butter
1 pound whitefish (cod, haddock, or halibut)
2 tablespoons fresh parsley, minced
Juice from 1 lemon

In heavy skillet, melt butter over low heat. Add fish and sauté 4-5 minutes on each side until it turns opaque and flakes easily with fork.

Squeeze lemon juice over fish and top with parsley. Divide into four equal portions and serve.

4 Servings

SIZZLING SHRIMP SCAMPI

1 pound large shrimp
⅔ cup olive oil
2 cloves garlic, chopped
2 cloves garlic, minced
2 dried hot chili peppers (do not chop)
1 tablespoon orange zest
1 tablespoon and 1 teaspoon dry sherry
Salt and pepper to taste

In large skillet, heat olive oil over medium heat. Add chopped garlic and sauté until garlic turns a light golden brown. Add shrimp, minced garlic, orange zest, and chili pepper. Cook without stirring until shrimp turns pink. Stir shrimp, adding sherry and salt and pepper to taste. Divide into 4 equal portions, counting shrimp if necessary, and serve immediately.

4 servings

STEAMED FISH

[1]

2 pounds whitefish (cod, haddock, or halibut)
3 tablespoons soy
2 tablespoons rice vinegar
1 pound bok choy
1 clove garlic
¾ cup shredded carrot
3 scallions, sliced

Combine soy, vinegar, ginger, and garlic in bowl.

Place carrots and bok choy in large skillet. Place fish fillets over vegetables. Pour soy mixture over fish. Cover with scallions. Cover and heat to boiling over high heat. Reduce heat to medium and cook until fish flakes easily with fork. Divide into six equal portions and serve.

6 servings

BEEF AND PORK

CARIBBEAN JERK PORK

4 boneless pork loin chops

2 tablespoons jerk seasoning

½ pineapple, cubed

1 tablespoon olive oil

2 limes

½ teaspoon red pepper

Mix juice from limes with jerk seasoning, toss pineapple in seasoning, spread seasoning on pork and grill or broil pork chops until done. Refrigerate or freeze leftovers.

4 servings

HEARTY PORK STEW

Serving Size

Approx. 1½ cups

1 pound pork tenderloin, cubed

1 tablespoon olive oil

2 cups sweet potatoes, peeled and cubed

1 cup red bell pepper, chopped

¾ cup coarsely chopped cabbage

1 14.5-ounce can organic chicken broth

3 cloves garlic, minced

1½ teaspoons Cajun seasoning

Heat oil in large Dutch oven. Add pork and cook, stirring occasionally, until brown. Add remaining ingredients and heat to boiling. Cover. Reduce heat and simmer 12-15 minutes or until sweet potatoes are tender. Refrigerate or freeze leftovers.

6 servings

MARINATED SICILIAN STEAK

   4 6-ounce fillets
   3 tablespoons olive oil
   2 large plum tomatoes, cubed
   ½ cup green olives, pitted and chopped
   1½ teaspoons red onion, chopped
   1 tablespoon fresh lemon peel

Mix all ingredients together and refrigerate for at least 24 hours. Grill or broil steak to taste. Refrigerate or freeze leftovers.

4 servings

PORK CHOP MEDLEY

   4 center cut pork chops, cubed
   2 tablespoons olive oil
   3 cloves garlic, chopped
   3 medium zucchini, cut into chunks
   1½ tablespoons fresh oregano, chopped
   2 cups cherry tomatoes, halved
   ½ cup black pitted olives, halved
   ¾ cup chicken broth
   Salt and pepper to taste

Heat oil in large skillet. Add cubed pork pieces. Salt and pepper to taste. Cook, stirring occasionally, until pork is pink (approximately 4–6 minutes). Remove pork from pan. Add 1 tablespoon oil. Add zucchini and cook until golden brown (approximately 3 minutes). Add garlic and cook for 1 more minute. Stir in chicken broth. Add pork and oregano. Stir all ingredients. Simmer until pork is cooked through.

Add tomatoes and olives. Stir gently until all ingredients are heated through. Divide into 4 equal portions and serve over rice. Refrigerate or freeze leftovers.

4 servings

STEAK WITH BLOCKBUSTER BLEU CHEESE BUTTER

4 6-ounce, boneless strip steaks
⅓ cup crumbled bleu cheese
⅓ cup unsalted butter

Combine bleu cheese and butter in bowl and set aside. Season steaks with salt and pepper to taste. Grill, broil, or roast to desired tenderness. When ready to serve, place several small mounds of bleu cheese butter on each steak. Refrigerate or freeze leftovers.

4 servings

SWEET SALSA SMOTHERED STEAK

4 6-ounce, boneless strip steaks
1½ teaspoons Caribbean jerk seasoning
¼ cup peaches, chopped (fresh is preferable; if using canned make sure they are packed in their own juices, not syrup)
1 tablespoon lime juice
¼ cup red pepper, finely chopped
1 cup mango, chopped
1 teaspoon gingerroot, grated
1 teaspoon jalapeño, finely chopped

Sprinkle both sides of steak with jerk seasoning. Broil 7-10 minutes or until steak reaches desired doneness. While steak is cooking, mix peaches, pepper, mango, lime juice, ginger, and jalapeño in bowl. Top cooked steak with salsa. Refrigerate or freeze leftovers.

4 servings

LAMB

CINNAMON LAMB CHOPS

 2 tablespoons olive oil
 4 medium lamb chops
 2 medium onions, chopped
 3 garlic cloves, minced
 1¼ teaspoons ground cinnamon
 1 28-ounce can whole tomatoes in juice, chopped

Season lamb chops with salt and pepper to taste.

Heat 1 tablespoon olive oil over medium heat. Add lamb chops and brown on each side (approximately 4 minutes per side). Set aside.

Add additional 1 tablespoon olive oil to skillet. Sauté onions over medium heat until they turn golden brown. Add minced garlic. Add tomatoes with juice and cinnamon. Reduce heat to medium low, return the lamb chops to skillet, and bring the sauce to a simmer. Cover and simmer until the chops reach desired doneness, 20–30 minutes. Uncover and cook until the sauce thickens (approximately 10–12 minutes). Refrigerate or freeze leftovers.

4 servings

GLAZED LAMB CHOPS

1½ pounds lamb chops (6-8 chops)
⅓ cup orange juice
⅔ cup balsamic vinegar
1½ teaspoons honey
2 tablespoons soy sauce
Salt and pepper to taste

Mix orange juice, vinegar, honey, and soy sauce in large bowl. Season lamb with salt and pepper to taste. Place chops in bowl with marinade and refrigerate for 6 hours or overnight.

Remove lamb and set aside. Pour remaining marinade into saucepan and bring to a boil. Reduce heat, then boil gently until liquid is thick and reduced to ½ cup. Grill or broil lamb chops. Cover with cooked marinade and serve. Refrigerate or freeze leftovers.

6 servings

ROSEMARY LAMB

4 medium lamb chops
4 cloves garlic
3 tablespoons fresh lemon
2 tablespoons fresh rosemary

Combine all ingredients in large bowl. Marinate chops for 2 hours or more. Broil chops 8-12 minutes or until meat reaches desired tenderness. Refrigerate or freeze leftovers.

4 servings

Referrals
and Resources

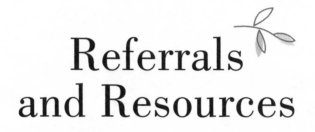

Alternative Medical Therapies

The following list gives a brief description of alternative and integrative medical therapies that have been used successfully for wellness and weight loss by my patients and others. There are unqualified or ineffective practitioners in both conventional and alternative medicine, so be cautious whenever you choose any health-care provider. (There are studies that indicate that medical error is among the top ten causes of death in America.) Outright quacks are rare, but they exist, too. Beware of extravagant claims. One of the problems is that certification standards vary so much from state to state. But almost every state now has some kind of certification process. Look for the following:

- Trained, licensed, and certified in their particular field

- Recommendations from other practitioners or friends

- The atmosphere and the practitioner feel safe and comfortable to you

- Your opinion is valued and your questions are fully answered

- Guidelines for the technique and length of the procedure are set at the first visit

- Some verifiable evidence of successful results in the treatment of your concern

- Ability to work with other health-care professionals in your life

Healing Modalities

Functional Medicine

Functional medicine is a comprehensive approach to health care that treats the patient first, not the disease. It integrates the best of Western and ancient modalities to treat the whole patient, with an emphasis on maintaining organ integrity and subtly shifting core physiology through nutrition and lifestyle. To find a functional medical practitioner near you, contact:

The Institute for Functional Medicine
4411 Pt. Fosdick Dr. NW, Suite 305
PO Box 1697
Gig Harbor, WA 98355
Phone: 800-228-0622
www.functionalmedicine.org

Traditional Chinese Medicine (TCM) / Traditional Oriental Medicine (TOM)

As the standard of care in the Orient for over 3000 years, TCM incorporates the use of acupuncture, diet, and herbal remedies with physical movement (qi gong and t'ai chi) and massage (known in Japan as shiatsu, "finger-pressure"). Oriental practitioners see the body as an intricate web of organs interconnected by channels (meridians) through which universal energy (*chi* or *qi*) flows. Healthy bodies have a dynamic balance of yin and yang energy, opposites that occur in nature (female/male, moon/sun, etc.). According to the tenets of Oriental medicine, disease (dis-ease) arises when the flow of *qi* is blocked and balance is disturbed, either within the body or between the body and its environment. Disease is prevented and health maintained by restoring the balance and flow. To find a practitioner contact:

American Association of Acupunture and Oriental Medicine (AAAOM)
P.O. Box 162340
Sacramento, CA 95816
Toll-Free: 866-455-7999
Phone: 916-443-4770
Fax: 916-443-4766
E-mail: info@aaaomonline.org
http://www.aaaomonline.org

Ayurveda

Originating over 5000 years ago in India, ayurvedic medicine predates all other known medical systems. This ancient form of healing stresses the mind-body-spirit connection. Ayurvedic practitioners believe that *prana*—or life force—responds to equivalent treatments in a different way in each person. Healing and preventative regimens are customized specifically around a person's body and spiritual type, or dosha. Ayurvedic medicine encompasses meditation, yoga, bodywork, aromatic oils, diet, and medicinal herbs to foster balance in the body and cleanse impurities.

American Academy of Ayurvedic Medicine, Inc. (AAAM)
100 Jersey Avenue
Building B, Suite 300
New Brunswick, NJ 08901
Phone: 732-317-8296
Fax: 732-317-8449
E-mail: info@ayurvedicacademy.com
http://www.ayurvedicacademy.com/

Biodentistry

Many chronic health problems may have been caused by damage from the mercury in dental fillings, root canals, and untreated tooth decay. In the practice of biological, or mercury-free, dentistry, practitioners use highly controlled sterilization and filtration techniques to remove and isolate the mercury from your mercury amalgam fillings. Mercury in fillings is controversial and most traditional dentists will tell you there's nothing to be concerned about, but mercury is highly toxic and may contribute to inflammation or an overburdened immune system.

To find a practitioner near you, contact:

Foundation for Toxic Free Dentistry
PO Box 608010
Orlando, FL 32860-8010

For more information, please read the newsletter furnished by Hal Huggins at Huggins Applied Healing:

Huggins Applied Healing
5082 List Drive
Colorado Springs, CO 80919
Phone: 866-948-4638
E-mail: Info@drhuggins.com
www.mercuryfreedentists.com

Homeopathy

Founded in early 19th-century Europe, homeopathy is a medical discipline based on the ancient law of similars: the same substances that cause an illness will cure it when administered in infinitesimally small doses. (Vaccines operate on a similar principle.) Using serially diluted remedies from natural sources, homeopaths (most of whom are also naturopaths) treat and prevent illness using one medicine at a time at the lowest dosage possible to create the required response. Licensing requirements vary from state to state, and you will often find acupuncturists, naturopaths, herbalists, DO's and MD's who are also licensed homeopaths. To find one, contact:

Natural Center for Homeopathy
801 North Fairfax Street, Suite 306
Alexandria, VA 22314
Phone: 703-548-7790
Fax: 703-548-7792
nationalcenterforhomeopathy.org

Naturopathy

Naturopathy applies to a belief system that holds the body as innately capable of recovering from injury and disease, and that health is the natural state. Most naturopaths implement elements from various alternative methods to create health, including homeopathy, herbal medicines, acupuncture, nutrition therapy, and bodywork. Naturopathy has its roots in ancient medicinal practices, but took form as a separate discipline in Germany in the 19th century. Founded on the precepts of a medical regimen of hydrotherapy, exercise, fresh air, sunlight, and herbal remedies, this system has evolved today to include a wide spectrum of holistic practitioners. To find one in your area, contact:

American Association of Naturopathic Physicians
4435 Wisconsin Avenue NW, Suite 403
Washington, DC 20016
Toll-Free: 866-538-2267
Phone: 202-237-8150
Fax: 202-237-8152
E-mail: member.services@naturopathic.org
www.naturopathic.org/

Body-Based Techniques

The following is a list of the most popular body-based techniques used by various health-care practitioners. They may be used alone or in combination. Again, the list is not comprehensive but should act as a good introduction.

Acupuncture: One of the main elements of Traditional Chinese Medicine, acupuncture is now widely accepted in Western medicine for the treatment of pain, nausea, and other conditions. (Insurance companies reimburse for the cost of acupuncture to treat dozens of diagnoses, a sure sign of acceptance in our culture.) Studies support its effectiveness for many other issues, such as cramps, dysmenorrhea, and menopausal symptoms.

Aromatherapy: Aromatherapy and flower essences are two separate and very different approaches to healing that utilize plants to effect changes and thereby heal our bodies. Aromatherapy utilizes volatile liquid plant materials, including essential oils and other aromatic compounds of plants, to relax our bodies or stimulate its function, especially our senses. Essential oils are very aromatic, but that is an added side benefit—their healing actions are quite physiological. For example, they can stimulate the limbic system and emotional centers of the brain, activate thermal receptors on the skin, act as natural antibiotics and fungicides, and possibly enhance the immune response in other ways not fully understood.

Bach Flower Essences: In the 1930s Edward Bach, a British bacteriologist and homeopath, developed a line of plant essences that he claimed would remedy negative emotional states, along with a system of matching a specific essence to a specific problem. Perhaps the most famous among these is a formulation called Rescue Remedy. Flower essences do not contain any of the actual molecular structure of the original plant but rather embody the very "spirit" of the healing qualities of the plant.

Chelation Therapy: Chelation therapy is an intravenously administered process used within the alternative medical community for many years to treat patients with dangerous levels of lead and other toxins in their system. In EDTA chelation therapy, a manmade amino acid known as ethylene diamine tetra-acetic acid acts as a "magnet" traveling throughout the body to bind (chelate) heavy metals and minerals, allowing them to be excreted through urination. In 2008, the National Institute of Health (NIH) completed a five-year $30 million study, called TACT (Trial to Assess Chelation Therapy), to evaluate the effectiveness of EDTA chelation therapy for the treatment of coronary artery disease (CAD). Prior to this, chelation therapy had not been well-studied, and it remains controversial.

Chiropractic: This is a system of treatment based on the concept that good health stems from the unimpeded flow of nerve impulses from the brain and spinal cord to other parts of the body. Misaligned vertebrae of the spine, which chiropractors call subluxations, disrupt this flow and are adjusted by the chiropractor along with other joints. All 50 states currently have licensing procedures for chiropractic practitioners. Many chiropractors use other natural remedies for adjunctive healing and prevention.

Herbal Remedies: The ancient practice of herbal medicine is utilized in all the schools of medicine described above. Of course, it is likewise the basis for many prescription drugs in the Western paradigm, once the active ingredient has been isolated and synthesized in a laboratory setting. Therapeutic herbal remedies are the specialty of herbalists, but they are a component of many other practices and can take the form of teas, tinctures, oils, creams, and pills. Many herbs can be poisonous or interact dangerously with prescription drugs, so it is best to use them only under the supervision of a qualified practitioner.

Hydrotherapy: Hydrotherapy encompasses a range of treatments involving water to prevent disease and promote healing. It may include cold and hot immersion baths, sitz baths, mud baths, steam baths, saunas, vigorous showers, salt rubs, hot/cold packs, foot baths, douches, or colonic irrigation. Patients may also be asked to drink restorative waters and teas for digestive ailments.

Massage: One of the oldest forms of healing, massage therapy is used alone or in conjunction with a variety of treatments to alleviate stress, tension, and soreness and to increase blood flow to the muscles. Some forms claim to detoxify, others to open blocked energy channels through applying pressure on certain points in the body. Types of massage include reflexology, Rolfing, shiatsu, Swedish massage, and sports massage, among others.

Movement and Exercise Therapy: Treatments include yoga, Pilates, physical therapy, Alexander Technique, and Feldenkrais Technique, among many others. These therapies promote circulation, elimination, and flexibility while easing chronic pain and any postural misalignment interfering with mobility.

Nutrition Therapy: This treatment promotes the links between your food, your metabolism, and your health. Depending on an individual's makeup, a regimen of certain foods, vitamins and minerals can cure and prevent disease—both physical and psychological. Treatments range from dietary prescriptions such as macrobiotics to megadoses of vitamins and minerals. Dieticians, doctors, and many other practitioners receive certification from the American Board of Nutrition. Nutritionists may be licensed or certified depending on their state requirements.

Osteopathy: Osteopathic physicians (DOs) are trained and licensed as rigorously as conventional medical practitioners (MDs), but the founding philosophy of osteopathic medicine is to treat the whole person, focusing on preventive care. In this regard osteopathy may be considered to be a holistic form of medicine, yet strictly speaking it is not an alternative modality. Osteopaths serve medical residencies, hold unrestricted licenses to prescribe drugs, and frequently perform surgery. Osteopathy is sometimes confused with chiropractic medicine because it involves osteopathic manipulative therapy (OMT), which includes spinal manipulation and craniosacral techniques. Emphasizing the neuromusculoskeletal system, osteopaths create health by balancing the energy between the organs and the connection between mind and body.

Reiki/Energy Medicine: This approach uses the vital energy of the body to enhance health. The Reiki practitioner has had his or her own energy channels cleared, and can thereby act as a funnel for the universal life force energy through touch to the patient. Energy medicine is frequently used in combination with diet therapy and herbal or homeopathic remedies to bring a person back into emotional and physical alignment.

Therapeutic Touch: This technique is a form of energy medicine in which the practitioner's hands are moved over a person's body, often without direct contact, to break up energy blockages and promote healing. Therapeutic touch works with a person's individual energy field, a concept that has its roots in the Chinese concept of *qi*, the Ayurvedic principle of *prana* (life force), and the ancient practice of laying on of hands. Numerous studies have shown its efficacy in decreasing pain and anxiety, reducing the need for medication post-surgery, and increasing hemoglobin levels. It is now part of the core curriculum at many nursing schools.

331

Mind-Body Connection Techniques

These techniques strive to create awareness of the connection between our conscious and unconscious mind, as well as our emotions, outlook and physical state. They are often used in combination with body-based therapies and address a much overlooked aspect of healing and prevention.

Biofeedback: This is a series of techniques developed to help people overcome various forms of stress-related habits, illnesses, symptoms, and phobias. Electronic monitors help a person gauge and alter facets of their stress response by altering the electric signals. By increasing a person's awareness of physiological activity in her muscles, she can be trained to control what are otherwise automatic physical responses to tension and stress, such as heartbeat, blood pressure, skin temperature, and brain-wave patterns. The efficacy of biofeedback for essential hypertension has been well established in clinical trials.

Emotional Freedom Techniques (EFT): Developed by Gary Craig from the tenets of acupuncture, EFT uses sequential tapping of the energy meridians rather than needles to unlock energy blockage and treat physical and emotional imbalance. EFT is surprisingly effective, regardless of one's belief system. Once the technique is learned, EFT can be used by anyone, just about anywhere, both to counter pain, cravings, negative emotions, and complex problems, as well as to reinforce positive behavior. Those with entrenched problems enjoy a higher success rate under the guidance of a trained practitioner.

Guided Imagery: Harnessing the imagination to create a "construct of reality" can give us powerful yet gentle insight into the unconscious mind. Using highly personalized themes, guided imagery invokes not just visualizations but taps into sounds, smells, and tactile experiences as well, to which the body responds as though they were the real thing. Studies show that a biophysical response to positive imagery can effectively override the hardwiring of engrained thought patterns and habits to help create better health and attain otherwise unreachable goals.

Hypnosis/Self-Hypnosis: A technique that renders an altered state of consciousness in the patient, hypnotherapy can be administered either through the help of a practitioner or on one's own accord. Hypnotherapy can be used for behavior modification (e.g., smoking cessation), to treat trauma and phobia, or to relieve chronic or symptomatic pain such as that of childbirth.

Meditation/Visualization: These techniques work by having the patient focus on one image or thought for a duration of time while practicing deep breathing. Meditation—a pillar of Ayurvedic medicine—is used to quiet the mind, often in tandem with physical exercise (yoga or other). Visualization works similarly, training the patient to gain control over pain or reduce anxiety by triggering deep relaxation.

The Relaxation Response: Pioneered by Herb Benson, MD, a Harvard internist, the Relaxation Response involves attaining a state of deep relaxation whereby a person can counteract the ill effects of pain, anxiety and stress. Employing a variety of mind/body exercises to achieve a meditative state, the Relaxation Response has been used for years to help people successfully overcome all sorts of physiologically and psychologically-based problems, including high blood pressure, addiction—even some stress-related infertility issues. Eliciting the Relaxation Response is a component of the high rate of success Dr. Alice Domar has achieved with patients in her Mind/Body Program for Infertility.

Spiritual/Psychic Healing: Using powers that are beyond our understanding—let alone medical knowledge—is an ancient practice. Prayer, touch, and other religious rituals have been successfully used throughout time to cure physical and mental illness. Practitioners work by channeling beliefs and creating a special link between the patient and a superior consciousness, thereby effecting change. Many studies documenting the efficacy of prayer in healing have been published in peer-reviewed journals over the years. In particular, the lifelong work of Dr. Larry Dossey has served to broaden our understanding of the links between spirituality and healing. By presenting solid scientific evidence, Dr. Dossey has helped to legitimize prayer's healing effects within conventional medical circles.

Glossary adapted with permission from Women to Women website at www.womento-women.com.

Clinical Labs

I rely on the following clinical laboratories for much of my diagnostic testing. Their Websites offer detailed, valuable information about the tests they provide, as well as additional references. Your medical professional can use this page as a resource as well. In some cases, if you are finding it difficult to get a specific test, you may be able to go through the labs to find a practitioner in your area whom they've worked with before.

Aeron LifeCycles Clinical Laboratory
1933 Davis Street Suite 310
San Leandro, CA 94577
Phone: 800-631-7900 option 6
Fax: 510-729-0383
www.aeron.com

Adrenal Testing/Hormone Panel
Aeron Lifecycles is one of the few labs accepted in the state of NY. (NY does not recognize many alternative tests)

ALCAT-Allergy Testing
Cell Science Systems
1239 East Newport Center Drive, Suite 101
Deerfield Beach, FL 33442
Phone: 800-US ALCAT (872-5228)
Fax: 954-428-8676
E-mail: info@alcat.com

DiagnosTEX, LLC
Phone: 817-514-MBS1 or 1-888-514-MBS1
Fax: 1-877-514-MBS8 or 1-877-514-MBS8
E-mail: info@dysphagiadiagnostex.com

Adrenal Testing/Hormonal/Digestive Testing

Genova Diagnostics (formerly Great Smokies)
63 Zillicoa Street
Asheville, NC 28801
Toll-Free: 800-522-4762
Phone: 828-253-0621
www.genovadiagnostics.com

A full-service lab that provides, among other tests, genetic profile, adrenal, function comprehensive parasitology, allergies, amino acid deficiency, stool testing, and liver detoxification (stage one and stage two)

Doctor's Data, Inc.
Customer Service
3755 Illinois Avenue
St. Charles, IL 60174-2420
Phone: 800-323-2784 (USA & Canada)
Phone: 0871-218-0052 (United Kingdom)
Phone: 630-377-8139 (Elsewhere)
www.doctorsdata.com

Tests for heavy metal toxicity, digestive issues, and adrenal function

Metametrix Clinical Laboratory
3425 Corporate Way
Duluth, GA 30096
Toll-Free: 800-221-4640
Phone: 770-446-5483
www.metametrix.com

Tests for amino acid deficiency, allergies, stool, and digestive issues

NeuroScience Inc.
373 280th St.
Osceola, WI 54020
Phone: 888-342-7272
E-mail: customerservice@neurorelief.com

Tests neurotransmitter levels, amino acids, and adrenal function

Parasitology Center, Inc. (PCI)
11445 East Via Linda, #2-419
Scottsdale, Arizona, 85259-2638
Phone: 480-767-2522
Fax: 480-767-5855
E-mail: omaramin@aol.com

Tests for parasites

ZRT Laboratory
8605 SW Creekside Place
Beaverton, OR 97008
Phone: 503-466-2445
Fax: 503-466-1636
E-mail: info@zrtlab.com

Tests hormonal function

Products

Gluten-Free Products

Here is a short list of delicious gluten-free products to enjoy while you are on the Core Balance Diet. Some of these products are used in the recipes, others are included to help those of you who are sensitive to gluten—and your families— to avoid it entirely. These products can be found at your local natural foods store or by ordering online at www. glutenfree.com or www.glutenfreemall.com. I've listed brands and products that I have personally used. If you decide to try another brand or product, please read the label to make sure it will work for you.

Bagels and Breads
Against the Grain Gourmet Sesame bagels
Better Bread Pizza
Glutino Frozen Bagels, breadsticks (pizza and sesame), biscuits, and original crackers
Enjoy Life Bagels
Food for Life Raisin Pecan Bread
Le Garden Old Fashioned Bread
Le Garden Seeded Croutons
Mary's Gone Crackers (all flavors)
Blue Diamond Nut-Things crackers

Cereal
Bakery on Main Apple Raisin Cereal
Cream Hill Estates Lara's Rolled Oats
Nature's Gate Mesa Sunrise

Condiments
Barkat Gravy Mix
Maxwell's Chicken Gravy
Esparaggo's Asparagus Guacamole
J & S Peabutter (nonpeanut butter)
Hempzel's Horseradish Hemp and Honey Mustard
Mr. Spice Indian Curry Sauce

Desserts

Envirokids cookies

Candy Tree Black Licorice Vines

Eragrain Frozen Natural Oatmeal Raisin Cookies

Barkat Ice Cream Cones

Arico Chocolate Chip Cookie Bar

Glutino Shortbread Dreams

Entrees

Amy's Frozen Entrees

Glutino Frozen Pizza

Chebe Frozen Pizza

Gillian's Frozen Pizza

George's Pizza

Mrs. Leepers Hamburger Entrees

Grains

Shiloh Farms Kasha

Shiloh Farms Millet

Shiloh Farms Brown Basmati Rice

Mixes

Namaste Baking Mixes

Pamela's Pantry Waffle/Pancake Mix

The Cravings Place All-Purpose Pancake Mix

Authentic Foods Pancake Mix

Authentic Foods Chocolate Cake Mix

Cause Your Special Cake Mix

Cause Your Special Sugar Cookie Mix

Enjoy Life Soft-Baked Double Chocolate Brownies

Pasta

Ancient Harvest Quinoa Pasta Elbows

Ancient Harvest Quinoa Linguine

Glutano Macaroni

Tinkyada Brown Rice Pasta (all shapes)

Tinkyada Spinach Brown Rice Spaghetti

Tinkyada Vegetable Brown Rice Spirals

Tinkyada Organic Brown Rice Pasta (all shapes)

Snacks

Envirokids Rice Bars

Barkat Sesame Pretzels

Glutino Bretzels

Soups

Celefibir Vegetable Bouillon Cubes

Full Flavor Foods Chicken Soup Stock

Yeast-Free Flour

Bob's Red Mill Gluten-Free Flour

Yogurt

Brown Cow Plain Yogurt

Recommended Household Products

I've included here a list of my favorite nontoxic kitchen, bed, bath, and baby products to help you replace those you clean out of your cupboards. I have tried to find you products that are attractive and durable and easy to find at your local natural foods store or on the Internet. I use these products at my clinic and in my home, and to the best of my knowledge they are as green as they claim to be. There are some great recipes for cleaning products listed on the Women to Women website. I also recommend the Gaiam catalog (www.gaiam.com) and the Whole Earth Catalog (www.wholeearth.com) as resources for nontoxic (or at least, less toxic) home products.

Kitchenware

Stainless Steel Water Bottles

Envirowave   (www.enviroproductsinc.com)

Rice Cookers/Pressure Cookers

Miracle SS Rice Cooker   (www.ultimate-weight-products.com)

Ghan Nabe Iron Rice Cooker from Iwachu   (www.store.zensuke.com

Small ceramic rice cooker/crock pressure cooker   (www.kushistore.com)

Aeternum Pressure Cooker   (www.healthclassics.com)

Vegetable Steamers

Welco's 3-piece stainless steel steamer   (www.target.com)

Stainless Vegetable Steamer

Pasta Cooker Veggie Steamer

Silicone Veggie Steamer

Stainless steel vegetable steamer with feet   (www.crateandbarrel.com)

Blenders

Vitamix Blender   (www.vitamix.com)

Tea Kettles and Teapots

Ceramic Tea Kettle   (www.theteacorner.com)

Glass Tea Kettle   (www.theteacorner.com)

KitchenAid Porcelain Teapot/stainless steel interior   (www.bedbathandbeyond.com)

Glass Storage Containers

Anchor Hocking Glass Refrigerator Storage Containers   (www.cooking.com)

Snapware Glass Lock Round storage container   (www.bedbathandbeyond.com)

Frioverre Round Glass Storage Containers with lid   (www.chefscatalog.com)

Crate and Barrel Rectangular Storage Container   (www.crateandbarrel.com)

Pyrex Round and Rectangle storage containers   (www.pyrex.com)

Williams-Sonoma Glass Storage dishes   (www.william-sonoma.com)

Non-Leaching Baking Pans

Cabela's Cast Iron Pan   (www.cabelas.com)

Tramontina Stainless Steel baking pan   (www.qvc.com)

Stainless steel baking pan   (www.thewebrestaurantstore.com)

Pyrex Glass baking pans   (www.pyrex.com)

New Era Solution's Waterless Cookware   (www.neweracookware.com)

Tap/Drinking Water Filters

K5 Drinking water station   (www.kinetico.com)

PiMag Agua Pour   (www.nikken.com)

PiMag Agua Pour Deluxe   (www.nikken.com)

PiMag Agua Pour Express   (www.nikken.com)
PiMag deluxe under counter water system   (www.nikken.com)
PiMag countertop water system   (www.nikken.com)
PiMag Optimizer   (www.nikken.com)

Recipe Savers/Cookbooks

The Family Generation Recipe Collection Book by Nittany Quill   (www.talusproducts.com)

Fruit and Veggie Washes

Seventh Generation Veggie Wash   (www.seventhgeneration.com)

Cleaning Products

Seventh Generation dishwashing liquids

Earth's Best laundry detergent, fabric softener,
furniture care, tough and tender wipes, tub and tile soap
scum cleanser, disinfectant spray (www.earthsbest.com).

Household and Bedroom

Whole-System Water Filters

Kinetico 4040 chlorine removal only   (www.kinetico.com)

Kinetico 4040 chlorine and iron removal   (www.kinetico.com)

Kinetico 1030 and 1060 Dechlorinators   (www.kinetico.com)

Air Filters

Austin Air Healthmate HM   (www.healthpurifiers.com)

Austin Air Healthmate JR   (www.healthpurifiers.com)

Air Wellness Power Pro   (www.nikken.com)

Air Wellness Traveler   (www.nikken.com)

Hypoallergenic Bedding

Allergy free and asthma bedding   (www.allergyasthmatech.com)

Allergy Proof Mattress and Pillow Covers   (www.allergystore.com)

Dust mite mattress and pillow covers   (www.allergysolution.com)

Bath and Beauty Products

Shower/Bathtub Water Filters

Showerhead filter   (www.santeforhealth.com)

Bathtub filter   (www.santeforhealth.com)

Crystal Quest Luxury Showerhead filter   (www.purewaterforless.com)

Sprite All in One showerhead   (www.bestfilters.com)

Sprite Slim Line shower filter   (www.bestfilters.com)

Envirowave Premium shower filter   (www.enviroproductsinc.com)

Envirowave Bathtub filter   (www.enviroproductsinc.com)

PiMag Ultra Shower System   (www.nikken.com)

Hair Products

La Bella Hair Mist   (www.labellamaria.com)

La Bella Mousse   (www.labellamaria.com)

La Bella Gelle   (www.labellamaria.com)

Makeup

Suki Rich Pigment Mascara   (www.saftronrouge.com)

NVEY Organic Moisturizing Mascara   (www.saftronrouge.com)

Dr. Hauschka Volume Mascara   (www.saftronrouge.com)

NVEY Organic Creative Eye Color System   (www.saftronrouge.com)

NVEY Organic Eye Shadow   (www.saftronrouge.com)

Dr. Hauschka Eye Shadow Solos   (www.saftronrouge.com)

Face and Body Lotions

Terralina 8-ounce body lotion and facial moisturizer   (www.terralina.com)

Terralina fragrance free 8-ounce body lotion   (www.terralina.com)

Kiss My Face Vitamin A&E Moisturizer   (www.kissmyface.com)

Sunless Tanners

Gibraltar's Puttin' on a Tan   (www.gibraltarproducts.com)

Kiss My Face Instant Sunless Tanner   (www.kissmyface.com)

He Shi Express Liquid Tan   (www.body-careshop.com)

Sunscreens

BADGER SPF 15 for Face and Body   (www.badgerbalm.com)

UV Natural Adult Broad Spectrum   (www.ecobathroom.com)

Soleo Organics Sunscreen   (www.soleoorganics.com)

Dr. Hauschka Sunscreen SPF 8   (www.amazon.com)

Burt's Bees Chemical-Free Sunscreeen SPF 15 and SPF 30   (www.burtsbees.com)

Aloe Vera Sunscreen SPF 15   (www.saffronrouge.com)

Kiss My Face Sun Spray with SPF 30   (www.kissmyface.com)

Kiss My Face Sunscreen SPF 18 with oat protein complex   (www.kissmyface.com)

Chemical Free Mini/Maxi Pads, Reusable Cups and Tampons

Pandora Organic Cotton tampons   (www.pandora.com)

Natracare Certified Organic all-cotton tampons   (www.pandora.com)

Seventh Generation chlorine-free tampons   (www.pandora.com)

Glad Rags reusable menstrual pads   (www.gladrags.com)

The Keeper Menstrual cups   (www.gladrags.com)

The Moon Menstrual cups   (www.gladrags.com)

Diva Menstrual cups   (www.gladrags.com)

Nail Polish and Removers

Acquarella chemical-free nail polish   (www.ulew.com)

Nubar noncarcinogenic nail polish   (www.bynubar.com)

Sun Coat   (www.thedailygreen.com)

No-Miss   (www.thedailygreen.com)

Butter London   (www.butterlondon.com)

Electric Magnetic Field Chips

BIOPRO Cell Chip   (www.mybiopro.com)

Heat and Therapy Packs

Grandpa's Garden Herbal (Lavender) Rice Paks   (www.grandpasgarden.com)

Exercise Equipment-Burst Machine

The X-CISER from Corrective Wellness   (www.xiser.com)

Baby Products

These products are available at most natural foods stores. The Earth's Best baby food line is now being sold at Babies R Us. If you have trouble finding any of these products, please see www.fitpregnancy.com/goinggreen/ for links to individual vendors who will give you information and contact numbers for a store near you.

General Baby Care

Born Free glass/plastic bottles and drinking cups

Whole Foods 365 white natural diapers and wipes, chlorine-free

Gold Bond talc free baby powder (not the original formula)

Earth's Best JASON baby care line

California Baby sunscreen and bath products

Bourdreaux's Butt Paste, for tough diaper rash (paraben-free)

Cereals and Prepared Food
(available at local natural foods stores)

Earth's Best organic formulas, rice and whole grain baby cereal,
barley teething biscuits, baby snacks, jarred baby food when needed (fresh is best)

Stoneyfield's whole-milk plain yogurt (sweeten
with apple sauce to avoid sugar in packaged baby yogurt)

Perky-Os gluten-free cereal that stays crunchy in milk

Oatio's wheat-free oat cereal

Sleepsacks, Wraps, and Other

Swaddleme Microfleece or Cotton Infant Wrap   (www.kiddopatomus.com)

Dreamsie Sleep Sack's loose and comfy gown for when child
is bigger and no longer swaddling   (www.kiddopatomus.com)

Nursing Bras and Pumps

Bravado Nursing Bras   (www.mommygear.com)

Medella Nursing Pumps   (www.mommygear.com)

Lanolin nipple and body cream from Lansinoh   (www.mommygear.com)

Appendices

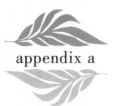

BODY MASS INDEX

To determine your Body Mass Index (BMI), use the table below or this simple calculation. Divide your weight in pounds by your height in inches. Divide that number by your height in inches and multiply the result by 703.

The BMI chart has caused some controversy over the years because it does not accommodate much wiggle room for people with a lot of muscle. Muscle weighs more than fat, so you can be extremely fit and have a higher BMI than appears healthy. The easy answer to this is to also measure your waist-to-hip ratio. If you have a BMI over 25 (some nutritionists are now saying 24) and less than 10 inches difference between your waist and hip measurements, it's a good bet you could help your health by taking off some weight.

BMI (kg/m2)	19	20	21	22	23	24	25	26	27	28	29	30	35	40
58	91	96	100	105	110	115	119	124	129	134	138	143	167	191
59	94	99	104	109	114	119	124	128	133	138	143	148	173	198
60	97	102	107	112	118	123	128	133	138	143	148	153	179	204
61	100	106	111	116	122	127	132	137	143	148	153	158	185	211
62	104	109	115	120	126	131	136	142	147	153	158	164	191	218
63	107	113	118	124	130	135	141	146	152	158	163	169	197	225
64	110	116	122	128	134	140	145	151	157	163	169	174	204	232
65	114	120	126	132	138	144	150	156	162	168	174	180	210	240
66	118	124	130	136	142	148	155	161	167	173	179	186	216	247
67	121	127	134	140	146	153	159	166	172	178	185	191	223	255
68	125	131	138	144	151	158	164	171	177	184	190	197	230	262
69	128	135	142	149	155	162	169	176	182	189	196	203	236	270
70	132	139	146	153	160	167	174	181	188	195	202	207	243	278
71	136	143	150	157	165	172	179	186	193	200	208	215	250	286
72	140	147	154	162	169	177	184	191	199	206	213	221	258	294
73	144	151	159	166	174	182	189	197	204	212	219	227	265	302
74	148	155	163	171	179	186	194	202	210	218	225	233	272	311
75	152	160	168	176	184	192	200	208	216	224	232	240	279	319
76	156	164	172	180	189	197	205	213	221	230	238	246	287	328

Height (in.)

Weight (lb.)

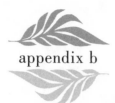

appendix b

GLYCEMIC INDEX
AND GLYCEMIC LOAD

Adapted from the Table of Glycemic Index and Glycemic Load Values 2002 from the *American Journal of Clinical Nutrition 2002*; 76:5-56. USA Copyright 2002 American Society for Clinical Nutrition

Glycemic Index (GI) and Glycemic Load (GL) Values for Selected Foods
(Relative to Glucose when Glucose = 100)

Food	GI	Serving Size	Carbs per serving (g)	GL
Fruits and Juices				
Apple	55	1 medium	21	12
Apricot	57	1 medium	9	5
Banana	51	1 medium	25	13
Carrots (raw)	131	1/2 cup	4	5
Cherries	40	1/2 cup	12	3
Cranberry Juice	105	4 ounces	18	19
Dates, dried	103	2 ounces	40	42
Orange (raw)	42	1 medium	11	5
Orange Juice	75	6 ounces	20	15
Mango	55	1 cup	17	8
Peach	55	1 medium	11	5
Pear	38	1 medium	11	4

Cereals & Grains				
All-Bran	72	1/2 cup	24	17
Cornflakes	81	1 cup	26	21
Oatmeal	82	1 cup	25	21
Raisin Bran	88	1 cup	47	41
Rice, white (boiled)	102	1 cup	45	45
Rice, brown (boiled)	55	1 cup	33	18
Spaghetti, white	58	1 1/2 cups	48	28
Spaghetti, whole wheat	40	1 1/2 cups	42	16
Vegetables				
Russet Potato (baked)	76	1 medium	30	23
Snack Food				
Corn Chips	46	1/2 cup	25	11
Doughnut	76	1 medium	23	17
Puffed Rice Cakes	52	2 cakes	14	12
Bread				
English Muffin	86	1 muffin	26	23
White Bread	100	1 large slice	12	12
Rye, Pumpernickel Bread	41	1 large slice	12	5
Gluten-Free Multigrain	76	1 slice	13	9
Whole Wheat Bread	60	1 slice	14	8
Dairy & Other				
Skim Milk	32	8 ounces	13	4
2% Yogurt	40	1 cup	9	3
Soy Milk	50	8 ounces	17	8
Legumes & Nuts				
Baked Beans	56	1 cup	15	7
Chickpeas	32	1 cup	30	3
Kidney Beans (dried/boiled)	28	1 cup	25	7
Lentils (dried/boiled)	29	1 cup	18	5
Cashew Nuts	22	1 ounce	9	2
Peanuts	14	1 ounce	6	1

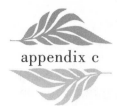

THE HPA AXIS AND MAJOR METABOLIC HORMONES

The hypothalamus stands at the apex of an important mood and weight loss pathway: the hypothalamus-pituitary-adrenal axis, or HPA. The pituitary and adrenal glands are major quarterbacks for the endocrine system; the pituitary is responsible for stimulating the release of thyroid stimulating hormone (TSH), which travels to the thyroid and causes the secretion of the thyroid hormones (T3, T4, and parathyroid, see also page 123) These hormones regulate energy production, heat generation, and oxygen uptake in your cells—in other words, your basic metabolic rate. As for the "A" in this alphabet soup—it stands for the adrenals, which are small walnut-shaped glands mounted on the top of your kidneys. When you are put under stress, the hypothalamus responds by releasing corticotropin-releasing factor (CRF), which activates adrenocorticotropic hormone (ACTH), which in turn stimulates the "fight-or-flight" response of the adrenal cortex, accompanied by a depression of the immune system and a surge of adrenaline (also called epinephrine) and cortisol. These hormones speed oxygen and glucose to the brain and blood to the essential organs to ready the body for action. Norepinephrine, another adrenal hormone, modulates the adrenaline/cortisol rush.

The higher the stress levels, the lower the blood levels of norephinephrine. But this action isn't always a defensive measure. The same cascade occurs every morning—albeit in much gentler form! As the sun rises, levels of the hormone melatonin ebb (triggered when your hypothalamus registers, via the optic nerves, a shift in light), along with norepinephrine. A dip in norepinephrine triggers the HPA axis—and the rise in adrenaline and cortisol that gets you up and moving. This (in very general terms) is the science behind your circadian rhythm—and jet lag! Interestingly, low levels of norepinephrine and correspondingly high levels of cortisol have long been considered factors in a depressed mood and seasonal affective disorder, or SAD. It's useful to note that when these chemicals are traveling in your blood, they are called hormones; when they travel synaptically, from nerve to nerve, they are called neurotransmitters, but they are structurally the same compound. Remember, the hypothalamus connects the nervous system to the endocrine system.

Stress, be it emotional or physical, stimulates the HPA axis each and every time. Chronic stress never lets it rest, which has far-reaching complications for all of your hormones and neurotransmitters!

Metabolic Hormones (Hunger Hormones)

Insulin is a primary hormone that is directly affected by your diet. It determines whether blood sugar gets used right away for immediate energy or stored as fat instead. Any disruption in the insulin-regulating mechanism, such as insulin resistance (see page 126 for more information), has an instant effect on some of the lesser metabolic hormones, the list of which grows longer every year as we uncover more of the inner workings of human metabolism.

The satiety hormone leptin, which is synthesized within fat cells, is just one part of a complex hunger-satiety network. Ghrelin, a hormone released by the cells lining the stomach, stimulates appetite when levels of leptin fall too low. Other signaling factors, like adiponectin and PYY3-36, are being studied now, both showing a definitive link between stress, insulin levels, and cravings.

Other Major Hormones

Human growth hormone (HGH) and DHEA are steroid hormones that play a role in ramping up metabolic function. One reason our metabolism slows as we age is the decline in these hormone levels. Chronically high or low levels of cortisol short-circuit the cross-talk between fat cells and insulin, leading to confused appetite signals and a higher percentage of fat accumulation— especially around the abdomen.

Melatonin, the hormone that regulates the circadian rhythm, also factors into your hunger time clock. Research shows that sleep deprivation throws off melatonin production, which in turn influences leptin and ghrelin production. In one study, subjects who were chronically sleep deprived had 15 percent more ghrelin than those who were well-rested. There is also some evidence that lack of sleep affects your levels of human growth hormone, because "pulses" of HGH are released at night.

TSH/Thyroid Hormones: Thyroid stimulating hormone from the pituitary gland initiates the release of the thyroid hormones, including the all-important triiodothyronine (T3) and thyroxin (T4). These hormones get oxygen into your cells and are crucial to your metabolism. Remember, your cells need oxygen to convert glucose into energy! Because of this, the thyroid is considered to be the foot on the pedal of your basic metabolic rate. The thyroid is also the only organ in the body that absorbs iodine, which it needs to manufacture its hormones. The thyroid makes 80 percent of your body's T4 and 20 percent of its T3. T3 increases the metabolic rate of individual cells and is the more biologically active hormone. Most T3 is created from inactive T4 in a process called the T4 to T3 conversion, which occurs in the thyroid, liver, and brain.

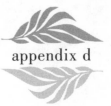

MAJOR FEMALE ENDOCRINE GLANDS AND THEIR HORMONES (A PARTIAL LISTING)

This table lists the major endocrine glands found in women and the hormones they release, as well as many of the diffuse endocrine organs and tissues in your body and their associated hormones. This list is not comprehensive; several of the hormones listed here are only newly described, and so much about hormonal function lies waiting to be discovered.

Hypothalamus
Thyrotropin-releasing hormone
Release-inhibiting hormones

Pituitary
Thyrotropin/thyroid-stimulating hormone (TSH)
Adrenocorticotropic hormone (ACTH)
Luteinizing hormone (LH)
Follicle-stimulating hormone (FSH)
Growth hormone (GH)
Prolactin
Melanocyte-stimulating hormone (MSH)
Oxytocin
Antidiuretic hormone (ADH, or vasopressin)

Pineal
Melatonin

Thyroid and Parathyroid

Thyroxine (T4)

Triiodothyronine (T3)

Calcitonin (CT)

Parathyroid hormone (PH)

Thymus

Thymosin

Thymopoietin

Serum thymic factor

Adrenals

Epinephrine

Norepinephrine

Testosterone

Estrogen

Dehydroepiandrosterone (DHEA)

Aldosterone

Cortisol

Corticosterone

Pancreas (Islets of Langerhans)

Insulin

Glucagon

Somatostatin (also secreted elsewhere)

Ovaries

Estrone

Estradiol

Estriol

Progesterone

Testosterone

Placenta

Human chorionic gonadotropin (HCG)

Breasts

Estrogen

The Diffuse Endocrine System (Other Organs and Tissues That Secrete Hormones)

Adipose Tissue (Fat) (Note that with development of abdominal/truncal obesity, adipose tissue begins to function as a major player in the endocrine system.)
Leptin
Adiponectin
Resistin
Plasminogen activating inhibitor–1 (PAI–1)
Estrogen
Others
Skin
Vitamin D3 (cholecalciferol)
Stomach and Small Intestine
Gastrin
Secretin
Cholecystokinin
Ghrelin
Motilin
Liver
25–hydroxycholecalciferol
Kidneys
Erythropoietin (EPO)
1,25-dihydroxycholecalciferol
Rennin
Heart
Atrial naturetic hormone

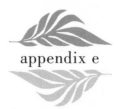

appendix e

NATURAL MENOPAUSE RELIEF

For the latter part of the 20th century, many women were prescribed hormone replacement therapy to help quell the symptoms of menopause, which include night sweats, hot flashes, vaginal dryness, irritability, anxiety, heart palpitations, weight gain, and loss of elasticity in hair and skin. Standard hormone replacement therapy (HRT) uses either a mixture of estrogens derived from the urine of a pregnant horse (Premarin) or a combination of horse estrogens and synthetic progesterone (Prempro) to replace the human sex hormones that naturally taper off in perimenopausal and menopausal women—primarily estrogen and progesterone.

At first, conventional HRT seemed heaven-sent. Not only did it soothe the symptoms of fluctuating hormones, but it supposedly guarded women against heart disease, built stronger bones, maintained supple skin and hair, and supported healthy brain function. But the 2002 Women's Health Initiative study results dealt this dream a blow. Health-care practitioners were shocked to learn that that this type of HRT might not protect a woman from getting heart disease, and actually increased her risk of breast cancer, blood clotting, and stroke. A reanalysis of this study completed in 2007 further suggested that actual heart disease risk depends on the age at which women begin HRT. But these results remain controversial, as yet another analysis in 2008 concluded that hormone therapy is associated with an increased risk of stroke regardless of when a woman starts the regime, unless the estrogen is used topically.

What concerns me and my colleague, noted breast surgeon Dr. Dixie Mills, is that the media and many practitioners are painting all HRT with the same tainted brush: women are now being advised in medical alerts that these risks apply regardless of the type of hormones involved. The reality is that the reanalysis showed associated risks only for conjugated equine estrogens and synthetic progestins—not for topical estrogen or for bioidentical hormones, which are manufactured in the lab to have the same molecular structure as the hormones made by your own body.

Customized bioidentical hormone therapy (bHRT) and USP progesterone in sublingual and topical supplements are a good natural alternative to equine-estrogen-based hormone therapy. At Women to Women, we use a supplement called Herbal Equilibrium with great success; it's a multibotanical tablet made from a proprietary blend of black cohosh, red clover, ashwaganda, passionflower, chaste tree berry, wild yam, and kudzu. We also recommend that patients increase their daily intake of soy isoflavones with our proprietary soy shake powder. If you would like to learn more or talk with a medical professional about any of these treatments, please read more at www.womentowomen.com or call to make an appointment at the Women to Women Clinic at 1-800-340-5382.

Adapted from copyrighted information previously published on the Women to Women Website.

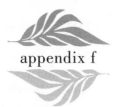

CAFFEINE–WHAT'S THE BUZZ?

One of the hardest things I've asked some of you to do this month is be vigilant about caffeine use—no more than a cup a day—and I'm asking those of you with adrenal imbalance to try and reduce this even more. Why? The results of many tests on caffeine have been confusing and inconclusive. It feels as if we can't go a month without hearing some new report weighing in on the relative dangers or health benefits of caffeine use, and the more we investigate caffeine, the hazier the picture gets. The AMA and the ADA suggest that one to two cups of coffee per day is a safe amount (approximately 100 to 200 mgs of caffeine), but in reality you may be sensitive to less or able to safely tolerate more. In my years of treating women, I've seen that even moderate caffeine use causes particular problems for three kinds of patients:

1. Women suffering from adrenal burnout and neurotransmitter deficits— that's those of you with adrenal or neurotransmitter imbalance!

2. Women who are insulin-resistant and aren't getting their energy from food—listen up if you've got hormonal imbalance or inflammatory issues!

3. Slow detoxifiers—a heads-up to those with digestive or detox issues!

And I might add that a caffeine addiction is like any other addiction and often has an emotional component. Let's face it, taking a caffeine holiday for this entire month will really help you achieve Core Balance; once you get there you can then decide how often to use caffeine.

Caffeine tolerance varies from woman to woman and depends largely on how caffeine interacts with her individual physiology and how efficiently she detoxifies—but there's the rub. In order for you to hear your body's real signals, you've got to remove caffeine long enough to tune in. And because it's addictive, even this temporary caffeine withdrawal can be a real source of anxiety and discomfort for many women. One way to begin to understand the part caffeine plays in your life—and your core imbalance—is to look at how it affects the inner workings of your body.

The molecular structure of caffeine resembles that of the neurotransmitter adenosine, but it has the opposite effect on brain cells. Adenosine helps you feel drowsy by slowing down nerve cell activity within the brain's arousal centers. This allows the brain's blood vessels to dilate, in turn allowing more oxygen in during sleep. Adequate adenosine levels are critical for good sleep cycles—a crucial requirement for detoxification. Because of its similar structure, caffeine binds to adenosine receptors on nerve cells, like a key in a lock, so that the nerve cells can't interact with real adenosine. Instead of slowing nerve cells down, caffeine speeds them up and constricts the blood vessels in the brain. This is how caffeine can impact sleep cycles, diminishing healing and detoxification efforts in the body. This also explains why caffeine is often used as a headache treatment, because it shuts down swelling blood vessels in the brains of some women (not all).

Caffeine increases the rate at which your neurons fire, stimulating our old friend the HPA (hypothalamic-pituitary-adrenal) axis. It also triggers an upswing in cortisol and the neurotransmitter dopamine, which activates the pleasure center in the brain. In this way caffeine is similar to, but less potent than, cocaine, amphetamines, and other psychoactive stimulants. As little as 100 to 200 mgs of caffeine in some women ups levels of norepinephrine and epinephrine/adrenaline, mimicking the fight-or-flight response—but most of the time you're sitting at your desk or in your car. When the rush is over and adrenaline levels drop, fatigue, irritability, inability to concentrate, headache, and weariness take over, setting the stage for a big caffeine—and sugar—craving. Caffeine is a habit-forming drug, and over time it takes more and more caffeine to produce the desired effect. It also enhances the effects of other stimulants, such as nicotine. Habitual users will experience real caffeine withdrawal symptoms within hours of reducing intake, usually headache and a drop in blood pressure, nausea, fatigue, irritability, anxiety, and depression. The half-life for caffeine in the body is anywhere from 3.5 to 6 hours, depending on the individual. So many of you can blame that afternoon slump on your morning coffee!

A subset of people who are slow detoxifiers may have a genetic variant of the caffeine-metabolizing enzyme CYP1A2. These people metabolize caffeine at a slower rate so it lingers longer, increasing the potential for negative effects. My point is that caffeine in and of itself may not be a problem if you are an efficient detoxifier. If, however, you have this genetic variant or your detoxification system is overloaded in other ways, caffeine use may tip your health over the edge. It's also possible that the myriad other chemicals in coffee and tea (like pesticide residues) are what tips the balance.

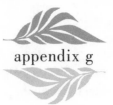

SELECTED SUPPLEMENTS

These supplements, among others, are central to the Core Balance Essential and Custom Plans. Here, you can read a little more about what they are and how they work and use the list that follows for ready reference. I have also included at the end the formulas for the medical foods I use in my practice to help support digestive, hormonal, and inflammatory imbalances. It is far easier to speak with your practitioner about a prepackaged source for medical foods to be used with their guidance, but if that is too difficult, you can learn here what nutrients and how much of each nutrient are in them.

5-HTTP: This naturally occurring amino acid is a precursor to the neurotransmitter serotonin and an intermediate in tryptophan metabolism. 5-HTP is found in small amounts in food (such as turkey and cheese) and is used in the treatment of depression.

ALA: Alpha-linoleic acid (ALA) is an omega-3 fatty acid proven to be effective in helping soothe symptoms of inflammation. Other essential fatty acids are readily available from fish, but these marine-derived fatty acids can also be synthesized by humans from ALA. ALA is only available through diet. Seed oils are the richest sources of ALA, notably the oils of rapeseed (canola), soybeans, walnuts, flaxseed (linseed), perilla, chia, and hemp.

Ashwaganda: Also spelled ashwagandha, this is a member of the pepper family known as *Withania somnifera*. Used as a general health tonic in Ayurvedic medicine, ashwaganda boosts energy, increases stamina, relieves fatigue, strengthens the immune system, soothes and calms, clarifies the mind, and slows the aging process. The powdered root of ashwaganda is normally used for whole-body tonics that improve general health and well-being. Ashwaganda is also called winter cherry, withania, asgandh, and Indian ginseng.

Astralagus: Also called huang qu, this is a powder made from the root of the *Astralagus membranaceus* plant and is used to strengthen the immune system. It aids in adrenal gland function and digestion and increases metabolism. Astralagus is contraindicated when fever is present.

Betaine HCl: A combination digestive aid made up of betaine, a vitaminlike substance, and hydrochloric acid, which helps boost stomach acidity. This digestive aid can be useful in treating patients with digestive issues such as acid reflux (GERD, or gastroesophageal reflux disease)—particularly those found to have hypochlorhydria, in which there is too little acid produced by the stomach. Betaine HCl is occasionally prescribed for patients with other forms of indigestion, such as heartburn and gas, as well as rosacea, asthma, yeast, allergies, and environmental sensitivities. The high acid content of betaine HCl can cause irritation of the stomach, so it should be taken only in the middle of a meal. Because it can significantly change stomach pH, I recommend that betaine HCl be used under the guidance of an experienced health-care practitioner.

Black Cohosh: An herb known to lower blood pressure and cholesterol levels, as well as to relieve menopausal symptoms and cramps related to menstruation.

Cayenne: From the pepper family, an herb that aids digestion, improves circulation, and acts as a catalyst for other herbs. Useful in calming inflammation and joint pain.

Calcium: The most abundant mineral in the human body because it is essential to so many important functions. More than 99 percent of total body calcium is stored in the bones and teeth, where it is used to support strength, density, and structure. The remaining 1 percent is found throughout the body in blood, muscle, and the fluid between cells. Calcium is needed for muscle contraction, blood vessel contraction, and expansion, the secretion of hormones and enzymes, and sending messages through the nervous system. The body will leach calcium from bones and teeth so that a constant level of calcium is maintained in body fluid and vital body processes function efficiently, which is why supplementation is so important.

Calcium D-Gluconate: The gluconate salt of calcium, this is used to help maintain calcium balance and prevent bone loss (when taken as an oral supplement). It may also be helpful as a cancer preventative, but much research still needs to be done to show these effects empirically.

Chromium: This mineral, needed in the body in trace amounts, has two forms: the first is biologically active and found in food, the second is a toxic form that comes from industrial pollution. Supplemental chromium is made from the former. Chromium enhances the action of insulin and the metabolism of protein, fat, and carbohydrates. Chromium can be found in broccoli, grapes, red wine, and complex carbohydrates.

CLA: As counterintuitive as it sounds, conjugated linoleic acid (CLA) is essentially a trans fatty acid, though the changes to its molecular structure happen naturally as a part of conjugation, as opposed to synthetically damaged fats. For this reason it is not referred to as a trans fat in the United States and it has not proven to be harmful. CLA is produced by microflora in the bellies of grazing mammals. CLA as a supplement helps with glucose and fat metabolism and has been shown to reduce belly fat and help manage insulin resistance. Eggs and grass-fed beef and lamb are good sources of CLA from food.

Cinnamon: A potent herb that aids in the metabolism of fats, warms the body, and helps with digestion and in fighting off infection. Current research is supporting the role of cinnamon in counteracting insulin resistance, diabetes, and other metabolic dysfunctions—including weight gain.

Cordyseps sinensis: This is a species of mushroom used throughout Asia to invigorate the lungs and kidneys. It is also beneficial in aiding fat metabolism and blood sugar levels by curbing the actions of cortisol.

CoQ10: Co-enzyme Q10 is present in the mitochondria of all cells and is essential to proper mitochondrial production of adenosine triphosphate (ATP), or cellular energy. CoQ10 aids in cardiovascular health and is a potent anti-aging compound.

DIM: Diindolylmethane (DIM) is a plant-based nutrient found only in cruciferous vegetables, such as broccoli, brussels sprouts, and cauliflower, When cruciferous vegetables are chewed, plant enzymes are released. Once these enzymes enter the stomach and are exposed to stomach acid (HCL), a compound called indole-3 carbinol is formed that, in turn, yields DIM. DIM affects estrogen and how it is metabolized. Studies show that the most effective amount of supplemental DIM is 30 mgs of absorbable DIM per dose, and two daily doses of 60 mgs each (i.e., taken twice a day) for women. DIM is not very well absorbed by the body, so I encourage you to do your due diligence here and buy the best supplement you can find that's packaged in a proven bio-delivery system.

Essential Fatty Acids: Essential fatty acids are just that—essential. They cannot be synthesized in the body and must come from dietary sources. However, while only two of the fatty acids are technically "essential," omega-3 and omega-6—they combine to make omega-9—all omega-3 fatty acids are in critically short supply in the average American diet for the following reasons. Some fatty acids, in particular the omega-3s, lower triglycerides and soothe inflammation, helping the liver convert pro-inflammatory blood acids like homocysteine into anti-inflammatory agents. The omega-6s generally play a pro-inflammatory role, but there is evidence that at least one omega-6 fatty acid (gamma linoleic acid, or GLA), found in black currant and evening primrose oils, also prevents negative inflammatory effects. For optimal health, humans need a ratio of omega-6 to omega-3 fatty acids somewhere between 1:1 and 4:1. Unfortunately, the typical modern diet provides us with a ratio of way too much omega-6—between 11 and 30 times the amount we need! Because we must feed these essential nutrients to our body in the correct proportions to support normal cell growth and repair, that means we must either radically change the source of fat in our diets or else supplement our intake of omega-3s to a significant degree. Healthy omega-3s are eicosapentaenoic acid (EPA) and docosahexaenoic acid (DHA), both found in fish oils and algae, and are most highly recommended in supplemental form—but make sure your supplements are top-notch and mercury-free.

Flax (seed and oil): A potent plant nutrient that promotes healthy skin and strong bones, nails, and teeth. Helps to soothe inflammation, hormonal imbalances, and constipation. Seeds are preferable to oil. Flax contains omega-3 fatty acids.

Ginseng: A healthful herb generally used as a tonic and energy booster. The most common species used as a supplement is *Panax ginseng,* but there are other varieties. Ginseng is helpful in managing digestive issues, hormonal balance, fatigue, and weakness. Ginseng is beneficial for people with insulin resistance, diabetes, and adrenal conditions because it aids in decreasing levels of cortisol. Ginseng is contraindicated for people with problems with low blood sugar.

GLA: Gamma-linoleic acid (GLA) is an essential fatty acid in the omega-6 family that is found primarily in plant-based oils. Linoleic acid (LA), another omega-6 fatty acid, is found in abundance in most vegetable-based, polyunsaturated oils. LA is converted to GLA in the body. GLA is then broken down to arachidonic acid (AA), which is a pro-inflammatory blood compound, and/or another competing substance called dihomog-amma-linoleic acid (DGLA), which is an anti-inflammatory. Arachidonic acid also rises in the blood when we eat red meat and charcoal-grilled foods, which are inflammatory. The good news is that when more GLA is consumed as a supplement, it helps reduce the inflammatory effects of AA. It's the ratio of the two that's important. GLA is available directly from evening primrose oil (EPO), black currant seed oil, and borage oil.

Green Drinks: Natural food formulas made from plants known for their clarifying and detoxifying properties, such as wheat grass, chlorophyll, kelp, alfalfa, barley, parsley, and mushrooms. Introduce these drinks slowly, as some people can have severe reactions.

Indole-3 Carbinol: Found in cabbage, cauliflower, and brussels sprouts. Indole-3 car-binol is converted in the gut to diindolylmethane (DIM). Supplemental indole-3 carbinol has the same beneficial effects as DIM on estrogen metabolism.

Kelp: A kind of seaweed that can be eaten raw but is usually dried or granulated or ground into a powder to take in capsules. Kelp provides a rich array of vitamins and minerals, including iodine, and can be very good for brain health, your thyroid, and weight loss.

Kudzu: A phytochemical that suppresses alcohol cravings, lowers blood pressure, and relieves head and neck aches, kudzu is useful in treating digestive issues, among other conditions.

L-Glutamine: The most abundant free amino acid found in the muscles of the body. It is important for brain function, the synthesis of muscle proteins, and maintaining the mucosal lining of the intestinal walls. For this reason, glutamine is widely used in supple-mental form for digestive disorders. In the body, the process of glutamine production helps clear ammonia from the tissues. Because of this, supplemental glutamine should not be taken if you suffer from cirrhosis of the liver, kidney problems, Reye's syndrome, or any condition that can result in an accumulation of ammonia in the blood. Additional glutamine may do more damage in these cases than good.

Licorice: A very potent herb that fights inflammation, hormonal imbalance, and the accumulation of mucus and plaque in the body. Licorice also stimulates the immune sys-tem and adrenal function. Use of licorice for more than seven days may result in higher blood pressure for those predisposed to the condition. If you have high blood pressure, check with your practitioner and use deglycerized licorice.

Magnesium: The fourth most abundant mineral in the body. Almost half of total body magnesium is found in bone; the other half is found predominantly inside cells of body tissues and organs. Only 1 percent of magnesium is found in blood, but the body will leach magnesium from other areas in order to keep blood levels of magnesium constant. Magnesium maintains normal muscle and nerve function, keeps heart rhythm steady, supports the immune system, and fortifies bone. It aids in the regulation of blood sugar levels and is known to be involved in energy metabolism and protein synthesis. Magnesium is believed to be helpful in healing chronic conditions, such as cardiovascular disease, diabetes, and high blood pressure. Magnesium is found in leafy green vegetables, potato skins, fish, nuts, and seeds.

Melatonin: A hormone naturally produced by the pineal gland in the brain. Melatonin is a potent antioxidant and anti-aging hormone that controls your circadian rhythms (among other functions). Melatonin is thought to play a pivotal role in the production and operation of other hormones, namely estrogen, progesterone, and testosterone, and to stimulate the immune system. Melatonin production occurs in response to the encroaching darkness of nightfall and helps our bodies stay in sync—an essential foundation of Core Balance.

Milk Thistle: An herb used for centuries to protect the liver and kidneys from toxins and help with liver detoxification. A concentrated tablet or capsule is more effective than a tea because milk thistle has difficulty dissolving in water.

Passionflower: An herb that has a gentle, sedative effect, useful for lowering blood pressure, relieving anxiety, insomnia, and other stress-related conditions.

Phosphatidyl Serine: This soothing phosphorus-containing fatty compound is required by every cell in the body for the maintenance of healthy cell membranes. It is abundant in the nervous system and is believed to reduce symptoms of depression and "fuzzy" thinking. It also helps decrease high cortisol levels.

Probiotics: The term *probiotics* (in contrast to antibiotics) refers to foods or supplements rich in live microbes—the beneficial gut flora that help us digest and absorb our food, shore up our immune systems, neutralize toxins, and aid in the production of essential vitamins. Probiotics are used regularly to fortify or rebuild our own natural flora. Scientists estimate we've only identified a minute fraction (1 to 2 percent) of our microflora, including the essential ones: *Escherichia, Lactobacillus,* and *Bifidobacterium.* Many species of beneficial bacteria—such as *Lactobacillus bulgaricus* and *L. thermophilus,* which are used in fermenting yogurt, as well as the near-ubiquitous *E. coli*—manufacture B vitamins and vitamin K. They also break down otherwise indigestible carbohydrates. Other forms of bacteria digest proteins, freeing up their amino acids for absorption. And some target the digestion and storage of fat, helping us normalize our cholesterol and triglyceride levels. *Acidophilus* and *Bifidobacterium* strains increase the bioavailability of minerals that need short-chain fatty acids for optimal absorption, such as magnesium, iron, copper, and manganese. High-quality probiotics are safe, natural, and effective and can be taken with other supplements without worry. The best general-purpose probiotic supplements are refrigerated or designed to be shelf-stable. Look for supplements that contain *Saccharomyces, Lactobacillus acidophilus,* and *Bifidobacteria* in the billions.

Progesterone Cream: A cream compounded with the hormone progesterone, which occurs naturally in the body. In women, progesterone is produced primarily in the ovaries and adrenal glands and works to regulate the menstrual cycle and protect pregnancy. Progesterone is essential for a myriad of functions, including bone growth. It is a precursor to other hormones, including DHEA, estrogen, testosterone, and cortisol. Supplementation for those who have a deficiency or an estrogen/progesterone imbalance has a calming, antidepressant effect and helps soothe symptoms of hormonal fluctuations, such as PMS, night sweats, and hot flashes.

Rhodiola rosea: Rhodiola is a plant that when used in supplemental form optimizes serotonin and dopamine levels and alleviates depression. It is generally taken to relieve stress and boost mood.

Soy Isoflavones: The benefits of soy are derived primarily from its isoflavones, compounds that mimic the molecular structure of human estrogen. Depending on the type of estrogen receptors on the cells, isoflavones may reduce or mimic estrogen activity, making soy supplementation a powerful balancing agent for hormonal fluctuations. The best way to get soy isoflavones is in your diet, but supplementing with 80 mgs per day seems to help many women with perimenopausal and menopausal symptoms. Soy is a controversial subject, so I encourage you to read as much as you can about it, including the articles on soy at womentowomen.com, which are substantiated with numerous (and readily available) research articles.

Taurine: An organic acid that is a primary constituent of bile. It is necessary for proper musculoskeletal growth and has been found to help stabilize glucose levels and promote fat metabolization. Taurine also appears to have a soothing effect on the central nervous system, helping to relieve symptoms of anxiety.

Turmeric: Or curcumin, the yellow ingredient is the active ingredient and helps fight free radicals and toxins in the body. A potent detox agent and immune booster, turmeric aids circulation, lowers cholesterol, and improves cardiovascular health. Very helpful for inflammation-related conditions, especially joint pain and arthritis.

Tyrosine: A nonessential amino acid acquired by ingesting protein, specifically the casein in cheese, that can also be formed by the amino acid phenylalanine. It is an important precursor for the neurotransmitters adrenaline and noradrenaline and the skin- and hair-darkening hormone melanin. It is also a precursor for thyroid hormones, including thyroxine.

Uva Ursi: A diuretic herb that supports immune function by strengthening the spleen, liver, pancreas, bladder, and kidney against infection. Uva ursi is also useful for diabetes and prostate disorders and has been used for years to treat specific GI bacteria.

Wild Yam: Relaxes muscle spasms, reduces inflammation, and promotes detoxification through perspiration. It has properties that mimic progesterone, which aids in soothing symptoms of menopause and hormone imbalance.

Medical Food Formulas

I have referred to medical foods throughout this book because I am a firm believer in their efficacy. With a little research, you should be able to find a practitioner who works with medical foods and—barring that—a purveyor from whom you can learn more. Most women don't like to take a basket full of supplements, but if you already have a cabinet full of vitamins and minerals and want to try your own formula, I've given you the basic breakdown of vitamins and minerals in the medical foods that I use, but please be aware that packaged medical foods also contain a custom, proprietary blend of other nutrients that is not reproducible here. For more information on medical foods, please visit my Website. Also note that it is always preferable to work with a health-care professional when managing a Core Imbalance; see the Resources and Referrals to help you find one. If you boost your supplement regime to mimic a medical food or decide to purchase a prepackaged variety (which comes with a host of other helpful herbs and fiber), discontinue use of a daily multivitamin. If you take a full dose of medical food during the last 14 days of your Custom Plan, please discontinue use of your multivitamin and substitute your medical food for breakfast and your afternoon snack.

Medical food to support the management of digestive and inflammatory issues, including joint pain, contains:

Element	Amount
Vitamin A	2500IUs
Vitamin A	2500IUs
Vitamin C	180mgs
Calcium	300mgs
Iron	1.4mgs
Vitamin D	45IUs
Vitamin E	100IUs
Thiamin	2mgs
Manganese	3mgs
Copper	1mg
Zinc	13mgs
Chromium	60mcgs
L-Glutamine	750mgs
Folate	80mcgs
Riboflavin	2mgs
Niacin	35mgs
Pantothenic Acid	5mgs
Magnesium	280mgs
Phosphorus	430mgs
Vitamin B6	5mgs
Vitamin B12	3mcgs
Biotin	150mcgs

L-Lysine	770mgs
L-Threonine	34mgs
Gingerroot Extract	100mgs
D-Limonene	100mgs
Rosemary Leaf Extract	200mgs
Turmeric Rhizome Extract	316mgs
Sulfate	50mgs

Medical Food to help the management of hormonal imbalance contains:

Element	Amount
Vitamin C	60mgs
Calcium	600mgs
Iron	2.5mgs
Vitamin D	40IUs
Vitamin E	11IUs
Thiamin	0.8mg
Riboflavin	0.9mg
Manganese	0.4mg
Copper	1mg
Zinc	9mgs
Chromium	100mcgs
Folate	400mcgs
Isoflavones	17mgs
Niacin	10mgs
Pantothenic Acid	5mgs
Magnesium	160mcgs
Phosphorus	500mgs

Vitamin B6	25mgs
Vitamin B12	30mcgs
Biotin	150mcgs
Iodine	75mcgs

Medical food to help support the healing of insulin resistance, heart disease, and metabolic syndrome contains:

Element	Amount
Vitamin A	1750IUs
Vitamin C	60mgs
Calcium	600mgs
Iron	3mgs
Vitamin D	40IUs
Vitamin E	11IUs
Thiamin	0.8mg
Riboflavin	0.9mg
Manganese	0.3mg
Copper	1mg
Zinc	7.5mgs
Chromium	100mcgs
Folate	400mcgs
Isoflavones	17mgs
Niacin	10mgs
Pantothenic Acid	5mgs
Magnesium	150mgs
Phosphorus	500mgs
Vitamin B6	25mgs

Vitamin B12	30mcgs
Biotin	150mcgs
Iodine	75mcgs
Plant Sterols	2000mgs

Medical Food to help support the management of adrenal fatigue and detoxification capabilities contains:

Element	Amount
Vitamin A	1000IUs
Vitamin A	4000IUs
Vitamin C	110mgs
Calcium	75mgs
Iron	3.6mgs
Vitamin D	35IUs
Vitamin E	80IUs
Thiamin	2mgs
Manganese	1.3mgs
Copper	1mg
Zinc	10mgs
Chromium	50mcgs
L-Glutamine	100mgs
Folate	80mcgs
Riboflavin	2mgs
Niacin	7mgs
Pantothenic Acid	3.5mgs
Magnesium	140mgs
Phosphorus	200mgs
Vitamin B6	3.4mgs
Vitamin B12	3.6mcgs

Biotin	135mcgs
Iodine	53mcgs
L-Cysteine	30mgs
L-Lysine	35mgs
L-Threonine	35mgs
DL-Methionine	50mgs
L-Glycine	100mgs

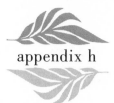

DIAGNOSTIC TESTS

Adrenal Stress Index (ASI): This test examines four saliva samples over a 24-hour period (testing cortisol levels at 7 Ė Ė 12 ι Ė ., 4 ι Ė ., and 10 ι Ė .–12 Ė) for levels of cortisol and DHEA hormones; it also evaluates gluten sensitivity.

ALCAT: This blood test analyzes serum levels of total immunoglobulin G (IgG) antibodies and immunoglobulin E (IgE) antibodies (depending on what you request), which reveal sensitivities and allergies to certain foods and combinations of foods. Antibodies are a kind of attack molecule created when a foreign body or other threat is detected by the immune system. There are five major classes of immunoglobulin, which are categorized depending on shape (an antibody's individual shape determines what threat it's going to fight). You can also ask for a chemical and mold panel and/or an intestine permeability test.

Breath Test for Small Intestine Bacterial and Fungal Overgrowth: Measures levels of hydrogen and methane gases that can indicate an overgrowth of bacteria, including yeast (candida), leading to overfermentation of food in the small intestine.

Comprehensive Digestive Stool Analysis (CDSA): This test evaluates digestion and absorption, bacterial balance and metabolism, yeast levels, and immune status for patients with irritable bowel syndrome, indigestion, malabsorption, and other gastrointestinal problems.

Comprehensive Metabolic Profile: At-home urine and blood test for amino acid deficiency.

Comprehensive Parasitology 2 (CP x 2): A stool test to identify abnormal intestinal microflora, such as yeast and other harmful bacteria and parasites.

C-Reactive Protein (CRP): A blood test to measure a protein in the blood called C-Reactive Protein (CRP), the presence of which indicates inflammation. I recommend asking for the newer high sensitivity CRP test (HS-CRP) instead of the older version. A reading greater than 1.0 means you are inflamed. If your test is normal, but you still have pain and other inflammatory symptoms, chances are good you have some low-grade inflammation happening somewhere.

Fasting Blood Sugar/Insulin and 2-Hour Postprandial Glucose/Insulin (FBS/2-Hour Glucose/Insulin): A blood test to measure glucose/insulin levels after fasting and then again two hours later after a meal high in simple carbohydrates and sugar (such as pancakes and syrup). I like to see fasting insulin levels below 14 and postprandial levels below 30. Fasting glucose levels should be around 85, postprandial glucose levels at 120 or lower.

Genetic Profile: A blood and urine test for predispositions to certain conditions, such as osteoporosis, cardiovascular disease, and breast cancer, which allows women to work with certain genetic proclivities through nutrition and targeted supplement use.

***H. pylori* Antigen:** A stool test for *Campylobacter*-like organisms, the presence of which has been correlated with gastritis and peptic ulcers, especially duodenal ulcers.

Hormone Panel: This panel uses saliva, blood, or urine samples to measure estriol, estrone, estradiol, progesterone, DHEA, testosterone, sex hormone-binding globulin (SHBG), and 2, 4, and 16 hydroxyestrones. The duration and timing of this test depend on whether or not you have gone through menopause. If you are menopausal, the test will evaluate your hormone status. A hormone panel will also tell you if your estrogen is being metabolized properly, which can influence your risk of developing breast cancer.

Iodine Patch Test: Self-administered at home with over-the-counter tincture of iodine. You paint a small patch on skin and observe it over 24 hours. Full absorption of iodine within four hours could indicate iodine insufficiency, suggesting further medical testing may be warranted.

Iodine Test: If the self-administered iodine patch indicates an iodine insufficiency, ask for a 24-hour urine test for iodine deficiency. Four iodide tablets are consumed and urine output collected for a 24-hour period. The urine is then tested for how much iodine is excreted. I like to see about 90 percent of the iodine that was consumed excreted, proof that the body has enough.

Liver Detoxification Profile: This test is conducted by Genova Diagnostic Labs and tests for phase one and phase two liver detoxification capabilities.

Neurotransmitter Test: This test uses a urine sample to evaluate serotonin, dopamine, norepinephrine, epinephrine (adrenaline), GABA, PEA, histamine, and creatinine levels. The neurotransmitter test is somewhat controversial, but can be used to give you a snapshot. You can ask for an amino acids profile at the same time, which will give you a good idea of any deficits.

Standard Comprehensive Metabolic Profile (CMP): Tests electrolytes, blood sugar, blood protein, pH level, and liver and kidney function. Available at most labs.

Urine Toxic Metals: A urine test for toxic metals, such as lead, mercury, and arsenic. The presence of heavy metals in your urine may reveal previously unknown heavy metal exposure.

References &
Further Reading

Introduction

Notes

1. J. Kaput and R. L. Rodrigues, "Nutritional Genomics: The Next Frontier in the Post-Genomic Era," *Physiological Genomics* 16, no. 2 (2004): 166–177.

2. L. Cordain, et al. "Origins and Evolution of the Western Diet: Health Implications for the 21st Century," *American Journal of Clinical Nutrition* 81, no. 2 (2005): 341–354.

3. A.S. Agaston "The End of Diet Debates? All Fats and Carbs Are Not Created Equal," *Cleveland Clinical Journal of Medicine* 72, no. 10 (2005): 946–950.

Further Reading

- For a great overall perspective on measuring weight and body mass, see Dr. Walter Willet's *Eat, Drink, and Be Healthy: The Harvard Medical School Guide to Healthy Eating.* (New York: Fireside Editions, 2001).

- If you are interested in reading a comprehensive textbook used by functional medical practitioners, see Jones, David, M.D., ed., *Textbook of Functional Medicine* (Gig Harbor, WA: Institute for Functional Medicine, 2005).

Chapter 1: Your Balancing Act

Notes

1. Kate Douglas, "Supersize Me?" *New Scientist,* no. 2588 (January 27, 2007).

2. Alex Spiegel "Hotel Maids Challenge the Placebo Effect," *Morning Edition,* NPR, January 3, 2008.

3. Thomas Holmes and Richard Rahe, "Holmes-Rahe Life Changes Scale," *Journal of Psychosomatic Research* 11 (1967): 213–218.

4. Dr. Herbert Benson, *The Mind/Body Effect* (New York: Simon and Schuster, 1979):35.

5. Tor Wager, Stephan F. Taylor, and Israel Liberzon, "Functional Neuroanatomy of Emotion: A Meta-Analysis of Emotion Activation Studies in PET and fMRI," *NeuroImage* 16 (2002): 331–348. Tor Wager and colleagues are presently conducting various other targeted studies into the neuro-imaging of emotions and pain sensations.

6. Jukka Westerbacka, et al., "Body Fat Distribution and Cortisol Metabolism in Healthy Men: Enhanced 5ß-Reductase and Lower Cortisol/Cortisone Metabolite Ratios in Men with Fatty Liver," in *Journal of Endocrinology & Metabolism* 88 (October 2003): 4924–4931.

7. C. S. Fox et al., "Abdominal Visceral and Subcutaneous Adipose Tissue Compartments: Association with Metabolic Risk Factors in the Framingham Heart Study" *Circulation* 116 (2007): 39–48.

8. "Mechanism Behind Mind-Body Connection Discovered," *ScienceDaily,* July 16, 2008. http://www.sciencedaily.com/releases/2008/07/080715152325.htm.

9. Eric Ravussin, "Rising Trend May Be Due to 'Pathoenvironment,'" *British Medican Journal* 311 (December 9, 1995): 1569.

10. F. Chaouloff et al., "Peripheral and Central Consequences of Immobilization Stress in Genetically Obese Zucker Rats," *American Journal of Physiology Regulatory, Integrative, and Comparative Physiology* 256, no. 2, (1989): 435–R442.

11. David Jones, M.D., ed., *Textbook of Functional Medicine,* (Gig Harbor, WA: The Institute for Functional Medicine 2005): 137–146.

Further Reading

- For more on the concept of individual metabolism, see Dr. Mark Hyman's *Ultrametabolism,* (New York: Scribner, 2006).

- For more data on the deleterious effects of stress on DNA see the article "Chronic Stress Accelerates Aging as Measured by Telomere Length," *Future Pundit,* November 30, 2004, www.futurepundit.com.

- Dr. Candace Pert is a pioneer in the field of psychosomatic research. Her discovery in the 1970s of endorphins and cell receptor sites revolutionized mind-body medicine. To read more about the "information-carrying molecules" in your body—otherwise known as hormones and peptides, or ligands—please see *Molecules of Emotion: The Science Behind Mind-Body Medicine* (New York: Scribner, 1997); Louise Hay's book *Heal Your Body* (Carlsbad, CA: Hay House, 1984), and Deepak Chopra's book *Ageless Body, Timeless Mind: The Quantum Alternative to Growing Old.* (New York: Harmony Books, 1993). Information about biological physics can be found at http://physics.wustl.edu/Research/ResearchInfoDocs/BiologicalPhysics.php.

Chapter 2: Your Core Physiology

Notes

1. Boyd Eaton, "The Ancestral Human Diet: What Was It and Should It Be a Paradigm for Contemporary Nutrition?" *Proceedings of the Nutrition Society* 65, no. 1 (2006):1–6.

2. Nicholas Wade, "Still Evolving, Human Genes tell new story;" *New York Times,* March 7, 2006.

3. L. Cordain et al., "Origins and Evolution of the Western Diet: Health Implications for the 21st Century," *American Journal of Clinical Nutrition* 81, no. 2 (2005): 341–354.

4. From a paper on "Mitochondrial Fuels" presented by Dr. Jeff Bland at the 2004 Institute for Functional Medicine Symposium.

5. Michael Schwartz, M.D. and Randy J. Seeley, Ph.D., "Neuroendocrine Responses to Starvation and Weight Loss," *New England Journal of Medicine* 336 (June 1997): 1802–1811.

6. Nicholas Wade, "Ice Age Ancestry May Keep Body Warmer and Healthier," *New York Times,* January 9, 2004.

7. Eduardo Ruiz-Resini et al., "Effects of Purifying and Adaptive Selection on Regional Variation in Human mtDNA," *Science* 303, no. 5655 (January 2004): 223–226.

8. Rhawn Joseph, Ph.D., from *Neuropsychiatry, Neuropsychology* (Philadelphia: Lippincott Williams & Wilkins, 1996), 161–270.

9. M. Bagnasco et al., "Evidence for the Existence of Distinct Central Appetite, Energy Expenditure, and Ghrelin Stimulation Pathways as Revealed by Hypothalamic Site-Specific Leptin Gene Therapy," *Endocrinology* 143 (2002): 4409–4421.

10. S. Q. Giraudo, C. J. Billington, and A. S. Levine, "Feeding Effects of Hypothalamic Injection of Melanocortin 4 Receptor Ligands," *Brain Research* 809 (1998): 302–306.

11. L. H. Storlien, "The Ventromedial Hypothalamic Area and the Vagus Are Neural Substrates for Anticipatory Insulin Release," *Journal of the Autonomic Nervous System* 13, no. 4 (August 1985): 303–310.

12. Dirk Hanson, "Neuroaddiction: The Reward Pathway," *Addiction,* http://www.dirkhanson.org/neuroaddiction.html.

Further Reading

- Some of the data in this chapter was culled from medical textbooks, specifically the *Textbook for Functional Medicine* (Gig Harbor, WA: The Institute for Functional Medicine, 2005) and *Harrison's Principles of Internal Medicine, 17th Edition* (New York: McGraw-Hill, 2008). Additional information about these systems may be found at www.womentowomen.com.

- For more on our evolving DNA, see Anderson S. Bankier et al., "Sequence and Organization of the Human Mitochondrial Genome," *Nature* 290 (1981): 457–465.

- See the following essential research papers on the hypothalamus for more basic information: Anand & Brobeck, 1951; Hoebel & Tetelbaum, 1966; Teitelbaum, 1961.

- For an in-depth explanation of hypothalamic control of appetite and relevant hormonal cross-talk discovered by researchers thus far, see the fascinating paper "Appetite Control" by Katie Wynne, Sarah Stanley, Barbara McGowan, and Steve Bloom in the *Journal of Endocrinology,* volume 184 (2005), pages 291–318.

Chapter 3: You Are What You Eat

Further Reading

- For an interesting look at modern nutrition, see Dr. Colin Campbell and Thomas M. Campbell's visionary book, *The China Study: Startling Implications for Diet, Weight Loss, and Long-Term Health,* (Dallas, TX: BenBella Press, 2006). I also recommend Eric Schlosser's *Fast Food Nation* (Boston: Houghton Mifflin, 2001) and Gary Taubes's, *Good Calorie, Bad Calorie* (New York: Knopf Publishing Group, 2007).

- For a comprehensive overview of micro and macronutrients and their relationship to our long-term health, see *Dietary Reference Intakes For Energy, Carbohydrate, Fiber, Fat, Fatty Acids, Cholesterol, Protein, and Amino Acids,* by the Institute of Medicine of the National Academies (Washington, DC: National Academies Press, 2005).

- The role of lipids and brain function is a fascinating subject; for more information see Toshio Ariga, W. David Jarvis, and Robert K. You's paper, "Role of Sphingolipid-Mediated Cell Death in Neurodegenerative Diseases," *Journal of Lipid Research,* volume 39 (1998). Also available at www.jir.org. In it, the authors discuss the role of lipid-signaling pathways and the regulation of cell survival as it relates to the brain and degenerative diseases such as Alzheimer's and Parkinson's.

Chapter 4: Getting Started

Notes

1. James W. Lyne and P. Barak, "Are Depleted Soils Causing a Reduction in the Mineral Content of Food Crops?" 2000 Annual Meetings of the ASA/CSSA/SSSA, November 5–9, 2000, Minneapolis MN, www.soils.wisc.edu.

2. Donald R. Davis et al., "Changes in USDA Food Composition Data for 43 Garden Crops, 1950 to 1999," *Journal of the American College of Nutrition* 23, no. 6 (2004): 669–682.

3. R. H. Fletcher and K. M. Fairfield, "Vitamins for Chronic Disease Prevention in Adults: Clinical Applications," *Journal of the American Medical Association* 287 (June 19, 2002): 3127–3129.

Further Reading

- Dr. Diana Schwarzbein's work has had a large influence on my thinking throughout the years. I recommend reading any of her excellent books, starting with *The Schwarzbein Principle* (Florida: Health Communications Inc., 1999).

- For an excellent reference book on nutrition, supplements, and nutritional values, see *The Nutrition Almanac, 5th Edition*, edited by Lavonne J. Dunne (New York: McGraw-Hill, 2002).

- For food value tables through the years, see the United States Department of Agriculture, Agricultural Research Service: USDA Nutrient Database for Standard Reference, Release 13, 1999. Nutrient Data Laboratory Home Page: http://www.nal.usda.gov/fnic/foodcomp.

- For more information on the degradation of our food supply, see also the article, "Our Decrepit Food Factories," by Michael Pollan, *New York Times,* December 16, 2007.

- Information on probiotics adapted from previously published material on my Website at www.womentowomen.com. Please subscribe to my free "Insight" newsletter for bimonthly newsletters and further reading. Probiotic references available at www.womentowomen.com/

digestionandgihealth/probiotics-references. See also "Probiotics: A Link to Permanent Weight Loss and Ultimate Health," by Ana Luque in *Well-Being Journal,* volume 17, no. 4 (July/August 2008): 3–7.

- For more reading on the biological significance of essential fatty acids, see "Links Biological Significance of Essential Fatty Acids" in the *Journal of Association of Physicians of India,* volume 54 (2006): 309–319.

- Many herbs and spices have an impact on the body's metabolism; an interesting study on the insulin-enhancing effects of cinnamon is reported in Richard Anderson et al., in "Isolation and Characterization of Polyphenol Type-A Polymers from Cinnamon with Insulin-Like Biological Activity," in the *Journal of Agricultural and Food Chemistry,* volume 52 (2004): 65–70.

Chapter 5: The Core Balance Essential Eating Plan

Notes

1. C. A. Daley et al., "A Literature Review of the Value-Added Nutrients Found in Grass-Fed Beef Products," 2004, www.csuchico.edu/agr/grassfedbeef/health-benefits.

2. P. J. H. Jones, N. G. Asp, and P. Silva, "Evidence for Health Claims on Foods: How Much is Enough? Introduction and General Remarks," *Journal of Nutrition* 138, no. 6 (June 1, 2008): 1189S–1191S.

Further Reading

- For more on the synergistic relationship between you and your food, see Michael Pollan's terrific article, "Unhappy Meals," in the *New York Times,* January 28, 2007.

Chapter 6: The Core Balance Essential Action Plan

Further Reading

- I'm not usually a huge fan of trendy diet books, but I have kept one on my shelf all these years because it has excellent information on exercise: Christopher V. Guerriero, *Maximize Your Metabolism* (San Diego, CA: Jodere Group, 2003).

- For an interesting and stunning look at the power of exercise, see Jonathan Shaw's article, "The Deadliest Sin: From Survival of the Fittest to Staying Fit Just to Survive: Scientists Probe the Benefits of Exercise—and the Dangers of Sloth," *Harvard Magazine* (March/April 2004): pages 36–43. Full article available at http://harvardmagazine.com/2004/03/the-deadliest-sin.html.

- For information on lack of sleep and weight gain, studies are numerous. To start, see R. Vorona et al., "Overweight and Obese Patients in a Primary Care Population Report Less Sleep Than Patients with a Normal Body Mass Index" in *Archives of Internal Medicine,* volume 165, no. 1 (2005), pages 25–30, and "Lack of Sleep Linked to Weight Gain" from Meridian Health, (01.26.2005) available at www.meridianhealth.com/index.cfm/NewsAnd-Media/HealthNews/MindBody/2008Jun.cfm.

- For scientific studies on the power of yogic breathing, see R. Brown and P. Gerbarg, "Sudarshan Kriya Yogic Breathing in the Treatment of Stress, Anxiety, and Depression: Part I—Neurophysiologic Model," in the *Journal of Alternative and Complementary Medicine,* volume 11, no.1 (2005): pages 189–201, and "Sudarshan Kriya Yogic Breathing in the Treatment of Stress, Anxiety, and Depression: Part II—Clinical Applications and Guidelines," in the *Journal of Alternative and Complementary Medicine,* volume 11, no. 4 (2005): pages 711–717.

- For more information on DHEA, vitamin D, serotonin, and the benefits of play, go to www.womentowomen.com and search the archives of the "Insight" newsletter.

Chapter 8: Digestive Imbalance Custom Plan

Notes

1. See the following articles: M. Kalliomaki, "Food Allergy and Irritable Bowel Syndrome" in *Current Opinion in Gastroenterology* 21, no. 6 (2005): 708–711, and I. Herzum et al., "Diagnostic and Analytical Performance of a Screening Panel for Allergy," *Clinical Chemical and Laboratory Medicine* 43, no. 9 (2005): 963–966.

2. T. S. Chen et al., "Effects of Sex Steroid Hormones on Gastric Emptying and Gastrointestinal Transit in Rats," *American Journal of Physiology: Gastrointestinal and Liver Physiology* 268 (1995): G171–G176.

Further Reading

- The following books are excellent reference reading on digestive sensitivities: Elizabeth Lipski's *Digestive Wellness, 3rd Edition* (New York: McGraw Hill, 2004); Michael Gershon's *The Second Brain* (New York: Harper Collins, 1989); Dr. Ellen Cutler's *The Food Allergy Cure* (New York: Random House, 2003); and Merla Zellerbach's *The Allergy Sourcebook: Everything You Need to Know* (New York: McGraw-Hill, 2000).

- See also B. N. Ames's articles "Delaying the Mitochondrial Decay of Aging," *National Academy of Science,* volume 1019, no. 1 (June 2004): pages 406–411. and "The Metabolic Tune-Up: Metabolic Harmony and Disease Prevention," in the *Journal of Nutrition,* volume 133, no. 5 (May 2003): pages 1544–1548.

Chapter 9: Hormonal Imbalance Custom Plan

Notes

1. Wake Forest University Baptist Medical Center, "Exercise Important in Reducing Size of Abdominal Fat Cells," *ScienceDaily* (August 7, 2006) http://www.sciencedaily.com /releases/2006/08/060807154847.htm.

2. L. R. Simkin-Silverman et al., "Lifestyle Intervention Can Prevent Weight Gain During Menopause: Results from a 5-Year Randomized Clinical Trial," *Annals of Behavioral Medicine* 26, no. 3 (December 2003): 212–220.

3. R. Azziz, "Reproductive Endocrinologic Alterations in Female Asymptomatic Obesity," *Fertility Sterility* 52, no. 5 (November 1989): 703–725.

4. J. Mann, "Meta-Analysis of Low-Glycemic Index Diets in the Management of Diabetes: Response to Franz," *Diabetes Care* 26 (2003): 3364–3365, http://care.diabetesjournals.org/cgi/content/full/26/12/3364.

5. D. Rogoff et al., "Abnormalities of Glucose Homeostasis and the Hypothalamic-Pituitary-Adrenal Axis in Mice Lacking Hexose-6-Phosphate Dehydrogenase," *Endocrinology* 148, no. 10 (October 2007): 5072–5080.

6. C. K. Sites et al., "Soy Linked to Less Belly Fat in Post-Menopausal Women," summarized from a study published in *Fertility and Sterility* 88, no. 6 (2007): 1609–1617. Soy has caused much controversy in the world of nutrition, but my research has led me to believe that the benefits outweigh the risks. For more on soy, as well as additional references, please go to www.womento-women.com and read the article and references entitled "Health Benefits of Soy—Why the Controversy" by my colleague, Dr. Dixie Mills.

Further Reading

- Books to enjoy: Dr. Susan Love's *Menopause & Hormone Book: Making Informed Choices,* (New York: Three Rivers Press, 1998); Dr. John Lee and Virginia Hopkins's *What Your Doctor May Not Tell You About Menopause: The Breakthrough Book on Natural Progesterone* (New York: TimeWarner, 1996); *The Glucose Revolution: The Authoritative Guide to the Glycemic Index* by Jennie Brand-Miller, Ph.D.; Thomas Wolever, M.D., Ph.D.; Kaye Foster-Powell; and Stephen Colagiuri, M.D. (New York: Marlowe & Co, 1999); and *Women's Bodies, Women's Wisdom* by Dr. Christiane Northrup (New York: Bantam, 1998).

- For a terrific overview of the female hormonal cascade, read Dr. Bethany Hays's chapter, "Hormonal Imbalances: Female Hormones: The Dance of the Hormones. Pt. I," in the *Textbook of Functional Medicine* (Gig Harbor, WA: Institute for Functional Medicine, 2005) 215–234.

Chapter 10: Adrenal Imbalance Custom Plan

Notes

1. D. Rogoff et al., "Abnormalities of Glucose Homeostasis and the Hypothalamic-Pituitary-Adrenal Axis in Mice Lacking Hexose-6-Phosphate Dehydrogenase," *Endocrinology* 148, no. 10 (October 2007): 5072–5080.

2. X. Belda et al., "The Effects of Chronic Food Restriction on Hypothalamic-Pituitary-Adrenal Activity Depend on Morning Versus Evening Availability of Food," *Pharmacology, Biochemistry and Behavior* 81 (2005): 41–45.

3. P. Björntorp, "Do Stress Reactions Cause Abdominal Obesity and Comorbidities?" *Obesity Reviews* 2, no. 2 (2001): 73–86.

4. Kate Ramsayer, "Sweet Relief: Comfort Food Calms, with Weighty Effect," *Science News* 164, no. 11 (September 13, 2003): 165.

5. M. E. Gluck, A. Geliebter, and M. Lorence, "Cortisol Stress Response is Positively Correlated with Central Obesity in Obese Women with Binge Eating Disorder (BED) Before and After Cognitive-Behavioral Treatment," *Annals of the New York Academy of Science* 1032 (December 2004): 202–207.

Further Reading

- Recommended books: *Feeling Fat, Fuzzy, or Frazzled?* by Dr. Richard Shames and Karilee Shames, Ph.D., R.N. (New York: Hudson Street Press, 2005) and *Your Fat Is Not Your Fault* by Carol M. Simontacchi with Margaret West (New York: Tarcher/Putnam,1997).

- I am also indebted to data collected on the deleterious biochemical effects of stress at the 14th International Symposium on Functional Medicine, entitled "The Weaver and the Web: Understanding the HPA and HPT Axes," which took place in Tucson, AZ, in May 2007.

Chapter 11: The Neurotransmitter Imbalance Custom Plan

Notes

1. E. G. Tafet, M. Toister-Achituv, and M. Shinitzky, "Enhancement of Serotonin Uptake by Cortisol: A Possible Link Between Stress and Depression," *Cognitive, Affective, & Behavioral Neuroscience* 1, no. 1 (March 2001): 96–104.

2. M. M. Hagan et al., "The Effect of Hypothalamic Peptide YY on Hippocampal Acetylcholine Release in Vivo: Implications for Limbic Function in Binge-Eating Behavior," *Brain Research*, volume 805 (1998): 20–28.

3. D.M. Makina et al., "Effect of Hypericum Extract on the Hypothalamic-Pituitary-Adrenal System in Rats," *Bulletin of Experimental Biology and Medicine* 132, no. 6 (December 2001): 1180–1181.

Further Reading

- If you are interested in reading more on this topic, I suggest the following books: *The Mood Cure* by Julia Ross (New York: Penguin Books, 2003); *Potatoes Not Prozac* by Kathleen Desmaisons, (New York: Simon & Schuster, 1999); and *The Food-Mood Solution* by Jack Challem and Dr. Melvyn R. Werbach (New York: Wiley, 2008). If you are struggling with compulsive eating that does not respond to diet and lifestyle changes, I also recommend *Fat Is a Family Affair* by Judy Hollis, Ph.D. (Minnesota: Hazelden, 2003) and any of Geneen Roth's work—a favorite of mine is *Breaking Free from Emotional Eating* (New York: Plume/Penguin USA, 2003).

- For more information on metabolism and mood, see the article by R. Morriss and F. A. Mohammed titled "Metabolism, Lifestyle, and Bipolar Affective Disorder," in the *Journal of Psychopharmacology*, volume 19, supplement 6 (November 2005): pages 94–101. For an interesting link between nutrition and depression, see the article by Frederick Cassidy, M.D., Eileen Ahearn, M.D., Ph.D., and J. Carroll, M.B., Ph.D., titled "Elevated Frequency of Diabetes Mellitus in Hospitalized Manic Depressive patients," in the *American Journal of Psychiatry*, volume 156 (September 1999): pages 1417–1420.

- DHEA has often been called the "joy" hormone by many in the wellness field. Since DHEA production begins to taper off in young adulthood, neurotransmitter imbalance at midlife can often be helped by DHEA supplementation (under medical guidance). For more information about DHEA's physiological effects, read H. A. Alhaj, A. E. Massey, and R. H. McAllister-Williams's paper, "Effects of DHEA Administration on Episodic Memory, Cortisol, and Mood in Healthy Young Men: A Double-Blind, Placebo-Controlled Study." *Psychopharmacologia,* (translated from French, published by Springer/Berlin) volume 188, no. 4 (November 2006): 541–551. In it, the authors conclude that DHEA administration leads to a reduction in evening cortisol levels and improved mood.

- General information for this chapter is supported by data presented by the 9th International Symposium of Functional Medicine, titled "Disorders of the Brain," and the 15th Symposium, titled "Neurobiology of Mood and Cognitive Disorders."

Chapter 12: The Inflammatory Imbalance Custom Plan

Notes

1. Andreas Festa, M.D. et al., "Inflammation in the Prediabetic State Is Related to Increased Insulin Resistance Rather Than Decreased Insulin Secretion," *Circulation* 108 (2003): 1822–1830.

2. Earl S. Ford, "Body Mass Index, Diabetes, and C-Reactive Protein Among U.S. Adults," *Diabetes Care* 22, no. 12 (December 1999): 1971–1977.

3. Kathryn E. Wellen, et al., "Obesity-Induced Inflammatory Changes in Adipose Tissue" published in the *Journal of Clinical Investigations* 112, no. 12 (December 2003): 1773–1914.

4. Zhuowei Wang et al., "Leptin Resistance of Adipocytes in Obesity: Role of Suppressors of Cytokine Signaling," *Biochemical and Biophysical Research Communications* 277 (2000): 20–26.

5. Nicoletta Botto et al., "Genetic Polymorphisms in Folate and Homocysteine Metabolism as Risk Factors for DNA Damage," *European Journal of Human Genetics* 11 (2003): 671–678.

6. Joseph L. Evans et al., "Oxidative Stress and Stress-Activated Signaling Pathways: A Unifying Hypothesis of Type 2 Diabetes," *Endocrinology Review* 23 (2002): 599–622.

7. Jennifer Acerman, "The Great Sunlight Standoff," *Psychology Today* (November/December 2007): 97–102.

Further Reading

- For further reading on this subject, I suggest the following books: *The Perricone Prescription* by Nicholas Perricone, M.D. (New York: HarperCollins, 2004); *The Inflammation Syndrome* by Jack Challem (New Jersey: Wiley, 2003); and *Ultra-Longevity* by Mark Liponis, M.D. (New York: Little Brown, 2007).

- The connection between adipose tissue, inflammation, and chronic disease is being closely studied by researchers across the globe. For more information, see Stuart P. Weisberg, et al., "Obesity Is Associated with Macrophage Accumulation in Adipose Tissue," published with the Wellen article referenced above in the *Journal of Clinical Investigations* 112, no. 12 (December 2003): 1773–1914. The researchers conclude that "Obesity alters adipose tissue metabolic and endocrine function and leads to an increased release of fatty acids, hormones, and pro-inflammatory molecules that contribute to obesity associated complications."

- To read more about inflammation's effect on our hunger hormones, read Peter Havel's paper, "Control of Energy, Homeostasis, and Insulin Action by Adipocyte Hormones: Leptin, Acylation Stimulating Protein, and Adiponectin," from the Department of Nutrition, University of California, Davis; published in *Current Opinion in Lipidology,* volume 13 (2002): pages 51–59.

- Information on helpful supplements and nutrients to soothe inflammation is adapted from data supplied at the 11th International Symposium on Functional Medicine, titled "The Coming Storm: The Rising Pandemic of Diabetes and Metabolic Syndrome."

- More information about the beneficial effect of vitamin D on our immunity, mood, and longevity, see Richard Hobday, *The Healing Sun* (Tallahassee, FL: Findhorn Press, 1999).

Chapter 13: Detoxification Imbalance Custom Plan

Notes

1. "National Report on Human Exposure to Environmental Chemicals," Department of Health & Human Services, Center for Disease Control, (July 2005) www.cdc.gov.

2. See the following research paper: C. Pelletier, P. Imbeault, and A. Tremblay's "Energy Balance and Pollution by Organochlorines and Polychlorinated Biphenyls," in the *Obesity Review,* volume 4, no. 1 (February 2003): pages 17–24.

Further Reading

- Detox is a very popular subject right now, with plenty of good sources to reference. For more information, I suggest reading any work by Sherry Rogers, M.D., including *Tired or Toxic: A Blueprint for Health* (New York: Prestige Publications, 1990) and my dear friend Dr. Frank Lipman's work, including *Total Renewal* (New York: Tarcher/Putnam, 2003); and *Ultra-Prevention: A Six-Week Plan That Will Make You Healthier for Life,* by Mark Hyman, M.D. and Mark Liponis, M.D. (New York: Scribner 2003). You can also find a lot of information about detox on my website: www.womentowomen.com.

- For more information on quantity of man-made chemicals and our exposure, see also G. Y. Nicolau's paper, "Pesticide Effects upon the Circadian Time Structure in the Thyroid, Adrenal, and Testis in Rats," in *Endocrinologie,* volume 20, no. 2 (April/June 1982): pages 73–90 and "Curbing the Toxic Onslaught" by Donald E. Colbert, M.D., *NutriNews* Newsletter (Autumn 2005): pages 1–5.

- To read more about toxins and metabolism, see the paper by C. Pelletier, P. Imbeault, and A. Tremblay entitled "Thermogenesis and Weight Loss in Obese Individuals: A Primary Association with Organochlorine Pollution," in the *International Journal of Obesity Obesity-Related Metabolic Disorders,* volume 28, no. 7 (July 2004): pages 936–939.

- For a scary look at the long-range impact of endocrine disrupting hormones, read W. Souder's fascinating article, "It's Not Easy Being Green: Are

Weed-Killers Turning Frogs into Hermaphrodites?" in *Harper's Magazine* (2006 August), 59–66.

- For more on the impact of heavy metals, read T. Eeva, E. Belskii E, and B. Kuranov's, "Environmental Pollution Affects Genetic Diversity in Wild Bird Populations," in *Mutation Research*, Volume 608, no. 1, (September 19, 2006): pages 8–15.

- Read the comprehensive paper, "Toxic Nation Report: A Report on Pollution in Canadians" from *Environmental Defense,* (November 2005) for a shocking overview of how much chemical residue circulates in the average Western-ized human body. Available as a PDF download at www.environmentalde-fence.com.

Now What?

Notes

1. For more information on HcG studies, see M. R. Stein, R. E. Julis, and C. C. Peck, "Ineffectiveness of Human Chorionic Gonadotropin in Weight Reduc-tion: A Double-Blind Study," *Journal of the American Medical Association* 236 (1976): 2495–2497.

Further Reading

- For even more information on HCG trials, read W. Hinshaw, J. E. Sawicki, and J. J. Deller, Jr., "Human Chorionic Gonadotropin (HCG) Treatment of Obesity" in the *Archives of Internal Medicine,* volume 137 (1977): pages 151–155; and "Dieters Take a Jab at Fat With Injections For Weight Loss," by Alexandra Horowitz, Resident Publications, (2008 March).

Chapter 14: Your Issues are in Your Tissues

Notes

1. Jeffrey Steingarten, *It Must've Been Something I Ate* (New York: Vintage Books, 2003): 6.

2. Dr. Alice Domar, *Healing Mind, Healthy Woman* (New York: Henry Holt, 1996): 11.

3. Andrew Harvey, The Direct Path: Creating a Journey to the Divine Using the World's Mystical Traditions, (New York: Broadway Books, 2000): 13.

4. Candace Pert, *Molecules of Emotion,* (New York: Scribner, 1997): 270.

5. For data on touch therapy, oxytocin, and hugging, see article by M. S. Carmichael, et al., entitled, "Plasma Oxytocin Increases in the Human Sexual Response" in the *Journal of Clinical Endocrinology & Metabolism,* volume 64 (1987): pages 27–31.

Further Reading

- One of my favorite books about the deleterious effects of hidden emotions is Karol Truman's *Feelings Alive Never Die* (Phoenix, AZ: Olympus Distributing, 1991). It describes how certain body parts are affected by different emotions.

- One of the pioneering studies into the connection between emotional trauma and physical health is the landmark ACE study conducted by Dr. Vincent J. Felitti titled "The Relation Between Adverse Childhood Experiences and Adult Health: Turning Gold into Lead," which was first published in *The Permanente Journal,* volume 6, no. 1 (Winter 2002). It is a fascinating read for anyone interested in the science behind this connection.

- Learn more about the power of hugging in the article, "A Hug A Day," by Jan McColm in *Endeavors* magazine (University of North Carolina at Chapel Hill, (Winter 2004).

Chapter 15: Revising your Negativity Script

Further Reading

- For more on cognitive distortions, read Dr. David Burns's book *Feeling Good: The New Mood Therapy* (New York: Harper, 1999).

- I also recommend all of Byron Katie's work, including the seminal *Loving What Is* (New York: Three Rivers Press, 2002) and *I Need Your Love—Is That True?* (New York: Three Rivers Press, 2005).

- *The Artist's Way: A Spiritual Path to Higher Creativity* (New York: Tarcher/Putnam, 1992/2002) by Julia Cameron is a must read for anyone interested in tapping into her creative source.

Chapter 16: Wrapping It Up

Further Reading

- For more on the dangers of chemicals in cosmetics, read "The Dark Side of Beauty" by Rosemary Carstens in *Alternative Medicine* (January 2006), available online in the archives at www.naturalsolutionsmag.com. You can also access the "Skin Deep Report" to research the safety of your cosmetics and beauty products at the Environmental Working Group Website found at www.ewg.org.

- For more on color analysis and image consulting, please contact Julie Cunningham at Julie Cunningham Color: 1717 Congress St., Portland, ME 04102 or call 207-773-5500.

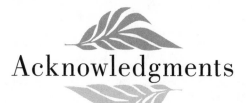

Acknowledgments

My own journey began with my mother, Sonja, who taught me how to look beyond what was in front of my eyes and always ask questions, and with my father, Thomas, who always encouraged me in my intellectual pursuits. I am eternally grateful to them for setting me on my path. I also thank my brothers, Ralph, for never giving up on me, and Evan, who loves and supports me unconditionally. I would have gotten lost along the way if not for Edgar Cayce and the Association for Research and Enlightenment, where I learned to ask bigger questions and not accept what I was told as dogma. At Pumpkin Hollow, Dora Kunz and Delores Krieger first taught me therapeutic touch and showed me that the body has an energetic realm—a priceless gift. I am indebted to Anne Rafter, with whom I first began looking at the possibility of starting a holistic health-care center for women when it was far from the norm. To that end, I send prayers of thanks to our pioneering sister, Christiane Northrup, M.D., who led the way for all of us to follow and who, along with our wonderful colleague Ellen Fenn, M.D., joined with Anne and me to start Women to Women in the 1980s. I also want to thank Dr. Northrup's assistant, Diane Grover. Thank you to my mentors, Dr. Jeff Bland and Dr. Candace Pert, for teaching me so much of what they know and to my esteemed colleagues Liz Lipski, Louise Hay, and Cheryl Richardson for their huge impact on my life and in this field. Much appreciation is due to Jeff McKinnon, Betsy Peters, and everyone at Concordia Partners for taking my message into cyberspace. I am grateful to Dixie Mills, M.D., for always being there to listen and for standing by me through so many transitions. I owe an immeasurable debt to Frank Lipman, M.D., for being a sounding board and my own personal pep team. To Fern Tsao, Frank Gentile, Eileen Beasley, Aita Passmore, Robert Deutsche, and Thea Fournier, who keep me healthy. And most importantly, thank you, thank you, a million times to Donna Poulin, my lifesaver, organizer, true friend, and the creative mind behind many of the recipes in this book. I am also so grateful to the hard-working practitioners at Women to Women for the difference they are making in women's lives: Marcy Holmes, Jay Reighley, Carrie Levine, and the rest of our energetic, dedicated staff; and of course, I would be nothing without my spectacular, brave, amazing patients. You are my inspiration.

A special thanks to my agent, Stephanie Tade, for all that she does, and to my editor, Patty Gift, her assistant Laura Koch, and Anne Barthel, copyeditor extraordinaire. And of course, a million thanks to Genevieve Morgan, a great writer, collaborator, and friend—I am so grateful to the universe for bringing us together. Thank you to Julie Cunningham for her undying support, advice, affection, and enthusiasm throughout the years. To my dear, dear friends Laurie Chandler, Jane Honeck, Sally McCue, and Linda Ward, thank you for standing by my side no matter what, for your support, and for your enduring love. It has meant so much. Love and thanks to my husband, Joseph, my stepson Joe, and my sons, Micah and Joshua, who have all sacrificed so much for the sake of women's health, and especially to my daughter, Katya. This book took shape with the dream that the world will soon be a different place for her and for all young women setting out on journeys of their own.

Marcelle Pick

On the road to this book, I've been lucky enough to meet several individuals who held their lamps high enough to light my way or who stopped to give me directions. Thank you to my grandmother and mother for encouraging me not to be afraid to travel alone; to my teachers, Gary Gurney, Kathleen Swinbourne, Brett Russman, Susan Conley, Aruni Nan Futoronsky, and Stephanie Tade for their insight; and, beyond measure, to Marcelle, whose lamp helped to alter my life's direction. I'm also sincerely grateful to the many courageous women who shared their personal—and often painful—stories with me. I owe a huge debt to Tess, Tabitha, Vicki, and Luanne, the amazing women who kept my life and house in order during the writing of this book, and to my father and stepmother for stepping up when the going got really rough. Thank you to all my wise, witty, big-hearted friends for having my back and making the trip so much fun. But above all, thank you to my beloved boys, Tom, Graham, and Wyeth, for being who they are and for being with me.

Genevieve Morgan

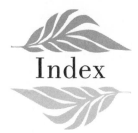

Index

INDEX OF RECIPES AND MENUS

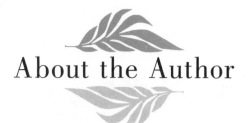

About the Author

Marcelle Pick, MSN, OB/GYN NP, co-founded Women to Women with a vision to change women's health care. The clinic pioneered the combination of alternative and conventional medicine, using a holistic approach that not only treats illness but also helps women make life choices to prevent disease. Women to Women continues seeing thousands of women from around the world each year.

Marcelle Pick earned a B.S. in Nursing and a B.A. in Psychology from the University of New Hampshire and an M.S. in Nursing from Boston College–Harvard Medical School. Certified as nurse practitioner for both OB/GYN and pediatrics, Pick has served as medical advisor to *Healthy Living Magazine,* lectured on a variety of topics, and appears regularly on television to discuss women's health.

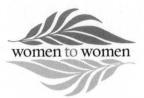

women to women

Twenty five years ago, Marcelle Pick and her partners began a revolution in health care that continues to this day. They founded one of the first medical clinics in the world devoted to health care for women by women. In early 2004, Marcelle launched Women to Women's Personal Program online to bring a guided, at-home version of her pioneering natural approach to women across the country.

Try the Personal Program for Core Balance at home

The Personal Program for Core Balance is an easy, at-home version of the sustainable weight-loss solutions offered in this book. Log in to *womentowomen.com/corebalance* and use the code above to access resources designed specifically to support the recommendations made in the book.

Special access code:

17437

womentowomen.com/corebalance

The Program has seven versions, each designed to give you the nutrients you need to support your body as you work with your individual core imbalance. Each version contains the pharmaceutical-grade supplements recommended in this book, bundled together for your convenience.

Members of the Personal Program can follow the Core Balance Diet step-by-step online with interactive tools, helpful strategies, and more. Members also receive free support by phone from our caring and experienced Wellness Coaches who provide encouragement and advice.

The Personal Program has helped tens of thousands of women regain a natural, balanced relationship with their bodies, and we can help you too. Call 800-593-2594 to find out more now.

Or become a patient at the Clinic

Women with entrenched core imbalances or special concerns are welcome to become patients at our clinic in Yarmouth, Maine. All of the practitioners at the clinic have been trained by Marcelle on the weight-loss/wellness protocols in this book. To make an appointment, call 800-340-5382. (Please note that as a medical practice we cannot answer medical questions or dispense medical advice outside of an appointment.)